Encyclopedia of Glaucoma: Essential Aspects

Volume III

Encyclopedia of Glaucoma: Essential Aspects
Volume III

Edited by **Abigail Gipe**

FOSTER ACADEMICS

New Jersey

Published by Foster Academics,
61 Van Reypen Street,
Jersey City, NJ 07306, USA
www.fosteracademics.com

Encyclopedia of Glaucoma: Essential Aspects
Volume III
Edited by Abigail Gipe

© 2015 Foster Academics

International Standard Book Number: 978-1-63242-150-0 (Hardback)

Contents

Preface

This book was inspired by the evolution of our times; to answer the curiosity of inquisitive minds. Many developments have occurred across the globe in the recent past which has transformed the progress in the field.

Glaucoma is a specialty in ophthalmology that consists of a group of diseases that affect the optic disc and visual fields and is often followed by elevated intraocular pressure. This book is summarised with new topics in glaucoma that have not been covered earlier and it has broadly highlighted some common topics on glaucoma. It is a well examined and balanced work inclusive of the essential aspects. This book is dedicated to glaucoma experts, general ophthalmologists, amateurs and researchers to increase their knowledge and understand these complex diseases to encourage further investigation for the benefit of the entire humanity.

This book was developed from a mere concept to drafts to chapters and finally compiled together as a complete text to benefit the readers across all nations. To ensure the quality of the content we instilled two significant steps in our procedure. The first was to appoint an editorial team that would verify the data and statistics provided in the book and also select the most appropriate and valuable contributions from the plentiful contributions we received from authors worldwide. The next step was to appoint an expert of the topic as the Editor-in-Chief, who would head the project and finally make the necessary amendments and modifications to make the text reader-friendly. I was then commissioned to examine all the material to present the topics in the most comprehensible and productive format.

I would like to take this opportunity to thank all the contributing authors who were supportive enough to contribute their time and knowledge to this project. I also wish to convey my regards to my family who have been extremely supportive during the entire project.

Editor

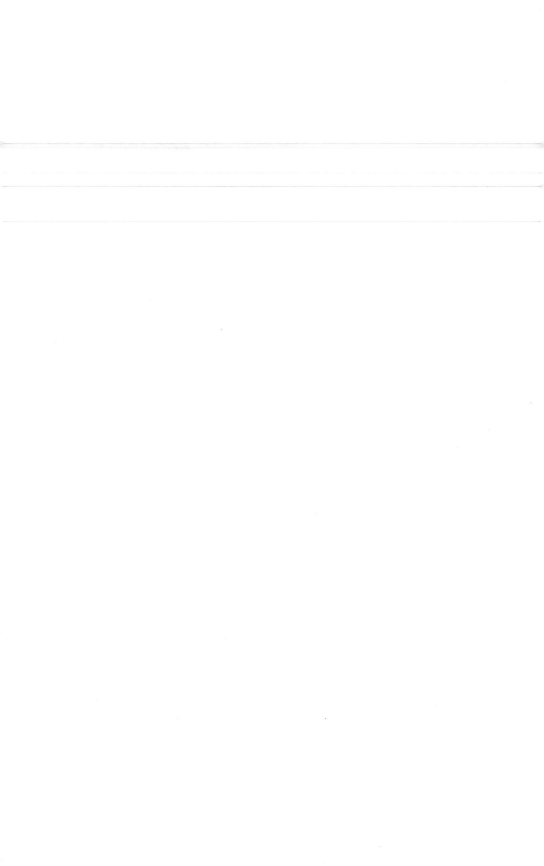

Basic Aspects

Experimental Glaucoma After Oxidative Stress and Modulation of the Consequent Apoptotic Events in a Rat Model

Nicola Calandrella, Simona Giorgini and
Gianfranco Risuleo

Additional information is available at the end of the chapter

1. Introduction

Glaucoma derives from an increase of the intra-ocular pressure (IOP) due to accumulation of the aqueous humor which causes degenerative events at the level of the retina and the optic nerve. This results in a progressive damage of the optic nerve that is paralleled by the gradual loss of retinal ganglion cells (RGC). The pathology causes increasing eyesight deterioration particularly in the peripheral areas of the visual field. The optic nerve papilla becomes paler and shows an augmented excavation as compared with a normal physiological situation. The increase of the IOP is to be ascribed, in the majority of cases, to an alteration of the ocular hydrodynamics: in particular the normal efflux of aqueous humor from the anterior chamber of the eye is severely hindered. The drainage system is located in the limbal regions or in the sclero-corneal junction. The inner surface presents a hollow (depression) known as inner scleral spur which is filled by the trabecular meshwork and the canal of Schlemm. Primary open angle glaucoma is caused by the failure of drainage from the trabecular meshwork, while the primary closed angle glaucoma consists in a modification of the iris-corneal angle. It is commonly accepted that glaucoma is the second cause of blindness in the world; as a matter of fact it has been estimated that 68 millions of patients are affected by this pathology and out of them, about 7 millions suffer complete bilateral blindness as a consequence of the glaucoma. The onset of the disease may occur at any age, also at childhood, but it is significantly more frequent in elderly people. Glaucoma is generally categorized in five different groups; two of them are the above mentioned open and closed angle primary glaucoma which are also the most widespread ones. A broad variety of pathological conditions may induce, as secondary event, the obstruction of the drainage system of the drainage angle which results in glaucoma. The primary open angle, which represents more than 60% of the cases, is a chronic condition. The outflow angle is not altered; the aqueous humor produced by the ciliary body reaches the trabecular meshwork, but its drainage is not efficient. This is possibly due to the decrease of diffusion towards the Schlemm's canal which causes a continuing increase of the IOP ending in the progressive degeneration of the optic nerve. Among the secondary factors contributing to the insurgence of glaucoma one should take into account: age (above 70), myopia and ethnic origin since the African populations seem to be more prone to develop the disease.

In the primary closed angle glaucoma which occurs in about 10% of patients, a closure of the filtration angle in the eye is observed and this is occasionally due to the trabecular obstruction by the iris. The mode of insurgence of this type of glaucoma, unlike other forms, is very rapid and is therefore also known as acute glaucoma. In this condition one of the main risk factors is also associated to familial and/or ethnic factors. As a matter of fact, East asian populations, the Chinese one in particular, show a significant aptitude towards this pathology, other risk factors being the patient's age (above 50 years of age the incidence of the pathology increases) and hypermetropia. To date a decisive therapy for neither open nor closed angle glaucoma is available, however some treatments exist allowing the slowing, and in some cases the arrest, of the progression of the disease.

Secondary glaucoma may develop as a consequence of other pathologies such as inflammation, cataract, traumas, pigments released from the iris and, finally, tumors. In this situation the eye activates its defense producing the hyper-secretion of aqueous humor thus leading to ocular hypertension. One of the main characteristics of glaucoma is the increased excavation of the optic disk which extends towards its margins. Even though some studies support the idea that the pathology may start at retinal level, some indications exist that the early lesions occur at the level of the head of the optic nerve, in particular on the *lamina cribrosa*. Investigations demonstrate that the death of RGC occurs by apoptosis [1, 2]; the activation of this process, most likely, causes a reduction of the number of axons forming the optic nerve and this would evolve to the clinical signs consisting in the characteristic increase of papilla excavation which results in a reduction of the optic visual field. The ganglion retinal cells are the first target of the damage, mainly those found in the temporal region of the retina where the *lamina cribrosa* is thinner and thus gives an inefficient structural support to the RGC axons [3].

Hypotheses on the mechanisms of cell degeneration are diverse, the mechanical stress and the ischemic model being two of the most corroborated ones. The mechanical stress theory purports that the increase of the IOP within the anterior chamber causes a direct hyper-pressure at the retina-vitreous interface. This mechanical stress would directly trigger cell death by physical compression. According to this theory the mechanical insult causes modifications of the cell function: with respect to this, it has been reported that this type of insult may alter gene expression in organs such as the heart and the endothelial vessels. Furthermore, by the activation of transduction pathways, different functional responses are induced in retinal cells and astrocytes [4]. This IOP-induced mechanical stress could also inhibit the retrograde transport along the ganglion cell axons. Regarding this particular point, it has been observed a block in the axonal transport at the level of the *lamina cribrosa* followed by a drastic reduction of neurotrophins required for the survival of the RGC [5]. Furthermore, a reduction of the axon-plasma transport and the accumulation of toxic level of neurotransmitters have been observed; also, an increase of nitric oxide and endothelins as well as remodeling of the extra-cellular matrix has been monitored. Studies validate, on the other hand, the theory of the ischemic model, i,e, the vascular model of ischemia, as a main cause of the increased mechanical compression and subsequent oxidative stress at cell level.

The ischemic hypothesis postulates that the high intraocular pressure and the deformation of the *lamina cribrosa* may generate a compression of the blood vessels at retina and/or optic nerve level with a subsequent ischemic damage. In the pathological ischemic condition a temporary interruption of blood perfusion occurs and this determines a lack of oxygen, glucose and trophic substances in general. In patients with normal pressure and open angle glaucoma it was reported a decrease of the blood flow at the head of the optic nerve and an increase of hemagglutination. In addition, in this type of glaucoma an alteration of endothelin-mediated blood flow occurs. This protein is expressed in the endothelial cells and constricts blood vessels thus raising the blood pressure; its action is mainly exerted on the smooth muscles of the blood vessels [6]. The raise of the IOP plays a crucial role in the etiology of the disease, however the observation of glaucoma patients with normal pressure values suggests that diverse factors act synergistically to the insurgence of the pathology.

The glaucoma neuropathy may be also due to an insufficient vascular perfusion of the optic nerve which causes an ischemic damage to this organ. The ischemia thus generated, ends in an oxidative stress at RGC level and causes apoptotic death. This phenomenon happens because when re-perfusion initiates, the presence of oxygen in the tissue exposed to ischemia, induces the formation of radical oxygen species (ROS). When the concentration of ROS is too high, the anti-oxidant systems of the cell become unable to inactivate them, due to a deficient homeostasis, thus the free radicals are no longer neutralized and may cause cell death either via apoptosis or necrosis. In conclusion both types of stress, the mechanical and the ischemic one, can contribute to the establishment of the disease [2].

1.1. Cellular targets of the ocular hypertension

A complex interaction between neural and glial cells exists during the differentiation and the life of the nervous system. As a matter of fact, neuroglia cells maintain the normal functions of the nervous system since they control the extra cellular environment, block the toxic agents and supply the trophic resources and, last but not least, provide a structural support to the neurons. In glaucoma, astrocytes play a very important role as far as the re-modeling of the *lamina cribrosa* is concerning. Actually, they may also have a role also in the onset of the disease. Studies conducted on human glaucoma have, in fact, evidenced that the disorganization at astrocyte level in the anterior areas of the optic nerve, is associated to hypertrophy and over-expression of the glial fibrillary acidic protein (GFAP) which also occurs in astrocyte cultures subjected to high hydrostatic pressure. Following ischemic episodes, traumas or neuro-degenerative disorders, the phenotype of the astrocyte cells and microglia, activates the production of cytokines, ROS, nitric oxide and tumor necrosis factor α (TNF-α); all these molecules are mediators involved in the tissue damage [2]. In a similar way, glial cells located in the retina and in the head of the optic nerve may carry out their normal physiological role as supporters of the cell bodies and their relative axons of the ganglion cells; on the contrary they may have a noxious role towards the same structures in pathological conditions.

1.2. Oxidative stress and retinal ganglion cell death in glaucoma

Oxidative stress is initiated by the imbalance between the production of ROS and their elimination by antioxidants. This phenomenon plays a key role in neuronal damage ending with neuron death which usually occurs by apoptosis. These reactive oxygen species are produced by mitochondria but can also derive from enzymatic degradation of neurotrans-mitters, neuroinflammatory mediators, and redox reactions [7]. Mitochondrial dysfunction can result in an increased level of ROS which is often found in neurodegenerative pathologies. Abnormal protein folding, defective ubiquitination and proteasome degradation systems may cause the production of ROS [8]. This promotes neuronal death *via* diverse molecular mecha-nisms including protein modification and DNA damage [9]. In any case, whether the oxidative stress triggers cell death is a component of a more complex neuro-degenerative process is yet to be elucidated [8]. Literature reports exist showing that neural damage occurs following oxidative stress in animal models of optic nerve injury and in human glaucoma. For example, DNA damage as well as protein and lipid peroxidation products, such as malonal-dihaldehyde accumulate in the trabecular meshwork and retina in animals with raised IOP [2, 10 - 16]. The high concentration of intra-cellular ROS has also been proposed as a crucial death signal after axonal injury, even though this may not directly cause a glaucoma, which would lead to RGC apoptosis [17 – 21]. Dysfunction of perfusion and reduced oxygen availability may play a role in the insurgence of an oxidative damage [22, 23]. The formation of ROS at mitochondrion level is required to activate a transcription factor known as hypoxia-inducible factor-1 alpha that induces the expression of several genes involved in the control of hypoxia, [24, 25]. Cells have a very effective protective antioxidant system including superoxide dismutase (SOD), catalase, glutathione peroxidase and glutathione reductase [26]; if this systems partially or totally fail in neutralizing the ROS in the RGCs population, the progression of glaucoma could be triggered. Evidence exists supporting this idea; as a matter of fact SOD activity is lower than normal in the trabecular meshwork of glaucoma patients [27, 28] and in the retina as monitored in experimental ocular model of hypertension [19]. A recent study *in vivo* showed a dramatic increase in RGCs after optic nerve axotomy which preceded apoptosis [19]. Reactive oxygen species alter the redox equilibrium in the cell and this produces cysteine sulfhydryl oxidation. As a consequence oxidative cross-linking leads to the formation of new disulfide bonds that result in conformational changes of the proteins and activation of apoptotic signals [29, 30]. To date many studies have shed light on the molecular events causing the death of RGC. These evidences were gathered from investigations on animal models where acute or chronic optic nerve damage was generated and in experimentally induced glaucoma. A number of cellular phenomena are involved in the apoptotic death of RGCs; just to mention some: deprivation of neurotrophic factor, loss of synaptic connectivity, oxidative stress, axonal transport failure (for an exhaustive review on this topics see [31]).

Apart from the elevated intraocular pressure, other risk factors such as genetic background, decreased corneal thickness, age and vascular dys-regulation may play an important role in the insurgence of glaucoma [32 - 39]. However, even if these factors may determine a risk to develop the disease, it remains difficult to establish a cause/effect relationship to develop this pathology: actually, one should consider that a high intraocular pressure is common among open-angle patients but many individuals showing this sign eventually will not develop glaucoma [40]. A further apparently paradoxical phenomenon is that a significant number of glaucoma patients progressively lose vision even though they react positively to drugs lowering the IOP [41 - 44]. In conclusion the cause of RGC in glaucoma still remains to be fully elucidated. Certainly the understanding of the apoptic death in RGC determined by the pathology is to be ascribed to the high complexity and the multifactorial character of the disease. The development of new neuroprotective therapies, even though will give a scant contribution to the elucidation of the molecular and cellular mechanisms underlying the disease, will certainly help to slow the development and progression of the pathology in glaucoma patients.

1.3. Mitochondrial malfunctions and ophthalmogical diseases

The association of ophthalmologic diseases to a mitochondrial etiology is assuming an increasingly interest: many authors consider, as a matter of fact, that the pathologies originate from impaired mitochondrial function, oxidative stress and enhanced apoptotic death. The mitochondrial role in the development of primary congenital glaucoma, characterized by trabecular dysgenesis, has been recently suggested. The formation of the trabecular meshwork during development is thought to have particular sensitivity to oxidative stress induced damage. Mitochondrial DNA (mtDNA) mutations, in particular, are emerging as causative agents of ophthalmologic disorders affecting mostly the optic nerve and the retina as well as the extra-ocular muscles. Also in these cases antioxidant therapy represents a good tool to treat these ophthalmologic conditions. Mitochondrial dysfunction is suggested, for example, to play an important role in age related macular degeneration, glaucoma and diabetes dependant retinopathy. Some biomarkers have been identified in the mitochondrial oxidative stress response: for instance, prohibitins also known as PHB may have diverse functions and are also involved in mitochondrial structure and functionality. These proteins present a ring-like structure with 16–20 alternating Phb1 and Phb2 subunits in the inner mitochondrial membrane [45]. The precise molecular function of the PHB molecular complex is not clear even though it has been hypothesized that they may have a role as chaperone for respiration chain proteins or as providers of a scaffold for the optimal mitochondrial morphology and function. Prohibitins have been demonstrated to stimulate cell proliferation both in plants and mammals such as rodents. As far as tissue re-modeling is concerned, the proteins of the matrix metalloproteinase (MMP) family could be a useful tool in gene therapy aimed at the protection/rescue of the RGCs. Therefore PHB and MMP could constitute an effective biomarker and/or a therapeutic target for ophthalmologic pathologies. (For a recent review see [46]).

2. A model of experimental glaucoma in rat

Several experimental animal models exist to investigate the ocular pathologies. In our laboratory we have developed a rat model of hypertension that mimics and reproduces the situation found in human glaucoma. This animal model will be briefly reviewed in the following sections [2].

2.1. Induction of the intra-ocular hypertension

To induce ocular hypertension *in vivo* [50] causing a condition of acute glaucoma in rat we injected in the anterior chamber of the right eye methylcellulose (MTC) suspended in physiological solution (the contra-lateral eye served as control). The IOP was monitored by tonometry. The hypertension induced by MTC was also performed in the presence of the antioxidant trolox [50]. The degree of animal sufferance was evaluated by the behavioral Irwin test and by the recovery of bodyweight. Ocular inflammation was assessed by the Drize test adapted to the rat, both approaches were described in detail in [49]. Intra-ocular pressure was monitored on 20 different animals that were finally sacrificed by hemorrhagic shock (decapitation). The eyes were removed and the cornea eliminated at limbus level; vitreous humor, and crystalline lens were discarded. The remaining samples of retina and optic nerve were fixed in paraformaldehyde, quickly washed in PBS finally included in freezing resin and cryostat-cut. Chromatin morphology and structure as well as DNA fragmentation was evidenced by terminal deoxynucleotidyl transferase dUTP nick end labeling (TUNEL) reaction and validated by the formation of the apoptotic ladder after agarose gel electrophoresis. The apoptotic ladder is generated by nucleolytic inter-nucleosomal DNA cleavage since during the late stages of apoptosis the enzyme DNase I is activated. This causes the formation of multiple nucleosomal DNA fragments which can be easily visualized, by gel electrophoresis, by fluorescence after ethidium bromide staining.

2.2. Lipoperoxidative damage of the membrane and apoptosis after induction of cell stress

The data obtained in our laboratory support the idea that ocular hypertension causes apoptotic death of retinal ganglion cells and over-expression of molecular markers typical of oxidative cell stress response and apoptosis. Glial cells may have a neuroprotective role in a pathological situation; in any case they may contribute protection from neuron damage. In particular, during progression of glaucoma, astrocytes are involved in the re-modeling of the *lamina cribrosa* and they could act as initiators of the pathology. With respect to this see the role of PHB and MMP mentioned in preceding section. Studies on experimental models of ocular hypertension and human glaucoma evidenced an astrocyte hypertrophy and a loss of organization both at retina and optic nerve level. The up-regulation of the GFAP was also observed, as mentioned in a previous section of this work, in cultured astrocytes grown at high hydrostatic pressure. The GFAP is considered a very important stress marker in diverse retinal pathologies. Activation of the glial cells may also have noxious consequences on neurons, as they may cause mechanical damages and alterations of the micro-enviroment also, they may fail to provide the structural/nutritionl support to the neural cells. This could trigger the release and/or production of neurotoxic and proapoptotic compounds such as nitric oxide synthase (NOS). The nitric oxide thus produced is a reactive free radical present in cells as a response to increased intracellular concentrations of Ca^{2+}. It is known that NOS increases in cerebral ischemia and the over-expression of this enzyme causes relevant damage: the overall result is a detrimental action on the cell membrane. Recent studies demonstrated that an excess of NO is toxic and this compound increases as a consequence of ocular hypertension. In glaucoma, the involvement of inducible NOS (iNOS) has also been suggested. The oxidative stress and the increase of IOP also cause up-regulation of ubiquitin (Ub) and stimulation of the Ub-proteasome pathway: this possibly derives from the activation of the apoptotic program. In any case it should be pointed out that we also demonstrated that a well-known natural substance, carnitine, endowed of antioxidant properties and improvement of muscle performance, can ameliorate the glaucomatous pathology in the rat model system developed in our laboratory [2, 16].

3. Conclusions

In conclusion, literature data imply that the RGCs are one of the main targets of the oxidative stress in the neural tissue. As shown in our studies, the injection of methylcellulose into the anterior chamber of the eye activates diverse signals of stress at the level of RGCs. Mainly, the up-regulation of the GFAP and DNA damage become evident. Methylcellulose hinders the efflux of fluids from the canals of Schlemm thus increasing the IOP. The consequent oxidative stress is shown by the overexpression of iNOS, which is an enzyme primarily involved in the mitochondrial lipid peroxidation, with consequent damage of the cell membrane. This is validated by the accumulation of intracellular malonal-dihaldehyde: a hallmark of lipoperoxidation. The ubiquitin-mediated proteasome pathway is also activated and this is directly related to the execution of the apoptotic death. The antiapoptotic role of carnitine plays a key role in the stabilization and function of the cell membrane, the mitochondrial one in particular. The contemporary treatment with methylcellulose and carnitine reduces the level of typical markers of cell sufferance and apoptotis, this enhances the mitochondrial performance, improves the overall homeostatic response to the hypertensive insult, and limits the apoptotic phenomena.

Author details

Nicola Calandrella, Simona Giorgini and Gianfranco Risuleo*

*Address all correspondence to: gianfranco.risuleo@uniroma1.it

Department of Biology and Biotechnology "Charles Darwin"- Sapienza University of Rome, Rome, Italy

References

[1] Capaccioli, S, Nucci, C, Quattrone, A, & Carella, E. Apoptosi nel glaucoma. In: Apoptosi in oftalmologia, Ed I.N.C. (1998). , 44-57.

[2] Calandrella, N, Scarsella, G, Pescosolido, N, & Risuleo, G. Degenerative and apoptotic events at retinal and optic nerve level after experimental induction of ocular hypertension. Mol Cell Biochem, (2007). , 301, 155-163.

[3] Quigley, H. A, Dunkelberger, G. R, & Green, W. R. Retinal ganglion cell atrophy correlated with automated perimetry in human eyes with glaucoma. Am. J. Ophthalmol (1989). , 107, 453-464.

[4] Wax, M. B, Tezel, G, Kobayashi, S, & Hernandez, M. R. Responses of different cells lines from ocular tissues to elevated hydrostatic pressure. Br. J. Ophthalmol (2000). , 84, 423-428.

[5] Quigley, H. A, Mckinnon, S. J, Zack, D. J, Pease, M. E, Kerrigan-baumrind, L. A, Kerrigan, F. D, & Mitchell, R. S. Retrograde axonal trasport of BDNF in retinal ganglion cell is blocked by acute IOP elevation in rat. Invest. Ophthalmol. Vis. Sci. (2000). , 41, 3460-3466.

[6] Morgan, J. E. Optic nerve head structure in glaucoma: astrocytes as mediators of axonal damage. Eye (2000). , 14, 437-444.

[7] Halliwell, B. Oxidative stress and neurodegeneration: where are we now? J. Neurochem. (2006). , 97, 1634-1658.

[8] Andersen, J. K. Oxidative stress in neurodegeneration: cause or consequence? Nat. Med. (2004). , 5, 18-25.

[9] Cross, J. V, & Templeton, D. J. Thiol oxidation of cell signaling proteins: controlling an apoptotic equilibrium. J. Cell. Biochem. (2004). , 93, 104-111.

[10] Babizhayev, M. A, & Bunin, A. Lipid peroxidation in open-angle glaucoma. Acta Ophthalmol. (Copenh) (1989). , 67, 371-77.

[11] Izzotti, A, Saccà, S. C, Cartiglia, C, & De Flora, S. Oxidative deoxyribonucleic acid damage in the eyes of glaucoma patients. Am. J. Med. (2003). , 114, 638-646.

[12] Ko, M. L, Peng, P. H, Ma, M. C, Ritch, R, & Chen, C. F. Dynamic changes in reactive oxygen species and antioxidant levels in retinas in experimental glaucoma. Free Radic. Biol. Med. (2005). , 39, 365-373.

[13] Moreno, M, Campanelli, J, Sande, P, Snez, D, & Keller-sarmiento, M. Rosenstein R Retinal oxidative stress induced by high intraocular pressure. Free Radic. Biol. Med. (2004). , 37, 803-812.

[14] Sacc, S, Pascott, A, Camicione, P, Capris, P, & Izzotti, A. Oxidative DNA damage in
      the human trabecular meshwork: clinical correlation in patients with primary open-
      angle glaucoma. Arch. Ophthalmol.(2005). , 123, 458-463.

[15] Tezel, G, Yang, X, & Cai, J. Proteomic identification of oxidatively modified retinal
      proteins in a chronic pressure-induced rat model of glaucoma. Invest. Ophthalmol.
      Vis. Sci. (2005). , 46, 3177-3187.

[16] Calandrella, N, De Seta, C, Scarsella, G, & Risuleo, G. Carnitine reduces the lipo-per-
      oxidative damage of the membrane and apoptosis after induction of cell stress in ex-
      perimental glaucoma. Cell Death Dis. (2010). e 62.

[17] Geiger, L. K, Kortuem, K. R, Alexejun, C, & Levin, L. A. Reduced redox state allows
      prolonged survival of axotomized neonatal retinal ganglion cells. Neuroscience
      (2002). , 109, 635-642.

[18] Kanamori, A, Catrinescu, M. M, Kanamori, N, Mears, K. A, Beaubien, R, & Levin, L.
      A. Superoxide is an associated signal for apoptosis in axonal injury. Brain (2010). ,
      133, 2612-2625.

[19] Lieven, C. J, Schlieve, C. R, Hoegger, M. J, & Levin, L. A. Retinal ganglion cell axoto-
      my induces an increase in intracellular superoxide anion. Invest. Ophthalmol. Vis.
      Sci. (2006). , 47, 1477-1485.

[20] Nguyen, S. M, Alexejun, C. N, & Levin, L. A. Amplification of a reactive oxygen spe-
      cies signal in axotomized retinal ganglion cells. Antioxid. Redox Signal. (2003). , 5,
      629-634.

[21] Swanson, K. I, Schlieve, C. R, Lieven, C. J, & Levin, L. A. Neuroprotective effect of
      sulfhydryl reduction in a rat optic nerve crush model. Invest. Ophthalmol. Vis. Sci.
      (2005). , 46, 3737-3741.

[22] Izzotti, A, Bagnis, A, & Sacc, S. The role of oxidative stress in glaucoma. Mutat. Res.
      (2006). , 612, 105-114.

[23] Tezel, G. Oxidative stress in glaucomatous neurodegeneration: mechanisms and con-
      sequences. Prog. Retin. Eye Res. (2006). , 5, 490-513.

[24] Chandel, N. S, Mcclintock, D. S, Feliciano, C. E, Wood, T. M, Melendez, J. A, Rodri-
      guez, A. M, & Schumacker, P. T. Reactive oxygen species generated at mitochondrial
      complex III stabilize hypoxia-inducible factor-1alpha during hypoxia: a mechanism
      of O2 sensing. J. Biol. Chem. (2000). , 275, 25130-25138.

[25] Duranteau, J, Chandel, N. S, Kulisz, A, Shao, Z, & Schumacker, P. T. Intracellular sig-
      naling by reactive oxygen species during hypoxia in cardiomyocytes. J. Biol. Chem.
      (1998). , 273, 11619-11624.

[26] Vendemiale, G, Grattagliano, I, & Altomare, E. An update on the role of free radicals
      and antioxidant defense in human disease. Int. J. Clin. Lab. Res. (1999). , 29, 49-55.

[27] Behndig, A, Svensson, B, Marklund, S. L, & Karlsson, K. Superoxide dismutase isoenzymes in the human eye. Invest. Ophthalmol. Vis. Sci. (1998). , 39, 471-475.

[28] [28] De La Paz, M. A, & Epstein, D. L. Effect of age on superoxide dismutase activity of human trabecular meshwork. Invest. Ophthalmol. Vis. Sci. (1996). , 37, 1849-1853.

[29] Carugo, O, Cemazar, M, Zahariev, S, Hudaky, I, Gaspari, Z, Perczel, A, & Pongor, S. Vicinal disulfide turns. Protein Eng. (2003). , 16, 637-639.

[30] Park, C, & Raines, R. T. Adjacent cysteine residues as a redox switch. Protein Eng. (2001). , 14, 939-942.

[31] Almasieh, M, Wilson, A. M, & Morquette, B. Cueva Vargas J.L., Di Polo A. The molecular basis of retinal ganglion cell death in glaucoma. Prog Retin Eye Res (2012). , 31, 152-181.

[32] Agis, I. The advanced glaucoma intervention study (AGIS): 7. the relationship between control of intraocular pressure and visual field deterioration. Am. J. Ophthalmol. (2000). , 130, 429-440.

[33] [33] Gordon, M, Beiser, J, Brandt, J, Heuer, D, Higginbotham, E, Johnson, C, Keltner, J, Miller, J, Parrish, R. N, Wilson, M, & Kass, M. The Ocular hypertension treatment study: baseline factors that predict the onset of primary open-angle glaucoma. Arch. Ophthalmol. (2002). , 120, 714-720.

[34] Leske, M. C, Heijl, A, Hyman, L, Bengtsson, B, Dong, L, & Yang, Z. EMGT Group. Predictors of long-term progression in the early manifest glaucoma trial. Ophthalmology (2007). , 114, 1965-1972.

[35] Leske, M. C, Connell, A. M, Wu, S. Y, Nemesure, B, Li, X, Schachat, A, & Hennis, A. Incidence of open-angle glaucoma: the Barbados eye studies. The Barbados Eye Studies Group. Arch. Ophthalmol. (2001). , 119, 89-95.

[36] Mukesh, B. N, Mccarty, C. A, Rait, J. L, & Taylor, H. R. Five-year incidence of open-angle glaucoma: the visual impairment project. Ophthalmology (2002). , 109, 1047-1051.

[37] Wolfs, R. C. W, Klaver, C. C. W, Ramrattan, R. S, Van Duijn, C. M, Hofman, A, & De Jong, P. T. V. M. Genetic risk of primary open-angle glaucoma: populationbased Familial aggregation study. Arch. Ophthalmol.(1998). , 116, 1640-1645.

[38] Medeiros, F. A, Sample, P. A, Zangwill, L. M, Bowd, C, Aihara, M, & Weinreb, R. N. Corneal thickness as a risk factor for visual field loss in patients with preperimetric glaucomatous optic neuropathy. Am. J. Ophthalmol. (2003). , 136, 805-813.

[39] Leske, M. C. Ocular perfusion pressure and glaucoma: clinical trial and epidemiologic findings. Curr. Opin. Ophthalmol. (2009). , 20, 73-78.

[40] Friedman, D. S, Wilson, M. R, Liebmann, J. M, Fechtner, R. D, & Weinreb, R. N. An evidence-based assessment of risk factors for the progression of ocular hypertension and glaucoma. Am. J. Ophthalmol. (2004). , 138, 19-31.

[41] Caprioli, J. Neuroprotection of the optic nerve in glaucoma. Acta Ophthalmol. Scand. (1997). , 75, 364-367.

[42] Georgopoulos, G, Andreanos, D, Liokis, N, Papakonstantinou, D, Vergados, J, & Theodossiadis, G. Risk factors in ocular hypertension. Eur. J. Ophthalmol. (1997). , 7, 357-363.

[43] Harbin, T. S, Podos, S. M, Kolker, A. E, & Becker, B. Visual field progression in open-angle glaucoma patients presenting with monocular field loss. Trans. Sect. Ophthalmol. Am. Acad. Ophthalmol. Otolaryngol. (1976). , 8, 253-257.

[44] Leske, M. C, Heijl, A, Hussein, M, Bengtsson, B, Hyman, L, & Komaroff, E. For the Early Manifest Glaucoma Trial Group,. Factors for glaucoma progression and the effect of treatment: the early manifest glaucoma trial. Arch. Ophthalmol. (2003). , 121, 48-56.

[45] Tatsuta, T, Model, K, & Langer, T. Formation of Membrane-bound Ring Complexes by Prohibitins in Mitochondria. Mol. Biol. Cell (2005). , 16, 248-259.

[46] Schrier, S. A, & Marni, J. F. Mitochondrial disorders and the eye. Current Opinion in Ophthalmology (2011). , 22, 325-331.

[47] Zhu, M. D, & Cai, F. Y. Development of experimental chronic intraocular hypertension in the rabbit. Austl Nw Z J Ophthalmol (1992). , 20, 225-234.

[48] Mcclain, D. E, Kalinich, J. F, & Ramakrishnan, N. Trolox inhibits apoptosis in irradiated MOLT-4 lymphocytes. FASEB J (1995). , 9, 1345-1354.

[49] Drize, J. H, Woodard, G, & Calvery, H. O. Methods for the study of irritation and toxicity of substances applied topically to the skin and mucous membranes. J Pharm Exp Ther (1944). , 82, 377-390.

Chapter 2

Genetics and Environmental Stress Factor Contributions to Anterior Segment Malformations and Glaucoma

Yoko A. Ito and Michael A. Walter

Additional information is available at the end of the chapter

1. Introduction

Glaucoma is one of the leading causes of irreversible blindness worldwide [1]. A gradual loss of retinal ganglion cells (RGCs) result in degeneration of the optic nerve head and visual field loss. Glaucoma is an age-related disease with a strong genetic basis. The risk of developing glaucoma significantly increases after age 40 [2,3]. An estimated 79.6 million people worldwide will have glaucoma by 2020 [1]. Patients with mutations in glaucoma-associated genes are more likely to develop juvenile-onset and early adult-onset glaucoma. In any case, early detection of glaucoma is essential to effectively manage the progression of the disease by preventing further loss of RGCs. Despite many years of research in this field, the precise cause(s) of RGC death remain unknown. The pathophysiology of glaucoma is complicated as environmental, genetic, and even stochastic factors all contribute to the pathology of glaucoma. Also, both the posterior segment, where the RGCs are located, and the anterior segment of the eye play key roles in the disease.

Glaucoma can be classified as being primary, secondary, or congenital. These groups can then be further categorized to be open-angle or closed-angle, depending on the anterior chamber angle. In closed-angle glaucoma, the angle between the iris and the cornea is closed resulting in obstruction of aqueous humor flow. Primary glaucoma is non-syndromic and is not associated with any underlying condition. Primary congenital glaucoma is a rare form of glaucoma present at birth or within the first two years after birth. Glaucoma that develops as a result of an underlying ocular or systemic condition or eye injury is categorized as secondary glaucoma. Pseudoexfoliative glaucoma is an example of secondary glaucoma whereby fibrillar extracellular material deposits and accumulates in various ocular tissues, predisposing the patient to developing glaucoma.

Primary open angle glaucoma (POAG) is a common type of glaucoma where the iridocorneal angle is unobstructed. Although POAG can occur in patients with normal intraocular pressure (IOP), sometimes referred to as normal-tension glaucoma, elevated IOP is a major risk factor of developing POAG. IOP is dependent on proper flow of aqueous humor from the site of production in the posterior chamber to the site of drainage in the anterior chamber of the eye. The anterior chamber structures that function in regulating the drainage of aqueous humor from the eye are the trabecular meshwork (TM) and Schlemm's canal. Disruptions of the aqueous humor flow pathway are predicted to result in elevated IOP.

In this chapter, the recent advances in research regarding the contribution of the TM in maintaining proper IOP will be reviewed. An overview of the anterior chamber drainage structures, the TM and Schlemm's canal, and how these structures maintain the aqueous humor outflow pathway will be provided. Also, the changes that occur in the TM during the normal aging process and in the glaucoma phenotype will be compared. Then, the specific types of stresses that TM cells are exposed to, mainly mechanical, oxidative, and phagocytic stresses, and the effects these stresses have on gene expression will be examined. Recent advances in technology have enabled the analysis of global gene expression profiles. These analyses have revealed that signal transduction pathways play an important role in the cellular adaptive response to environmental stresses. Finally, the effect that environmental stresses have on glaucoma-associated genes will be considered.

2. Trabecular meshwork and aqueous humor outflow pathway

Aqueous humor is a colourless and transparent fluid that makes contact with various structures in both the anterior and posterior chambers of the eye including the lens, iris, and cornea. The lens and the cornea are clear and avascular, which enables light to be effectively transmitted to the photoreceptors in the back of the eye. Aqueous humor provides nutrients to the avascular lens and cornea and also removes metabolic waste products. The composition of aqueous humor has been of great interest due to the potential regulatory effects on all the structures to which it makes contact. For example, the presence of antioxidants such as glutathione and ascorbic acid [4,5] in the aqueous humor suggest that this fluid affects the ability of cells to respond and adapt to stress.

Aqueous humor flows from the site of production, which is the non-pigmented ciliary epithelial cells [6,7] in the posterior chamber, to the site of drainage, which is the TM and Schlemm's canal in the anterior chamber (Figure 1). Production and drainage of aqueous humor is a continuous and dynamic process. Diurnal variations in aqueous humor turnover rates occur ranging from 3.0μL/min in the morning to 1.5μL/min at night [8]. The balance between aqueous humor production and drainage is essential for maintaining a healthy IOP of approximately 15mmHg within the eye [9]. Abnormalities in aqueous humor drainage due to increased resistance at the TM are thought to result in elevated IOP, which is a major risk factor for developing glaucoma [10].

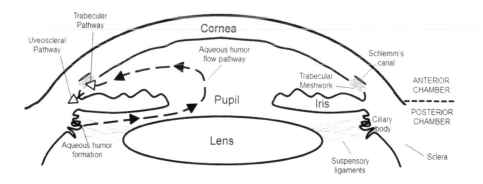

Figure 1. Schematic diagram of aqueous humor flow pathway. Aqueous humor is produced by the ciliary body in the posterior chamber and then flows into the anterior chamber. The majority of the aqueous humor will be drained from the eye via the trabecular pathway through the trabecular meshwork (TM) and Schlemm's canal. The rest of the aqueous humor is drained via the uveoscleral pathway. Increased resistance occurs when the TM and Schlemm's canal malfunctions. This disruption in aqueous humor outflow leads to increased intraocular pressure (IOP), which is a major risk factor for developing glaucoma.

Aqueous humor is drained from the eye by two distinct outflow pathways: the trabecular (aka conventional) pathway and the uveoscleral (aka unconventional) pathway. The uveoscleral pathway is an IOP-independent pathway in which the aqueous humor leaves the anterior chamber by passing through the ciliary muscle bundles into the supraciliary and suprachoroidal spaces and eventually into the sclera [11,12]. Direct measurement of the percentage of aqueous humor leaving the human eye via the uveoscleral pathway has proven to be difficult [13]. There appears to be great variation between individuals with values ranging from 36% to 54% in healthy young subjects [14,15]. The percentage of aqueous humor leaving the eye via the uveoscleral pathway decreases with age with values ranging from 4% to 46% in older subjects [15,16]. Thus, as aging progresses, a larger portion of aqueous humor is drained via the trabecular pathway.

Despite the individual variations, it is generally accepted that in humans, the majority of aqueous humor is transported through the TM via the trabecular pathway. Disruption of aqueous humor drainage through the trabecular pathway is thought to be the major contributing factor to alteration of IOP. The TM is a multi-layered tissue located in the anterior chamber angle. From the anterior chamber the aqueous humor passes through the multiple layers of the TM: the uveal meshwork, the corneoscleral meshwork, and the juxtacanalicular meshwork (also known as the cribriform plexus). Each layer consists of a central connective tissue (aka beam) surrounded by an outer endothelial layer. Connecting fibrils tightly connect the network of elastic fibres in the juxtacanalicular meshwork to the inner endothelial wall of Schlemm's canal [17-20]. As the aqueous humor passes through each layer of the TM, the intercellular space narrows resulting in increased resistance. Then, aqueous humor progresses through the inner endothelial cell layer of Schlemm's canal. The endothelial cells of Schlemm's canal express the tight junction protein Zona occludens-1 (ZO-1), which allows aqueous humor to be transported via the intercellular route [21]. The aqueous humor is also transported via the transcellular route through giant vacuoles [22-24]. Aqueous humor passes through Schlemm's canal and returns to the general circulation via the aqueous and episcleral veins [23,25]. IOP is affected by the episcleral venous pressure and the resistance to aqueous humor flow within the TM. Episcleral venous pressure directly affects IOP because aqueous humor must flow out of the eye against the pressure in the episcleral veins. The main source of resistance to aqueous humor flow is thought to be located in the intercellular (aka subendo-thelial) region of the juxtacanalicular network [26-29].

Extracellular matrix (ECM) occupies the intercellular space between the beams of TM cells. The ECM consists of glycosaminoglycans (GAGs), proteoglycans, laminin, various collagens, fibronectin, and vitronectin (reviewed in [30]). The constant turnover of this ECM has been proposed to play a role in maintaining proper aqueous humor resistance. The family of matrix metalloproteinases (MMPs) are secreted zinc proteinases that initiate ECM turnover [31,32]. MMP activity is inhibited by the family of tissue inhibitors of metalloproteinases (TIMPs). MMP activity is suggested to be important in regulating aqueous humor outflow facility by proteolytic alterations. Using perfused human anterior segment, Bradley *et al.* observed that increasing MMP activity increased the outflow rate while inhibiting MMP activity by the addition of TIMP decreased outflow rate [32]. MMP activity is suggested to have various functional consequences including degradation of ECM components, cleavage and modifica-tion of signaling molecules, and cleavage of intercellular junctions and basement membrane (reviewed in [33]).

Another factor that affects resistance is the ciliary muscle. The elastic anterior tendons of the ciliary muscle insert into the network of elastic fibres in the juxtacanalicular meshwork and corneoscleral meshwork [19,20,34]. The elastic fibres are surrounded by a collagen-based sheath [20]. Ciliary muscle contractions result in increased aqueous humor outflow facility [35]. Upon ciliary muscle contraction, the connecting fibres straighten. Since the ciliary muscle is connected to the TM and the inner wall of Schlemm's canal by the connecting fibrils, ciliary muscle contraction widens the intercellular space in the juxtacanalicular meshwork allowing aqueous humor to flow against less resistance [35]. In contrast, relaxation of the ciliary muscles results in the opposite effect where there is increased resistance to aqueous flow [36].

As outlined above, the aqueous humor flow pathway is a complex process regulated by structures in both the posterior and anterior chambers of the eye. The TM is a highly specialized tissue that is able to adapt to the dynamic nature of aqueous humor outflow. The ability to adapt is an essential characteristic of the TM, especially because these cells are located in an environment that is constantly changing (Figure 2).

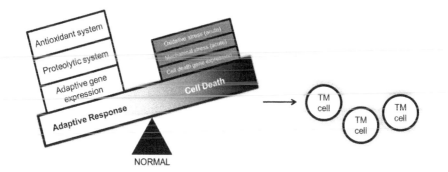

Figure 2. Trabecular meshwork under normal conditions. Even under normal conditions, the cells of the trabecular meshwork (TM) are constantly exposed to mechanical and oxidative stresses. TM cells have defense mechanisms including the antioxidant and proteolytic systems to protect the cells from these stresses. Also, specific changes in global gene expression occur in response to the specific stress, which enables TM cells to adapt to the environment and survive.

3. Change in trabecular meshwork during the normal aging process

Aging is a major risk factor for developing glaucoma. However, at the physiological level, minimal changes in aqueous humor flow dynamics occur in normal healthy subjects as aging progresses (reviewed in reference [37]). Using tonography, many studies have observed that aqueous humor outflow facility decreases with age [15,38-40]. The tonographic procedure measures outflow facility. IOP is first increased by applying force to the cornea using a tonometer probe. The subsequent decrease in IOP over the time of the test is used to determine aqueous humor outflow via the trabecular pathway. However, interpretation of results using the tonographic technique is limited because ocular rigidity is not taken into account. Since ocular rigidity increases with age [39,41], older subjects may appear to have a reduction in aqueous humor outflow facility because the stiffer eyes are less responsive to the tonographic technique, which involves applying force to the cornea. Also, the tonographic measurements do not take into account the change in pseudofacility, which refers to the probe-induced change in aqueous humor flow into the anterior chamber. In contrast to tonography, fluorophotometry is not affected by ocular rigidity and pseudofacility because no force is applied to the cornea. The outflow facility measured by fluorophotometry was 0.23±0.10µL/min/mmHg in 20-30 year old subjects (n=51) and 0.27±0.13µL/min/mmHg in subjects 60 years and older (n=53) [15]. Thus, fluorophotometric measurements indicate that there is in fact no difference in outflow facility as aging progresses [15]. Many studies using tonographic and fluorophotometric measurements have consistently shown that with age, aqueous humor production decreases [15,38,39,42-44]. Although outflow facility remains stable and aqueous humor production decreases, IOP remains stable in normal healthy subjects as aging progresses. Toris *et al.* have recently measured IOP to be 14.7±2.5mmHg in 20-30 year old subjects (n=51) and 14.3±2.6mmHg in subjects 60 years and older (n=53) [15]. A decrease in anterior chamber depth [15,45,46] with aging may account for the lack of change in IOP.

Interestingly, prominent changes at the structural and cellular levels occur with age. Connecting fibrils ensure that contact is maintained between the juxtacanalicular meshwork and the inner endothelial wall of Schlemm's canal [19,20]. The sheath surrounding these elastic fibres thickens with age [47]. The intercellular space narrows due to an increase in the amount of extracellular material from the thickened sheath, resulting in increased resistance [48,49]. Also, as aging progresses, the number of TM cells decrease [50,51]. Grierson and Howes estimate that at age 20, there are approximately 763 000 cells in the TM. By age 80, approximately 403 000 cells remain [51]]. The outer TM layers lose more TM cells while the least number of TM cells are lost from the inner juxtacanalicular layer [51,52]. This decline in TM cells appears to be a continuous and linear process with an estimated 0.58% loss of cells annually [50,52]. The linear decrease in TM cellularity is intriguing because the mechanism of cell loss may be different between the ages [52]. Age-related mechanisms such as accumulation of reactive oxygen species (ROS) and misfolded proteins are likely to contribute to cell loss in older subjects. However, other non-age-related mechanisms, such as exposure to mechanical stress, are likely responsible for cell death in the TM in younger subjects. Interestingly, Alvarado *et al.* noted that TM cells may have a reduced reparative capacity, which would further contribute to the decreased cellularity with age [52]. The loss of TM cells with age could have a more severe consequence in some individuals because there appears to be great variation in the absolute number of TM cells between individuals [53]. Therefore, individuals with less TM cells would be predicted to be less efficient in fulfilling the function of TM cells (Figure 3).

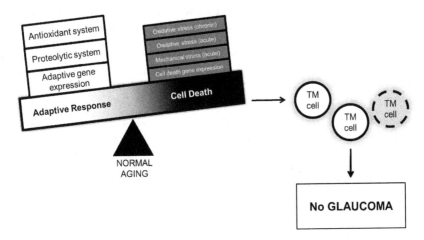

Figure 3. Trabecular meshwork during normal aging. During normal aging, the cellular defense mechanisms of the trabecular meshwork (TM) cells become less efficient. As in normal conditions (see Figure 2), the TM cells are exposed to a variety of stresses. However, the TM cells will also be exposed to other types of stresses such as chronic oxidative stress because there is an accumulation of reactive oxygen species (ROS) as aging progresses. Since the TM cells are no longer able to adapt to the environment, there will be increased TM cell death (dotted circle). However, the TM tissue still functions, preventing the onset of glaucoma.

Regardless of the individual variation in TM cell number, the consequence of losing TM cells in all aging individuals can be predicted. As avid phagocytes, TM cells are thought to clear debris from the aqueous humor outflow pathway [54-58]]. Although TM cells have the ability to ingest particulate matters rapidly, the phagocytic process may have detrimental effects on the overall health of the cell, even leading to necrosis [59]. Zhou *et al.* also showed that after phagocytosis, temporary alteration of TM cells occurred including rearrangement of the cytoskeleton and increased migratory activity [60]. These alterations, although temporary, have been speculated to be linked to the age-related loss of TM cells [60]. TM cells also maintain aqueous humor outflow by releasing factors that regulate permeability of the endothelial cells of Schlemm's canal [61]. TM cells release various enzymes and cytokines both in the presence and absence of stimulation such as mechanical stretching and exposure to pro-inflammatory cytokines [61,62]. TM endothelial cells constitutively secrete cytokines such as Interleukin 8 (IL8], Chemokine, CXC motif, ligand 6 (CXCL6), and Monocyte chemotactic protein 1 (MCP1], strengthening the notion that the release of cytokines is important in maintaining aqueous humor outflow [62].

4. Change in trabecular meshwork in glaucoma disease phenotype

Even with the age-related structural and cellular changes, the TM effectively functions to drain aqueous humor. However, in patients with glaucoma, the structural and cellular changes are more pronounced and as a result, TM function is disrupted. In glaucomataous eyes, there is more prominent and irregular thickening of the sheaths of the elastic fibers. Also, there is increased deposition of sheath-derived plaques compared with normal eyes [47,63]. This increase in extracellular material in the TM is predicted to block aqueous humor outflow [20] contributing to the development of disease. As in normal aging, there is a linear decrease in cellularity as aging progresses in the TM of POAG patients. Moreover, Alvarado *et al.* observed fewer cells in the glaucomatous TM compared with the non-glaucomatous TM over a wide range of ages [50].

The risk of developing glaucoma significantly increases after age 40. Despite the fact that glaucoma is an age-related disease, aging in most people does not result in this disease (Figure 3). The changes that occur in the TM during the normal aging process may make the tissue more susceptible to malfunction. However, other unknown factors and even stochastic factors must be present for the TM to fail to a point that the glaucoma phenotype develops (Figure 4).

5. Exposure of trabecular meshwork to mechanical stress

In order to survive, TM cells must be able to constantly adapt to their continuously changing environment. Similar to any other cell in the body, TM cells are exposed to a variety of environmental stresses. Due to the location of cells of the TM, one of the major types of stress these cells are exposed to is mechanical stress. IOP continuously fluctuates throughout the day with a higher IOP occurring during the nocturnal period. The fluctuation in IOP is part of a normal physiological process and is unavoidable. Fluctuations in IOP occur with blinking, eye

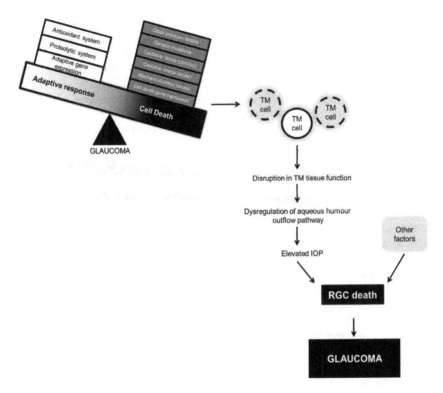

Figure 4. Trabecular meshwork of glaucoma phenotype. Similar to normal non-aging and aging conditions, trabecular meshwork (TM) cells are exposed to a variety of stresses. However, other unknown factors are present to initiate the cascade of events that lead to the development of glaucoma. Also, genetic mutations could compromise normal TM cell function. All of these factors are predicted to result in TM cell death (dotted circles) to the extent that the TM tissue is no longer able to function properly. Consequently, there will be dysregulation of aqueous humor drainage resulting in increased intraocular pressure (IOP), which would ultimately lead to retinal ganglion cell (RGC) death and glaucoma.

movements, and even with a change in body position. A supine body position has been shown to result in higher IOP compared with an upright body position [64,65]. The temporary fluctuation in IOP can vary up to 10mmHg [66]. This change in IOP results in distortions (including stretching and compression) of the cells and is sensed by the cells of the TM as mechanical stress.

6. Exposure of trabecular meshwork to oxidative stress

Another type of environmental stress that TM cells are exposed to is oxidative stress. Cells are constantly exposed to free radicals that are the by-products of normal cellular metabolism. In addition, the aqueous humor is itself a source of free radicals. Hydrogen peroxide (H_2O_2) is normally present in the aqueous humor and is suggested to be the key source of oxidative stress for the TM [67]. Initially, the concentration of H_2O_2, a reactive oxygen species (ROS), was reported to be between 25-60 μM in the aqueous humor using the dichloropheno-indopheno (DCPIP) assay [5,68-70]. However, technical issues with the DCPIP method, including the interference of ascorbic acid with the assay [70] and the spontaneous auto-oxidization of DCPIP in the presence of oxygen [71], has resulted in the re-examination of H_2O_2 in the aqueous humor. Different methods have indicated that H_2O_2 is present in the aqueous humor, but at much lower concentrations than previously thought [70,71]. An accurate concentration of H_2O_2 is still difficult to obtain and may vary greatly between individuals. Since cells of the TM are in direct contact with aqueous humor, these cells are exposed both intracellularly and extracellularly to oxidative stress.

Free radicals at lower concentrations are beneficial to the cell (reviewed in [72,73]). Low concentrations of ROS act as second messengers for signal transduction and gene regulation. For example, low concentrations of ROS activate the Nuclear factor kappa-B (NF-κB) transcription factor, which plays a key role in many cellular processes including inflammation, cell proliferation, and apoptosis (reviewed in [74]) However, higher concentrations of free radicals can have negative effects on the cell (Figure 5). Free radicals can damage proteins and DNA, promote lipid peroxidation, disrupt mitochondrial function, and trigger cell death (reviewed in [73]). Cells have an antioxidant defense mechanism to counter the deleterious effects of ROS. For example, superoxide dismutase (SOD) is an antioxidant enzyme that converts superoxide free radical anion (O_2^-) into H_2O_2 and molecular oxygen (O_2) [75]. H_2O_2 must then be converted into H_2O by two other antioxidant enzymes: peroxisomal catalases and the family of glutathione peroxidases (GPx). In the event that H_2O_2 is not converted, then it may split into the hydroxyl radical (OH•), which can be dangerous because it can react with almost any macromolecule within a short diffusion distance. Cells, through the activity of nitric oxide synthase, are able to produce the free radical nitric oxide (NO). NO itself is hardly toxic and is in fact important in regulating various cellular functions. In fact NO has been suggested to increase aqueous humor outflow by relaxing the ciliary smooth muscles [76,77]. However, NO becomes dangerous when it spontaneously reacts with superoxide O_2^- , forming the powerful oxidant peroxynitrite (ONOO-) [78]. Peroxynitrite is highly reactive and can damage biological molecules resulting in cell death (reviewed in [79]). In this way, the antioxidant defense mechanism also functions in minimizing the deleterious effects of reactive nitrogen species (RNS).

Chronic oxidative stress is recognized to be a major contributor to the aging process and various diseases including neurodegenerative diseases such as Parkinson's [80,81] and Alzheimer [82-84], cancer [72,85], and cardiovascular diseases [86]. Since POAG is an age-related disease, chronic oxidative stress is also suggested to have a role in the pathophysiology of this disease (reviewed in [87]). In POAG, both the RGCs and the anterior segment structures such as the TM are exposed to chronic oxidative stress conditions. TM cells are exposed to acute oxidative stress under normal physiological conditions [67]. The presence of cellular defense mechanisms in TM cells enables TM cells to quickly and effectively respond and adapt to their environment (Figure 2). Two cellular defense mechanisms present in TM cells are the antioxidant system, which defends against ROS, and the proteolytic system, which removes unwanted biomaterials from the cell, many of which are products of oxidative stress-related damage. However, as aging progresses, the normal cellular defense mechanisms become less effective and the cell is less able to remove potential toxic materials such as ROS and misfolded proteins (Figure 3). The gradual accumulation of toxic materials will lead to an environment where the cells are exposed to chronic oxidative stress. We hypothesize that the cellular defense mechanisms, already compromised due to the aging process, become completely over-whelmed under such chronic oxidative stress conditions. Cell death will occur when the cells are no longer able to adapt to the environment. Since accumulation of ROS occurs with age, the loss of TM cells during the aging process may also be in part due to exposure of TM cells to chronic oxidative stress conditions. The presence of fewer TM cells as aging progresses could also be detrimental to the TM tissue as there are fewer cells to protect against ROS in the aqueous humor. Although it remains a likely possibility, evidence that chronic oxidative stress directly contributes to the loss of TM cells with age is currently lacking.

In comparison to non-glaucomatous individuals, the TM cells of glaucoma patients appear to have more oxidative stress-related damages, including the accumulation of oxidatively damaged DNA[88,89], proteins[90], and organelles, as well as lipid peroxidation products [91,92] (Figure 5). Oxidative stress can damage DNA, resulting in the formation of 8-hy-

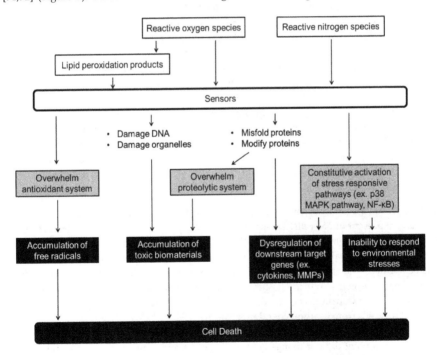

Figure 5. Overview of various oxidative stress-related effects on the cell, which would contribute to cell death.

droxy-2`-deoxyguanosine (8-OHdG). The levels of 8-OHdG were increased in DNA extracts from glaucomatous TM cells compared with healthy controls [88,89]. Also, aqueous humor and serum levels of 8-OHdG were significantly higher in glaucoma patients (n=28] compared with the age-matched control group of senile cataract patients (n=27) [93].

Despite having more oxidative stress-related damages, TM cells of glaucoma patients appear to have increased activity of some components of the antioxidant defense mechanism. Increased levels of glutathione peroxidase (GPx) and superoxide dismutase (SOD) activities were measured in aqueous humor of glaucomatous patients compared with the control group of senile cataract patients [94,95]. However, no apparent change in catalase activity levels have been detected [94,95]. Thus, at least some components of the antioxidant defense mechanism are functioning to prevent TM cell death under glaucomatous conditions.

Aqueous humor is both a source of free radicals and a source of antioxidants. Since low concentrations of free radicals are necessary for normal cellular function, TM cells rely on the very high content of antioxidants in the aqueous humor to achieve a balance that maximizes cell survival. High aqueous humor concentration of the antioxidant ascorbic acid (aka Vitamin C), which is about 20 times higher than in plasma [70], suggests that this antioxidant may be a major protector against free radicals in the eye [96-98]. Ascorbic acid has also been suggested to protect cells against ultraviolet light [98,99]. In addition to being an antioxidant, ascorbic acid is suggested to also have a role regulating the ECM of the TM. TM cells synthesize many types of glycosaminoglycans (GAGs) into the ECM including hyaluronic acid [100]. Ascorbic acid can increase hyaluronic acid synthesis [100]. Since hyaluronic acid has been shown to increase the expression of several MMPs [101], altered levels of this GAG would affect ECM turnover. Interestingly, Knepper et al. has shown that there is significantly less hyaluronic acid in the TM of POAG patients compared with the TM of normal subjects [102,103]. Thus, ascorbic acid is predicted to affect the aqueous outflow pathway by acting as an antioxidant and by regulating the ECM components that are important in maintaining the aqueous humor outflow pathway. Although some groups observed no difference in aqueous ascorbic acid levels between POAG patients and senile cataract patients [104,105], Lee et al. observed greater levels of ascorbic acid in the aqueous humor of POAG patients [106]. The difference in observation may be due to the great individual variation in ascorbic acid levels [105]. Nevertheless, ascorbic acid appears to play a protective role for TM cells.

In addition to the antioxidant system, the proteolytic system is another cellular defense mechanism present in TM cells. The proteolytic system is essential for the removal of oxidatively damaged proteins and organelles. The 20S proteasome, 26S proteasome, and immunoproteasome are the main cellular systems in eukaryotic cells that eliminate damaged proteins. The 20S proteasome tends to degrade oxidized proteins while the 26S proteasome degrade ubiquitynated proteins. In many tissues, including the TM, there is a decline in proteasomal activity with age. Caballero et al. reported that primary cultures of human trabecular meshwork (HTM) cells from healthy older donors (ages 66, 70, and 73) had decreased proteasomal activity compared with healthy young donors (ages 9, 14, and 25) [90]. Since the overall proteasomal content did not change between the older and younger donors, the decrease in proteasomal activity is most likely due to oxidation of the proteasomal subunits and the overload of the proteasomal machinery with damaged proteins. Caballero *et al.* observed an increase in oxidized proteins in the older donors [90]. Accumulation of oxidized protein is not the only biomolecule detrimental to proteasomal function.

The accumulation of lipid peroxidation products in the TM is suggested to also contribute to proteasomal dysfunction [107]. Lipid peroxidation occurs when a ROS attacks a polyunsaturated fatty acid, thus initiating the lipid peroxidation chain reaction, which results in highly reactive aldehydes [108,109]. Lipid peroxidation products interact with protein, which results in modification to the protein structure and activity [109]. Accumulation of lipid peroxidation end products have been observed in many neurodegenerative diseases including Alzheimer's disease [110] and Parkinson's disease [111]. In glaucoma, an increase in lipid peroxidation end products, including diene and triene conjugates, and Schiff's bases, were observed in glaucomatous TM tissue (n=17) and aqueous humor (n=16) compared to age-matched controls (n=13 and n=17, respectively) [91]. In addition, Fernandez-Durango *et al.* measured increased levels of the lipid peroxidation mediator, malondialdehyde (MDA), in the aqueous humor of patients with terminal cases of POAG (n=38) compared to the cataract control group (n=48) [92]. Accumulation of lipid peroxidation products is predicted to have severe consequences on the TM by modifying proteins such as calpain-1. The calpains are a family of calcium-activated non-lysosomal cysteine proteases. In glaucomatous TM tissue, aggregated and degraded calpain-1 is present, but calpain-1 activity is lower compared with normal TM tissue [107]. In the TM of glaucomatous eyes, the lipid peroxidation products isolevuglandins, specifically iso[4]levuglandin E2, modifies calpain-1, thereby inhibiting calpain-1 activity. Although the physiological function of calpain-1 in the TM remains to be elucidated, calpain-1 modified by isolevuglandins is more prone to form larger aggregates. One of the major consequences of this modification is a disruption in the proteasomal machinery. This type of malfunction of the proteasomal machinery appears to be specific to the TM and does not occur in the posterior segment of the eye. Thus, accumulation of oxidative stress-related biomolecules along with a decrease in proteasomal activity with age perpetuates a vicious cycle that is postulated to greatly hinder cell survival.

7. Global change in gene expression in response to stress

As reviewed in the previous sections, cells of the TM are exposed to a variety of environmental stresses. The stresses can vary in form (mechanical, phagocytic, and oxidative), magnitude, and duration (acute or chronic). The antioxidant system and the proteolytic system are effective cellular defense mechanisms that protect cells. Recent advances in technology have shown that a change in the global gene expression profile is another major part of a cell's adaptive response to stress (reviewed in [112]. The change in gene expression profile in response to stress has revealed that signal transduction pathways are a necessary means of integrating complex signals and propagating these signals to effectors. In the next section, we will examine the specific sensors and signal transduction pathways that result in an appropriate response to stress in TM cells.

8. Sensors of TM cells

Cells have stress sensors that are highly specialized for survival in a particular environment. The specific mechanism of how TM cells sense various stimuli is largely unknown [48]. Mechanosensitive ion channels, specifically calcium-dependent maxi-K+ channels, are present in TM cells [113]. Stretch-activated channels located on the TM cell membrane are predicted to increase intracellular calcium levels. Another potential mechanism through which TM cells sense mechanical stress is the ECM. ECM receptors such as integrins are connected to the cytoskeleton, which is attached to the nuclear membrane. Thus, signals may be propagated from the extracellular environment where the mechanical stress occurs to the nucleus where gene expression can be altered in response to the stress [114]. Although the consequences of oxidative stress-related damages have been extensively studied, how the cell initially senses oxidative stress remains largely unknown [48,115]. In fact, the identification of oxidative stress sensors in any cell type has proven to be very difficult. In the future, identifying more sensors in TM cells will give insight into how TM cells achieve specificity in responding to specific stresses such as mechanical and oxidative stresses.

9. Global change in gene expression in response to mechanical stress

Exposure of TM cells to acute mechanical stress requires a quick and specific adaptive response to ensure maximal survival occurs. Recent studies examining the change in the global gene expression profile of TM cells has given insight into how TM cells are able to adapt and respond to the constant exposure to mechanical stress.

Several groups have examined the change in global gene expression profile of TM cells in response to mechanical stress [116-119]. Vittitow *et al.* and Vittal *et al.* both observed a change in expression of a large number of genes in response to mechanical stress. In TM from postmortem human donors, application of mechanical stress resulted in the upregulation of 40 genes and the downregulation of 14 genes [116]. Mechanical stretching of cultured porcine TM cells resulted in the upregulation of 126 genes and downregulation of 29 genes [117]. However, there was very little overlap in genes between the studies most likely due to the use of different experimental models as well of stochastic factors. Nevertheless, these studies reveal that TM cells appear to respond specifically to the *type* of stress. A large number of genes that changed expression levels were involved in ECM and cytoskeletal function, which is predicted to function in response to mechanical-stretch related changed to the cell and extracellular environment [117,118]. Several studies have shown that exposure of TM cells to mechanical stress results in increased levels of active MMPs, specifically MMP2 [120-123]. The MMP family of zinc proteases initiate ECM turnover, which has been predicted to regulate aqueous humor outflow facility by altering resistance. Furthermore, temporal variation of mechanical stretching resulted in a different gene expression profile indicating that TM cells are also able to respond specifically to the *magnitude* of mechanical stress.

Induction of stress response is thought to result in conditions that are detrimental to cell growth due in part to activation of cell cycle checkpoints [115,124]. Also, during stress response, the cell diverts energy to the adaptive response and as a result, less energy is available for cell growth-related functions [112,125]. Thus, there is a continuous balance between cell growth and stress response. In order to achieve this balance, stress responses must be transient and be temporally restricted. Consistent with this theory, exposure to mechanical stress resulted in a change in expression of a large number of stress-related genes while few growth-related genes were affected [117]. Another related characteristic of stress response is the highly reversible nature of the global change in gene expression. After removal of stress, inactivation of the stress-induced signal transduction pathway occurs, likely because constitutive activation of stress response would be detrimental to the overall health of the cell. Although the specific reversal of the gene expression profile in TM cells after the removal of mechanical stress has not been examined, TM cells appear to physiologically return to the pre-stress state after a period of time. Perfusion of anterior segment cultures is an effective experimental model for examining TM function [126].In this model, anterior segment explants are perfused with culture medium at a constant pressure, resulting in a stable and physiologically relevant flow rate [122,127]. Using perfused human anterior segment culture, Bradley *et al.* observed that doubling the flow rate resulted in immediate doubling of IOP [122]. However, after two days, TM cells lowered outflow resistance and thus, restored the IOP to pre-stress levels even under conditions where the flow rate remained doubled. In this study, the TM cells appear to reach a new homeostatic condition even when the stress is not removed.

Cells use multiple signal transduction pathways to integrate various input signals and coordinate an appropriate stress response. In TM cells, activation of signal transduction pathways appears to be important in mediating an appropriate stress response. Vittitow *et al.* observed that nearly 32% of genes altered in the global gene expression profile in response to mechanical stretch of TM cells functioned in various signal transduction pathways [116]. One particularly interesting signal transduction pathway is the stress-activated protein kinase (SAPK) pathways, a highly conserved signalling pathway in eukaryotes that are activated by many different environmental stresses. A rapid response to stress is essential to maximize cell survival. Thus, the SAPK pathway enables rapid phosphorylation of components of various signal transduction pathway so that a response occurs within minutes of initial exposure to the stress [128,129]. In mammals, the SAPKs are the p38 mitogen-activated protein kinases (MAPKs). There is evidence that the MAPK signal transduction pathway is involved in the TM cell response to mechanical stress [130]. In TM cells, the p38 MAPK pathway is suggested to modulate the regulation of stretch-induced cytokines such as TGF-β1 and IL-6 [131]. Thus, the p38 MAPK pathway functions in co-ordinating and regulating signal transduction pathways in response to stress. However, in primary glaucomatous TM cells, Zhang *et al.* demonstrated that the p38 MAPK pathway is unresponsive to exogenous manipulation, including the administration of Interleukin 1 (IL1), which has been shown to activate the p38 MAPK pathway in non-glaucomatous TM cells [132]. Although examination of the p38 MAPK pathway *in vivo* is required, this pathway may be unresponsive in glaucomatous TM cells because it is already maximally activated [132]. The cause of this constitutive activation remains unknown. Nevertheless, the constitutive activation of the stress-responsive MAPK pathway is predicted to have serious consequences as the TM cells will lose its ability to mediate the stress response through the stress-dependent activation of the p38 MAPK pathway.

10. Global change in gene expression in response to oxidative stress

Despite the evidence that TM cells are exposed to oxidative stress, not much is currently known about the change in global gene expression profile in TM cells in response to chronic oxidative stress. Examining the effects of chronic oxidative stress on TM cells is especially challenging because it is difficult to experimentally create an environment where TM cells are exposed to chronic oxidative stress.

Porter *et al.* examined the global gene expression profile of phagocytically challenged TM cells under normal and acute oxidative stress conditions [133]. As avid phagocytes, TM cells are predicted to keep the aqueous humor outflow pathway clear of debris [55]. When TM cells were phagocytically challenged to *E. coli* under normal conditions, 1190 genes were upregulated and 728 genes were downregulated [133]. When TM cells were phagocytically challenged to E. coli under oxidatively stressed conditions at 40% O_2, 976 genes were upregulated and 383 genes were downregulated. Although many of the altered genes were involved in immune response, cell adhesion, and regulation of ECM, there were only 6 genes that were altered in both the normal and oxidatively stressed conditions. TM cells therefore appear to have distinct gene expression profiles specific to the type of stress. Under experimental conditions, different types of stresses tend to be examined one at a time to elucidate the response of the cells to that particular stress. However, TM cells under physiological conditions are simultaneously exposed to different stresses. Studies in yeast have shown that cells are able to combine and integrate these different signals and produce an adaptive response [128]. Thus, analyzing a combination of stresses in TM cells will possibly reveal the role that cross-protection plays in these cells. Cross-protection refers to the ability of cells to become resistant to stress after first being exposed to a sub-lethal stress [134].

Transcription factors are essential regulators of signal transduction pathway components. NF-κB was identified as the transcription factor responsible for activation of many of the genes in the gene expression profile of phagocytically challenged TM cells including MMP1 and MMP3 [133]. The NF-κB transcription factor has also been shown to mediate the activation of endothelial leukocyte adhesion molecule (ELAM1) and the inflammatory cytokine IL1 [135]. ELAM1 is a cell adhesion molecule that is readily expressed in glaucomatous TM cells [135-137]. Activation of ELAM1 and IL1 by the NF-κB transcription factor in response to oxidative stress promotes cell survival. However, constitutive activation of NF-κB is predicted to be detrimental to cell survival and even contribute to the development of glaucoma [135]. The NF-κB transcription factor regulates the expression of numerous downstream target genes with varying functions including MMPs that regulate ECM turnover. Dysregulation of these downstream target genes is predicted to cause disruptions to TM cell function. In many situations, the altered gene expression returns to a steady-state level that is comparable to unstressed conditions even when the cells remain exposed to a particular stress [125]. As mentioned previously, activation of stress-related genes during a stress response diverts energy and resources from cell growth. Thus, situations where steady state levels are not achieved can pose a great risk to the overall health of the cell, ultimately affecting its ability to survive.

11. Unspecific gene expression response

Studying the change in the global gene expression profile of TM cells reveals that a large number of genes are either upregulated or downregulated in response to various environmental stresses. Many of the genes that have altered expression do not appear to have any relevant function in the adaptive response to the specific stress. Analysis of global gene expression profiles in other systems such as *S. cerevisiae* yield similar findings of an unspecific gene expression response [138-140]. Furthermore, studies in *E. coli* have revealed that when cells are exposed to an unknown stress that the cell would not encounter under normal biological conditions, an unspecific and stochastic gene expression response was triggered [141,142]. Since cells may not have specific sensors to detect multiple stresses simultaneously, the unspecific stress response has been suggested to protect cells under multiple stress conditions by changing the expression of a large number of genes, some of which function in promoting a general adaptive response [125]. Furthermore, this unspecific and stochastic gene expression response may be an important evolutionary mechanism, thereby allowing cells to adapt to an unpredictable challenge [125]. Even though cells of the TM are in a dynamic environment with a multitude of challenges, the unspecific gene expression response may enable these cells to quickly and effectively adapt to a new steady state. In the future, distinguishing between stress-essential genes (necessary for immediate response) and stress-induced genes (most likely necessary for unspecific or long-term response) in TM cells is critical in understanding how TM cells adapt to stress in the long-term and prepare for subsequent stresses. Finally, although examining a particular stress-induced gene is important in elucidating its role in aqueous humor regulation, examining the *network* of genes altered in response to stress will provide further insight into the complex nature of the adaptive response of TM cells.

12. Effect of environmental stress on glaucoma-associated genes

Exposure of anterior segment structures, specifically the TM, to environmental stresses disrupts the aqueous humor outflow pathway and contributes to the development of glaucoma. Glaucoma, however, has a complex etiology. In addition to the environmental stress factors, genetic factors contribute to the development of this disease. At least 14 chromosomal loci have been identified for POAG (GLC1A to GLC1N) [143]. Currently three genes from these loci have been associated with glaucoma: *myocilin* (*MYOC*), *optineurin* (*OPTN*), and *WD repeat domain 36* (*WDR36*). Mutations in these three genes account for less than 5% of POAG cases [144]. Glaucoma is also a major consequence for many anterior segment dysgenesis disorders including Axenfeld-Rieger Syndrome (ARS) and Peter's anomaly. Mutations in the transcription factor genes, FOXC1 and PITX2, are associated with ARS [145-147]. How mutations in FOXC1 and PITX2 cause disease is not well understood. Recent findings have suggested that patients with these types of mutations may be more sensitive to environmental stresses [148,149]. The cells of the TM may be less tolerant when exposed to various stresses, resulting in dysregulation of aqueous humor outflow. In this section, we will take a closer look at the effects of environmental stresses on two genes, MYOC, which is associated with POAG, and FOXC1, which is associated with ARS.

MYOC was the first POAG gene to be reported [150-152]. Patients with MYOC mutations tend to present with juvenile and early adult-onset forms of POAG. However, the most commonly reported MYOC mutation, Q368X, is associated with later adult-onset POAG. MYOC is expressed in most ocular tissues [153] including the TM and is secreted into the aqueous humor [154,155]. The release of MYOC is associated with the release of exosomes. Signaling molecules within these exosomes is predicted to function in maintaining TM homeostasis [156]. Specific MYOC mutations appear to sensitize cells to oxidative stress. Joe et al. observed that Human Embryonic Kidney 293 (HEK293) cells stably transfected with the Y437H MYOC mutation have decreased expression of antioxidant genes and produced more ROS [156,157]. Also, more H_2O_2-induced cell death occurred in HEK293 cells overexpressing various MYOC mutations compared with wild type. The extent of cell death differed between mutants. Furthermore, 18 month old Y437H mutant mice had increased expression of ER stress markers and decreased levels of antioxidant proteins [157]. These findings suggest that patients with MYOC mutations are more sensitive to oxidative stress. The decreased ability to response to oxidative stress may contribute to the development of glaucoma earlier on in these patients' lives.

Anterior segment dysgenesis covers a wide spectrum of developmental anomalies that can affect the iris, cornea, lens, TM, and Schlemm's canal. We have already discussed the importance of the TM and Schlemm's canal in maintaining the aqueous humor outflow pathway. Disruptions in this pathway may result in increased IOP, which is a major risk factor of developing glaucoma. Glaucoma is estimated to develop in approximately 50% of patients with anterior segment dysgenesis [158-160]. Although the mechanism that leads to glaucoma may vary between different anterior segment dysgenesis disorders and even between individuals with the same disorder, recent findings suggest that environmental stresses affect the normal functioning of the disease-associated gene. Patients with ARS can present with a variety of ocular anomalies and systemic anomalies. Ocular anomalies include iris hypoplasia, corectopia, polycoria, and posterior embryotoxon while systemic anomalies include dental anomalies and redundant periumbilical skin. ARS patients with FOXC1 mutations have a 50-80% risk of developing earlier-onset glaucoma [161]. As a transcription factor, FOXC1 regulates the expression of a myriad of genes including genes that function in proteolysis, cell matrix adhesion, apoptosis, signal transduction, and stress response [148]. Berry et al. observed that FOXC1 plays a role in TM cell viability by directly regulating the transcription factor FOXO1A which is involved in the cellular stress response pathway and apoptosis. Decreasing the expression of FOXC1 increased the sensitivity of TM cells to oxidative stress. Tight regulation of the FOXC1 transcription factor is essential because both a high (FOXC1 duplications) and low FOXC1 (loss of function mutations) gene dose results in anterior segment dysgenesis phenotypes associated with glaucoma. Interestingly, FOXC1 itself appears to be responsive to stress as well (Y.A.I. and M.A.W. personal observations). Thus, the FOXC1 transcription factor appears to play an important role in responding to environmental stresses. Disruptions to normal FOXC1 function are predicted to disrupt the regulation of downstream target genes that are involved in executing a rapid and effective adaptive response. Therefore, ARS patients with FOXC1 mutations may have a compromised ability to respond to environmental stresses resulting in the early age of development of glaucoma. Thus, even in the case of anterior segment developmental disorders, oxidative stress appears to have an impact on the TM. Studying genes that are associated with both the primary and secondary glaucomas provide an invaluable tool to understanding the contribution of environmental stresses on the development of glaucoma.

13. Conclusion

The functional nature of the TM inevitably results in exposure of this tissue to a highly dynamic environment. Examining the functional roles of single genes have provided invaluable insight into how specific genes contribute to normal TM cell function and how these TM cells are able to respond to specific stresses. However, the recent analyses of global gene expression profiles have indicated that an extensive number of genes are involved in mediating the TM cell stress response. We are beginning to piece together how these singles genes function as part of a 'network' of genes. Individual components of this network of genes are potential therapeutic targets for promoting cell survival and maintaining TM cell function. However, future research needs to examine how these genes interact with each other and the environment in a more physiologically relevant context; as part of a TM stress-response network. Understanding the network of genes that are involved in executing the adaptive response is complicated, but essential to developing effective treatments for anterior segment malformations and glaucoma.

Acknowledgements

We would like to thank Dr. Fred Berry and Mr. Tim Footz for critically reviewing this manuscript. Y.A.I. is supported by the Sir Frederick Banting and Dr. Charles Best Canada Graduate Scholarship provided by the Canadian Institutes of Health Research.

Author details

Yoko A. Ito and Michael A. Walter*

*Address all correspondence to: mwalter@ualberta.ca

Department of Medical Genetics, University of Alberta, Edmonton, AB, Canada

References

[1] Quigley, H. A, & Broman, A. T. The number of people with glaucoma worldwide in 2010 and 2020. Br J Ophthalmol (2006). , 90, 262-267.

[2] Rudnicka, A. R, Mt-isa, S, Owen, C. G, Cook, D. G, & Ashby, D. Variations in primary open-angle glaucoma prevalence by age, gender, and race: a Bayesian meta-analysis. Invest Ophthalmol Vis Sci (2006). , 47, 4254-4261.

[3] Leske, M. C. Open-angle glaucoma-- an epidemiologic overview. Ophthalmic Epidemiol 200;, 14, 166-172.

[4] Giblin, F. J, Mccready, J. P, Kodama, T, & Reddy, V. N. A direct correlation between the levels of ascorbic acid and H2O2 in aqueous humor. Exp Eye Res (1984). , 38, 87-93.

[5] Bhuyan, K. C, & Bhuyan, D. K. Regulation of hydrogen peroxide in eye humors. Effect of 3-amino-1H-triazole on catalase and glutathione peroxidase of rabbit eye. Biochim Biophys Acta (1977). , 1(2), 4.

[6] Mark, H. H. Aqueous humor dynamics in historical perspective. Surv Ophthalmol (2010). , 55, 89-100.

[7] Goel, M, Picciani, R. G, Lee, R. K, & Bhattacharya, S. K. Aqueous humor dynamics: a review. Open Ophthalmol J (2010). , 4, 52-59.

[8] Brubaker, R. F. Measurement of Aqueous Flow By Fluorophotometry. The Glaucomas; (1989). , 337.

[9] Millar, C, & Kaufman, P. L. Aqueous humor: Secretion and dynamics. In: Jaeger EA, Tasman W, editors. DUANE'S FOUNDATIONS OF CLINICAL OPHTHALMOLOGY: Philadelphia: Lippincott; (1995). , 1.

[10] Hollows, F. C, & Graham, P. A. Intra-ocular pressure, glaucoma, and glaucoma suspects in a defined population. Br J Ophthalmol (1966t). , 50, 570-586.

[11] Bill, A. The aqueous humor drainage mechanism in the cynomolgus monkey (Macaca irus) with evidence for unconventional routes. Invest Ophthalmol (1965). , 4, 911-919.

[12] Bill, A, & Hellsing, K. Production and drainage of aqueous humor in the cynomolgus monkey (Macaca irus). Invest Ophthalmol (1965). , 4, 920-926.

[13] Fautsch, M. P, & Johnson, D. H. Aqueous humor outflow: what do we know? Where will it lead us? Invest Ophthalmol Vis Sci (2006). , 47, 4181-4187.

[14] Townsend, D. J, & Brubaker, R. F. Immediate effect of epinephrine on aqueous formation in the normal human eye as measured by fluorophotometry. Invest Ophthalmol Vis Sci (1980). , 19, 256-266.

[15] Toris, C. B, Yablonski, M. E, Wang, Y. L, & Camras, C. B. Aqueous humor dynamics in the aging human eye. Am J Ophthalmol (1999). , 127, 407-412.

[16] Bill, A, & Phillips, C. I. Uveoscleral drainage of aqueous humor in human eyes. Exp Eye Res (1971). , 12, 275-281.

[17] Fine, B. S. Observations on the Drainage Angle in Man and Rhesus Monkey: a Concept of the Pathogenesis of Chronic Simple Glaucoma. a Light and Electron Microscopic Study. Invest Ophthalmol (1964). , 3, 609-646.

[18] Fine, B. S. Structure of the trabecular meshwork and the canal of Schlemm. Trans Am Acad Ophthalmol Otolaryngol (1966). , 70, 777-790.

[19] Rohen, J. W, Futa, R, & Lutjen-drecoll, E. The fine structure of the cribriform meshwork in normal and glaucomatous eyes as seen in tangential sections. Invest Ophthalmol Vis Sci (1981). , 21, 574-585.

[20] Lutjen-drecoll, E, Futa, R, & Rohen, J. W. Ultrahistochemical studies on tangential sections of the trabecular meshwork in normal and glaucomatous eyes. Invest Ophthalmol Vis Sci (1981). , 21, 563-573.

[21] Underwood, J. L, Murphy, C. G, Chen, J, Franse-carman, L, Wood, I, Epstein, D. L, et al. Glucocorticoids regulate transendothelial fluid flow resistance and formation of intercellular junctions. Am J Physiol (1999). C, 330-42.

[22] Tripathi, R. Tracing the bulk outflow route of cerebrospinal fluid by transmission and scanning electron microscopy. Brain Res (1974). , 80, 503-506.

[23] Epstein, D. L, & Rohen, J. W. Morphology of the trabecular meshwork and inner-wall endothelium after cationized ferritin perfusion in the monkey eye. Invest Ophthalmol Vis Sci (1991). , 32, 160-171.

[24] Brilakis, H. S, & Johnson, D. H. Giant vacuole survival time and implications for aqueous humor outflow. J Glaucoma (2001). , 10, 277-283.

[25] Ascher, K. W. The aqueous veins: I. Physiologic importance of the visible elimination of intraocular fluid. Am J Ophthalmol. (1942). , 25, 1174-1209.

[26] Lutjen-drecoll, E. New findings on the functional structure of the region of the angle of the chamber and its changes after glaucoma surgery (author's transl). Klin Monbl Augenheilkd (1973). , 163, 410-419.

[27] Maepea, O, & Bill, A. Pressures in the juxtacanalicular tissue and Schlemm's canal in monkeys. Exp Eye Res (1992). , 54, 879-883.

[28] Ethier, C. R, Kamm, R. D, Palaszewski, B. A, Johnson, M. C, & Richardson, T. M. Calculations of flow resistance in the juxtacanalicular meshwork. Invest Ophthalmol Vis Sci (1986). , 27, 1741-1750.

[29] Seiler, T, & Wollensak, J. The resistance of the trabecular meshwork to aqueous hu-
      mor outflow. Graefes Arch Clin Exp Ophthalmol (1985). , 223, 88-91.

[30] Acott, T. S, & Kelley, M. J. Extracellular matrix in the trabecular meshwork. Exp Eye
      Res (2008). , 86, 543-561.

[31] Woessner, J. F. Jr. Matrix metalloproteinases and their inhibitors in connective tissue
      remodeling. FASEB J (1991). , 5, 2145-2154.

[32] Bradley, J. M, Vranka, J, Colvis, C. M, Conger, D. M, Alexander, J. P, Fisk, A. S, et al.
      Effect of matrix metalloproteinases activity on outflow in perfused human organ cul-
      ture. Invest Ophthalmol Vis Sci (1998). , 39, 2649-2658.

[33] Page-McCaw A., Ewald AJ, Werb Z.Matrix metalloproteinases and the regulation of
      tissue remodelling. Nat Rev Mol Cell Biol (2007). , 8, 221-233.

[34] Rohen, J. W, Lutjen, E, & Barany, E. The relation between the ciliary muscle and the
      trabecular meshwork and its importance for the effect of miotics on aqueous outflow
      resistance. A study in two contrasting monkey species, Macaca irus and Cercopithe-
      cus aethiops. Albrecht Von Graefes Arch Klin Exp Ophthalmol (1967). , 172, 23-47.

[35] Lutjen-drecoll, E, Wiendl, H, & Kaufman, P. L. Acute and chronic structural effects of
      pilocarpine on monkey outflow tissues. Trans Am Ophthalmol Soc (1998). , 96,
      171-95.

[36] Barany, E. H. The mode of action of miotics on outflow resistance. A study of pilocar-
      pine in the vervet monkey Cercopithecus ethiops. Trans Ophthalmol Soc U K
      (1966). , 86, 539-578.

[37] Gabelt, B. T, & Kaufman, P. L. Changes in aqueous humor dynamics with age and
      glaucoma. Prog Retin Eye Res (2005). , 24, 612-637.

[38] Becker, B. The decline in aqueous secretion and outflow facility with age. Am J Oph-
      thalmol (1958). , 46, 731-736.

[39] Gaasterland, D, Kupfer, C, Milton, R, Ross, K, & Mccain, L. MacLellan H. Studies of
      aqueous humor dynamics in man. VI. Effect of age upon parameters of intraocular
      pressure in normal human eyes. Exp Eye Res (1978). , 26, 651-656.

[40] Croft, M. A, Oyen, M. J, Gange, S. J, Fisher, M. R, & Kaufman, P. L. Aging effects on
      accommodation and outflow facility responses to pilocarpine in humans. Arch Oph-
      thalmol (1996). , 114, 586-592.

[41] Armaly, M. F. The consistency of the 1955 calibration for various tonometer weights.
      Am J Ophthalmol (1959). , 48, 602-611.

[42] Bloom, J. N, Levene, R. Z, Thomas, G, & Kimura, R. Fluorophotometry and the rate
      of aqueous flow in man. I. Instrumentation and normal values. Arch Ophthalmol
      (1976). , 94, 435-443.

[43] Brubaker, R. F, Nagataki, S, Townsend, D. J, Burns, R. R, Higgins, R. G, & Wentworth, W. The effect of age on aqueous humor formation in man. Ophthalmology (1981). , 88, 283-288.

[44] Kupfer, C. Clinical significance of pseudofacility. Sanford R. Gifford Memorial Lecture. Am J Ophthalmol (1973). , 75, 193-204.

[45] Foster, P. J, Alsbirk, P. H, Baasanhu, J, Munkhbayar, D, Uranchimeg, D, & Johnson, G. J. Anterior chamber depth in Mongolians: variation with age, sex, and method of measurement. Am J Ophthalmol (1997). , 124, 53-60.

[46] Rufer, F, Schroder, A, Klettner, A, Frimpong-boateng, A, Roider, J. B, & Erb, C. Anterior chamber depth and iridocorneal angle in healthy White subjects: effects of age, gender and refraction. Acta Ophthalmol (2010). , 88, 885-890.

[47] Lutjen-drecoll, E, Kaufman, P. L, & Eichhorn, M. Long-term timolol and epinephrine in monkeys. I. Functional morphology of the ciliary processes. Trans Ophthalmol Soc U K (1986). , 105, 180-195.

[48] Llobet, A, Gasull, X, & Gual, A. Understanding trabecular meshwork physiology: a key to the control of intraocular pressure? News Physiol Sci (2003). , 18, 205-209.

[49] Lutjen-drecoll, E. Morphological changes in glaucomatous eyes and the role of TGFbeta2 for the pathogenesis of the disease. Exp Eye Res (2005). , 81, 1-4.

[50] Alvarado, J, Murphy, C, & Juster, R. Trabecular meshwork cellularity in primary open-angle glaucoma and nonglaucomatous normals. Ophthalmology (1984). , 91, 564-579.

[51] Grierson, I, & Howes, R. C. Age-related depletion of the cell population in the human trabecular meshwork. Eye (Lond) (1987). , 1, 204-210.

[52] Alvarado, J, Murphy, C, Polansky, J, & Juster, R. Age-related changes in trabecular meshwork cellularity. Invest Ophthalmol Vis Sci (1981). , 21, 714-727.

[53] Tschumper, R. C, & Johnson, D. H. Trabecular meshwork cellularity. Differences between fellow eyes. Invest Ophthalmol Vis Sci (1990). , 31, 1327-1331.

[54] Buller, C, Johnson, D. H, & Tschumper, R. C. Human trabecular meshwork phagocytosis. Observations in an organ culture system. Invest Ophthalmol Vis Sci (1990). , 31, 2156-2163.

[55] Grierson, I, & Chisholm, I. A. Clearance of debris from the iris through the drainage angle of the rabbit's eye. Br J Ophthalmol (1978). , 62, 694-704.

[56] Grierson, I, & Lee, W. R. Erythrocyte phagocytosis in the human trabecular meshwork. Br J Ophthalmol (1973). , 57, 400-415.

[57] Johnson, D. H, Richardson, T. M, & Epstein, D. L. Trabecular meshwork recovery after phagocytic challenge. Curr Eye Res (1989). , 8, 1121-1130.

[58] Rohen, J. W, & Van Der Zypen, E. The phagocytic activity of the trabecularmeshwork endothelium. An electron-microscopic study of the vervet (Cercopithecus aethiops). Albrecht Von Graefes Arch Klin Exp Ophthalmol (1968). , 175, 143-160.

[59] Shirato, S, Murphy, C. G, Bloom, E, Franse-carman, L, Maglio, M. T, Polansky, J. R, et al. Kinetics of phagocytosis in trabecular meshwork cells. Flow cytometry and morphometry. Invest Ophthalmol Vis Sci (1989). , 30, 2499-2511.

[60] Zhou, L, Li, Y, & Yue, B. Y. Alteration of cytoskeletal structure, integrin distribution, and migratory activity by phagocytic challenge in cells from an ocular tissue--the trabecular meshwork. In Vitro Cell Dev Biol Anim (1999). , 35, 144-149.

[61] Alvarado, J. A, Alvarado, R. G, Yeh, R. F, Franse-carman, L, Marcellino, G. R, & Brownstein, M. J. A new insight into the cellular regulation of aqueous outflow: how trabecular meshwork endothelial cells drive a mechanism that regulates the permeability of Schlemm's canal endothelial cells. Br J Ophthalmol (2005). , 89, 1500-1505.

[62] Shifera, A. S, Trivedi, S, Chau, P, Bonnemaison, L. H, Iguchi, R, & Alvarado, J. A. Constitutive secretion of chemokines by cultured human trabecular meshwork cells. Exp Eye Res (2010). , 91, 42-47.

[63] Rohen, J. W, & Witmer, R. Electrn microscopic studies on the trabecular meshwork in glaucoma simplex. Albrecht Von Graefes Arch Klin Exp Ophthalmol (1972). , 183, 251-266.

[64] Liu, J. H, Zhang, X, Kripke, D. F, & Weinreb, R. N. Twenty-four-hour intraocular pressure pattern associated with early glaucomatous changes. Invest Ophthalmol Vis Sci (2003). , 44, 1586-1590.

[65] Liu, J. H, Bouligny, R. P, Kripke, D. F, & Weinreb, R. N. Nocturnal elevation of intraocular pressure is detectable in the sitting position. Invest Ophthalmol Vis Sci (2003). , 44, 4439-4442.

[66] Coleman, D. J, & Trokel, S. Direct-recorded intraocular pressure variations in a human subject. Arch Ophthalmol (1969). , 82, 637-640.

[67] Rose, R. C, Richer, S. P, & Bode, A. M. Ocular oxidants and antioxidant protection. Proc Soc Exp Biol Med (1998). , 217, 397-407.

[68] Spector, A, & Garner, W. H. Hydrogen peroxide and human cataract. Exp Eye Res (1981). , 33, 673-681.

[69] Garcia-castineiras, S, Velazquez, S, Martinez, P, & Torres, N. Aqueous humor hydrogen peroxide analysis with dichlorophenol-indophenol. Exp Eye Res (1992). , 55, 9-19.

[70] Bleau, G, Giasson, C, & Brunette, I. Measurement of hydrogen peroxide in biological samples containing high levels of ascorbic acid. Anal Biochem (1998). , 263, 13-17.

[71] García-castiñeiras, S. Hydrogen peroxide in the aqueous humor: 1992-1997. (1998). , 17, 335-343.

[72] Valko, M, Rhodes, C. J, Moncol, J, Izakovic, M, & Mazur, M. Free radicals, metals and antioxidants in oxidative stress-induced cancer. Chem Biol Interact (2006). , 160, 1-40.

[73] Valko, M, Leibfritz, D, Moncol, J, Cronin, M. T, Mazur, M, & Telser, J. Free radicals and antioxidants in normal physiological functions and human disease. Int J Biochem Cell Biol (2007). , 39, 44-84.

[74] Gloire, G, Legrand-poels, S, & Piette, J. NF-kappaB activation by reactive oxygen species: fifteen years later. Biochem Pharmacol (2006). , 72, 1493-1505.

[75] Mccord, J. M, & Fridovich, I. Superoxide dismutase. An enzymic function for erythrocuprein (hemocuprein). J Biol Chem (1969). , 244, 6049-6055.

[76] Wiederholt, M, Sturm, A, & Lepple-wienhues, A. Relaxation of trabecular meshwork and ciliary muscle by release of nitric oxide. Invest Ophthalmol Vis Sci (1994). , 35, 2515-2520.

[77] Kamikawatoko, S, Tokoro, T, Ishida, A, Masuda, H, Hamasaki, H, Sato, J, et al. Nitric oxide relaxes bovine ciliary muscle contracted by carbachol through elevation of cyclic GMP. Exp Eye Res (1998). , 66(1), 1-7.

[78] Huie, R. E, & Padmaja, S. The reaction of NO with superoxide. Free Rad. Res. Com. (1993). , 18, 195-199.

[79] Pacher, P, Beckman, J. S, & Liaudet, L. Nitric oxide and peroxynitrite in health and disease. Physiol Rev (2007). , 87, 315-424.

[80] Jenner, P. Oxidative stress in Parkinson's disease. Ann Neurol (2003). Suppl 3:Sdiscussion S36-8., 26-36.

[81] Zhou, C, Huang, Y, & Przedborski, S. Oxidative stress in Parkinson's disease: a mechanism of pathogenic and therapeutic significance. Ann N Y Acad Sci (2008). , 1147, 93-104.

[82] Nunomura, A, Perry, G, Aliev, G, Hirai, K, Takeda, A, Balraj, E. K, et al. Oxidative damage is the earliest event in Alzheimer disease. J Neuropathol Exp Neurol (2001). , 60, 759-767.

[83] Pratico, D, Uryu, K, Leight, S, Trojanoswki, J. Q, & Lee, V. M. Increased lipid peroxidation precedes amyloid plaque formation in an animal model of Alzheimer amyloidosis. J Neurosci (2001). , 21, 4183-4187.

[84] Reddy, P. H, Mcweeney, S, Park, B. S, Manczak, M, Gutala, R. V, Partovi, D, et al. Gene expression profiles of transcripts in amyloid precursor protein transgenic mice: up-regulation of mitochondrial metabolism and apoptotic genes is an early cellular change in Alzheimer's disease. Hum Mol Genet (2004). , 13, 1225-1240.

5r>t>5
555555555555555555555555555555555555555555555555555555555555555555555555555555

[85] Wiseman, H, & Halliwell, B. Damage to DNA by reactive oxygen and nitrogen species: role in inflammatory disease and progression to cancer. Biochem J (1996). , 313, 17-29.

[86] Cai, H, & Harrison, D. G. Endothelial dysfunction in cardiovascular diseases: the role of oxidant stress. Circ Res (2000). , 87, 840-844.

[87] Kumar, D. M, & Agarwal, N. Oxidative stress in glaucoma: a burden of evidence. J Glaucoma (2007). , 16, 334-343.

[88] Izzotti, A, Sacca, S. C, Cartiglia, C, & De Flora, S. Oxidative deoxyribonucleic acid damage in the eyes of glaucoma patients. Am J Med (2003). , 114, 638-646.

[89] Sacca, S. C, Pascotto, A, Camicione, P, Capris, P, & Izzotti, A. Oxidative DNA damage in the human trabecular meshwork: clinical correlation in patients with primary open-angle glaucoma. Arch Ophthalmol (2005). , 123, 458-463.

[90] Caballero, M, Liton, P. B, Challa, P, Epstein, D. L, & Gonzalez, P. Effects of donor age on proteasome activity and senescence in trabecular meshwork cells. Biochem Biophys Res Commun (2004). , 323, 1048-1054.

[91] Babizhayev, M. A, & Bunin, A. Y. Lipid peroxidation in open-angle glaucoma. Acta Ophthalmol (Copenh) (1989). , 67, 371-377.

[92] Fernandez-durango, R, Fernandez-martinez, A, Garcia-feijoo, J, Castillo, A, De La Casa, J. M, Garcia-bueno, B, et al. Expression of nitrotyrosine and oxidative consequences in the trabecular meshwork of patients with primary open-angle glaucoma. Invest Ophthalmol Vis Sci (2008). , 49, 2506-2511.

[93] Sorkhabi, R, Ghorbanihaghjo, A, Javadzadeh, A, Rashtchizadeh, N, & Moharrery, M. Oxidative DNA damage and total antioxidant status in glaucoma patients. Mol Vis (2011). , 17, 41-46.

[94] Ferreira, S. M, Lerner, S. F, Brunzini, R, Evelson, P. A, & Llesuy, S. F. Oxidative stress markers in aqueous humor of glaucoma patients. Am J Ophthalmol (2004). , 137, 62-69.

[95] Ghanem, A. A, Arafa, L. F, & Baz, A. Oxidative stress markers in patients with primary open-angle glaucoma. Curr Eye Res (2010). , 35, 295-301.

[96] Kinsey, V. E. Transfer of ascorbic acid and related compounds across the blood-aqueous barrier. Am J Ophthalmol (1947). , 30, 1262-1266.

[97] Becker, B. Chemical composition of human aqueous humor; effects of acetazoleamide. AMA Arch Ophthalmol (1957). , 57, 793-800.

[98] Reiss, G. R, Werness, P. G, Zollman, P. E, & Brubaker, R. F. Ascorbic acid levels in the aqueous humor of nocturnal and diurnal mammals. Arch Ophthalmol (1986). , 104, 753-755.

[99] Reddy, V. N, Giblin, F. J, Lin, L. R, & Chakrapani, B. The effect of aqueous humor ascorbate on ultraviolet-B-induced DNA damage in lens epithelium. Invest Ophthalmol Vis Sci (1998). , 39, 344-350.

[100] Schachtschabel, D. O, Binninger, E. A, & Rohen, J. W. In vitro cultures of trabecular meshwork cells of the human eye as a model system for the study of cellular aging. Arch Gerontol Geriatr (1989). , 9, 251-262.

[101] Guo, M. S, Wu, Y. Y, & Liang, Z. B. Hyaluronic acid increases MMP-2 and MMP-9 expressions in cultured trabecular meshwork cells from patients with primary open-angle glaucoma. Mol Vis (2012). , 18, 1175-1181.

[102] Knepper, P. A, Goossens, W, & Palmberg, P. F. Glycosaminoglycan stratification of the juxtacanalicular tissue in normal and primary open-angle glaucoma. Invest Ophthalmol Vis Sci (1996). , 37, 2414-2425.

[103] Knepper, P. A, Goossens, W, Hvizd, M, & Palmberg, P. F. Glycosaminoglycans of the human trabecular meshwork in primary open-angle glaucoma. Invest Ophthalmol Vis Sci (1996). , 37, 1360-1367.

[104] Jampel, H. D, Moon, J. I, Quigley, H. A, Barron, Y, & Lam, K. W. Aqueous humor uric acid and ascorbic acid concentrations and outcome of trabeculectomy. Arch Ophthalmol (1998). , 116, 281-285.

[105] Leite, M. T, Prata, T. S, Kera, C. Z, & Miranda, D. V. de Moraes Barros SB, Melo LA,Jr. Ascorbic acid concentration is reduced in the secondary aqueous humor of glaucomatous patients. Clin Experiment Ophthalmol (2009). , 37, 402-406.

[106] Lee, P, Lam, K. W, & Lai, M. Aqueous humor ascorbate concentration and open-angle glaucoma. Arch Ophthalmol (1977). , 95, 308-310.

[107] Govindarajan, B, Laird, J, Salomon, R. G, & Bhattacharya, S. K. Isolevuglandin-modified proteins, including elevated levels of inactive calpain-1, accumulate in glaucomatous trabecular meshwork. Biochemistry (2008). , 47, 817-825.

[108] Gutteridge, J. M. Lipid peroxidation and antioxidants as biomarkers of tissue damage. Clin Chem (1995). , 41, 1819-1828.

[109] Reed, T. T. Lipid peroxidation and neurodegenerative disease. Free Radic Biol Med (2011). , 51, 1302-1319.

[110] Subbarao, K. V, Richardson, J. S, & Ang, L. C. Autopsy samples of Alzheimer's cortex show increased peroxidation in vitro. J Neurochem (1990). , 55, 342-345.

[111] Tsang, A. H, & Chung, K. K. Oxidative and nitrosative stress in Parkinson's disease. Biochim Biophys Acta (2009). , 1792, 643-650.

[112] De Nadal, E, Ammerer, G, & Posas, F. Controlling gene expression in response to stress. Nat Rev Genet (2011). , 12, 833-845.

[113] Irnaten, M, Barry, R. C, Quill, B, Clark, A. F, Harvey, B. J, & Brien, O. CJ. Activation of stretch-activated channels and maxi-K+ channels by membrane stress of human lamina cribrosa cells. Invest Ophthalmol Vis Sci (2009). , 50, 194-202.

[114] Clark, A. F. The cell and molecular biology of glaucoma: biomechanical factors in glaucoma. Invest Ophthalmol Vis Sci (2012). , 53, 2473-2475.

[115] Zhou, B. B, & Elledge, S. J. The DNA damage response: putting checkpoints in perspective. Nature (2000). , 408, 433-439.

[116] Vittitow, J, & Borras, T. Genes expressed in the human trabecular meshwork during pressure-induced homeostatic response. J Cell Physiol (2004). , 201, 126-137.

[117] Vittal, V, Rose, A, Gregory, K. E, Kelley, M. J, & Acott, T. S. Changes in gene expression by trabecular meshwork cells in response to mechanical stretching. Invest Ophthalmol Vis Sci (2005). Aug;, 46(8), 2857-2868.

[118] Gonzalez, P, Epstein, D. L, & Borras, T. Genes upregulated in the human trabecular meshwork in response to elevated intraocular pressure. Invest Ophthalmol Vis Sci (2000). , 41, 352-361.

[119] Borras, T. Gene expression in the trabecular meshwork and the influence of intraocular pressure. Prog Retin Eye Res (2003). , 22, 435-463.

[120] Okada, Y, Matsuo, T, & Ohtsuki, H. Bovine trabecular cells produce TIMP-1 and MMP-2 in response to mechanical stretching. Jpn J Ophthalmol (1998). , 42, 90-94.

[121] Kim, C. Y, Kim, S. S, Koh, H. J, You, Y. S, Seong, G. J, & Hong, Y. J. Effect of IOP elevation on matrix metalloproteinase-2 in rabbit anterior chamber. Korean J Ophthalmol (2000). , 14, 27-31.

[122] Bradley, J. M, Kelley, M. J, Zhu, X, Anderssohn, A. M, Alexander, J. P, & Acott, T. S. Effects of mechanical stretching on trabecular matrix metalloproteinases. Invest Ophthalmol Vis Sci (2001). , 42, 1505-1513.

[123] Bradley, J. M, Kelley, M. J, Rose, A, & Acott, T. S. Signaling pathways used in trabecular matrix metalloproteinase response to mechanical stretch. Invest Ophthalmol Vis Sci (2003). , 44, 5174-5181.

[124] George, J, Castellazzi, M, & Buttin, G. Prophage induction and cell division in E. coli. III. Mutations sfiA and sfiB restore division in tif and lon strains and permit the expression of mutator properties of tif. Mol Gen Genet (1975). , 140, 309-332.

[125] Lopez-maury, L, Marguerat, S, & Bahler, J. Tuning gene expression to changing environments: from rapid responses to evolutionary adaptation. Nat Rev Genet (2008). , 9, 583-593.

[126] Johnson, D. H, & Tschumper, R. C. Human trabecular meshwork organ culture. A new method. Invest Ophthalmol Vis Sci (1987). , 28, 945-953.

[127]   Keller, K. E, Bradley, J. M, & Acott, T. S. Differential effects of ADAMTS-1,-4, and-5 in the trabecular meshwork. Invest Ophthalmol Vis Sci (2009). , 50, 5769-5777.

[128]   Gasch, A. P, Spellman, P. T, Kao, C. M, Carmel-harel, O, Eisen, M. B, Storz, G, et al. Genomic expression programs in the response of yeast cells to environmental changes. Mol Biol Cell (2000). , 11, 4241-4257.

[129]   Boehm, A. K, Saunders, A, Werner, J, & Lis, J. T. Transcription factor and polymerase recruitment, modification, and movement on dhsp70 in vivo in the minutes following heat shock. Mol Cell Biol (2003). , 23, 7628-7637.

[130]   Tumminia, S. J, Mitton, K. P, Arora, J, Zelenka, P, Epstein, D. L, & Russell, P. Mechanical stretch alters the actin cytoskeletal network and signal transduction in human trabecular meshwork cells. Invest Ophthalmol Vis Sci (1998). , 39, 1361-1371.

[131]   Liton, P. B, Li, G, Luna, C, Gonzalez, P, & Epstein, D. L. Cross-talk between TGF-beta1 and IL-6 in human trabecular meshwork cells. Mol Vis (2009). , 15, 326-334.

[132]   Zhang, X, Schroeder, A, Callahan, E. M, Coyle, B. M, Wang, N, Erickson, K. A, et al. Constitutive signalling pathway activity in trabecular meshwork cells from glaucomatous eyes. Exp Eye Res (2006). , 82, 968-973.

[133]   Porter, K. M, Epstein, D. L, & Liton, P. B. Up-regulated expression of extracellular matrix remodeling genes in phagocytically challenged trabecular meshwork cells. PLoS One (2012). e34792.

[134]   Kultz, D. Molecular and evolutionary basis of the cellular stress response. Annu Rev Physiol (2005). , 67, 225-257.

[135]   Wang, N, Chintala, S. K, Fini, M. E, & Schuman, J. S. Activation of a tissue-specific stress response in the aqueous outflow pathway of the eye defines the glaucoma disease phenotype. Nat Med (2001). , 7, 304-309.

[136]   Zhou, Q, Liu, Y. Q, Zhao, J. L, & Zhang, H. Effects of oxidative stress on the expression of endothelial-leukocyte adhesion molecule-1 in porcine trabecular meshwork cells. Zhongguo Yi Xue Ke Xue Yuan Xue Bao (2007). , 29, 394-397.

[137]   Liton, P. B, Luna, C, Challa, P, Epstein, D. L, & Gonzalez, P. Genome-wide expression profile of human trabecular meshwork cultured cells, nonglaucomatous and primary open angle glaucoma tissue. Mol Vis (2006). , 12, 774-790.

[138]   Giaever, G, Chu, A. M, Ni, L, Connelly, C, Riles, L, Veronneau, S, et al. Functional profiling of the Saccharomyces cerevisiae genome. Nature (2002). , 418, 387-391.

[139]   Thorpe, G. W, Fong, C. S, Alic, N, Higgins, V. J, & Dawes, I. W. Cells have distinct mechanisms to maintain protection against different reactive oxygen species: oxidative-stress-response genes. Proc Natl Acad Sci U S A (2004). , 101, 6564-6569.

[140] Warringer, J, Ericson, E, Fernandez, L, Nerman, O, & Blomberg, A. High-resolution yeast phenomics resolves different physiological features in the saline response. Proc Natl Acad Sci U S A (2003). , 100, 15724-15729.

[141] Koonin, E. V. Chance and necessity in cellular response to challenge. Mol Syst Biol (2007).

[142] Stern, S, Dror, T, Stolovicki, E, Brenner, N, & Braun, E. Genome-wide transcriptional plasticity underlies cellular adaptation to novel challenge. Mol Syst Biol (2007).

[143] Hugo Gene Nomenclature CommitteeAvailable at: http://www.genenames.org/index.html.Accessed 08/14, (2012).

[144] Fingert, J. H. Primary open-angle glaucoma genes. Eye (Lond) (2011). , 25, 587-595.

[145] Nishimura, D. Y, Swiderski, R. E, Alward, W. L, Searby, C. C, Patil, S. R, Bennet, S. R, et al. The forkhead transcription factor gene FKHL7 is responsible for glaucoma phenotypes which map to 6Nat Genet (1998). , 25.

[146] Mears, A. J, Jordan, T, Mirzayans, F, Dubois, S, Kume, T, Parlee, M, et al. Mutations of the forkhead/winged-helix gene, FKHL7, in patients with Axenfeld-Rieger anomaly. Am J Hum Genet (1998). , 63, 1316-1328.

[147] Semina, E. V, Reiter, R, Leysens, N. J, Alward, W. L, Small, K. W, Datson, N. A, et al. Cloning and characterization of a novel bicoid-related homeobox transcription factor gene, RIEG, involved in Rieger syndrome. Nat Genet (1996). , 14, 392-399.

[148] Berry, F. B, Skarie, J. M, Mirzayans, F, Fortin, Y, Hudson, T. J, Raymond, V, et al. FOXC1 is required for cell viability and resistance to oxidative stress in the eye through the transcriptional regulation of FOXO1A. Hum Mol Genet 200815;, 17, 490-505.

[149] Strungaru, M. H, Footz, T, Liu, Y, Berry, F. B, Belleau, P, Semina, E. V, et al. PITX2 is involved in stress response in cultured human trabecular meshwork cells through regulation of SLC13A3. Invest Ophthalmol Vis Sci (2011). , 52, 7625-7633.

[150] Morissette, J, Cote, G, Anctil, J. L, Plante, M, Amyot, M, Heon, E, et al. A common gene for juvenile and adult-onset primary open-angle glaucomas confined on chromosome 1q. Am J Hum Genet (1995). , 56, 1431-1442.

[151] Sheffield, V. C, Stone, E. M, Alward, W. L, Drack, A. V, Johnson, A. T, Streb, L. M, et al. Genetic linkage of familial open angle glaucoma to chromosome 1q21-q31. Nat Genet (1993). , 4, 47-50.

[152] Stone, E. M, Fingert, J. H, Alward, W. L, Nguyen, T. D, Polansky, J. R, Sunden, S. L, et al. Identification of a gene that causes primary open angle glaucoma. Science (1997). , 275, 668-670.

[153] Karali, A, Russell, P, Stefani, F. H, & Tamm, E. R. Localization of myocilin/trabecular meshwork--inducible glucocorticoid response protein in the human eye. Invest Oph-thalmol Vis Sci (2000). , 41, 729-740.

[154] Resch, Z. T, & Fautsch, M. P. Glaucoma-associated myocilin: a better understanding but much more to learn. Exp Eye Res (2009). , 88, 704-712.

[155] Resch, Z. T, Hann, C. R, Cook, K. A, & Fautsch, M. P. Aqueous humor rapidly stimu-lates myocilin secretion from human trabecular meshwork cells. Exp Eye Res 201;, 91, 901-908.

[156] Hardy, K. M, Hoffman, E. A, Gonzalez, P, Mckay, B. S, & Stamer, W. D. Extracellular trafficking of myocilin in human trabecular meshwork cells. J Biol Chem (2005). , 280, 28917-28926.

[157] Joe, M. K, & Tomarev, S. I. Expression of myocilin mutants sensitizes cells to oxida-tive stress-induced apoptosis: implication for glaucoma pathogenesis. Am J Pathol (2010). , 176, 2880-2890.

[158] Alward, W. L. Axenfeld-Rieger syndrome in the age of molecular genetics. Am J Ophthalmol (2000). , 130, 107-115.

[159] Sowden, J. C. Molecular and developmental mechanisms of anterior segment dys-genesis. Eye (Lond) (2007). , 21, 1310-1318.

[160] Reis, L. M, & Semina, E. V. Genetics of anterior segment dysgenesis disorders. Curr Opin Ophthalmol (2011). , 22, 314-324.

[161] Strungaru, M. H, Dinu, I, & Walter, M. A. Genotype-phenotype correlations in Axen-feld-Rieger malformation and glaucoma patients with FOXC1 and PITX2 mutations. Invest Ophthalmol Vis Sci (2007). , 48, 228-237.

Chapter 3

Anatomy of Ciliary Body, Ciliary Processes, Anterior Chamber Angle and Collector Vessels

Adriana Silva Borges- Giampani and
Jair Giampani Junior

Additional information is available at the end of the chapter

1. Introduction

1.1. Anatomy of the ciliary body

The ciliary body is the site of aqueous humor production and it is totally involved in aqueous humor dynamics. The ciliary body is the anterior portion of the uveal tract, which is located between the iris and the choroid. (figure 1)

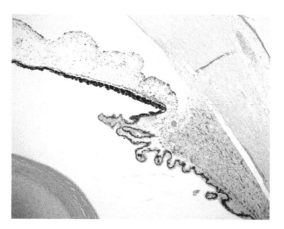

Figure 1. Histology of human ciliary body (courtesy Prof. Ruth Santo)

On cross-section, the ciliary body has the shape of a right triangle, approximately 6 mm in length, where its apex is contiguous with the choroid and the base close to the iris. Externally, it attaches to the scleral spur creating a potential space, the supraciliary space, between it and the sclera. The external surface forms the anterior insertion of the uveal tract. The internal surface of the ciliary body comes in contact with the vitreous surface and is continuous with the retina [1].

The anterior portion of the ciliary body is called the *pars plicata* or *corona ciliaris* and is characterized by ciliary processes, which consist of approximately 70 radial ridges (major ciliary processes) and an equal number of smaller ridges (minor or intermediate ciliary processes) between them [2].

The *pars plicata* is contiguous with the iris posterior surface and is approximately 2 mm in length, 0.5 mm in width, and 0.8-1 mm in height [2,3].

Thus, the ciliary processes have a large surface area, estimated to be 6 cm^2, for ultrafiltration and active fluid transport, this being the actual site of aqueous production; the *pars plicata* accounts for approximately 25% of the total length of the ciliary body (2 mm) [4] (figure 2)

The posterior portion of the ciliary body is called the *pars plana* or *orbicularis ciliaris*, which has a relatively flat and very pigmented inner surface, and is continuous with the choroid at the ora serrata.

In the adult eye, the anterior-posterior length of the ciliary body ranges 4.5-5.2 mm nasally and 5.6 -6.3 mm temporally [5].

The ciliary body is composed of muscle, vessels and epithelium.

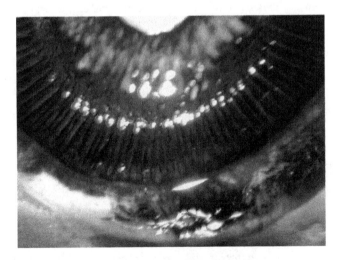

Figure 2. Pars plicata of rabbit ciliary body (courtesy of Prof. Durval Carvalho Jr.)

1.2. Ciliary muscle

The ciliary muscle consists of three separate muscle fibers: longitudinal, circular and oblique.

The longitudinal fibers (meridional), which are the most external, attach the ciliary body anteriorly to the scleral spur and trabecular meshwork at the limbus, and posteriorly to the supracoroidal lamina (fibers connecting choroid and sclera) as far back as the equator of the eye [6].

The contraction of the longitudinal muscle, opens the trabecular meshwork and Schlemm`s canal.

The circular fibers (sphincteric) make up the more anterior and inner portion, and run parallel to the limbus. This insertion is in the posterior iris. When these fibers contract, the zonules relax, increasing the lens axial diameter and its convexity.

The oblique fibers (radial or intermediate) connect the longitudinal and circular fibers. The contraction of these fibers may widen the uveal trabecular spaces.

1.3. Ciliary vessels

Traditional views hold that the vasculature of the ciliary body is supplied by the anterior ciliary arteries and the long posterior ciliary arteries, forming the major arterial circle near the root of the iris, wherefrom branches supply the iris, ciliary body and the anterior choroid. Recent studies in primates have shown a complex vascular arrangement with collateral circulation on at least three levels [7,8]: an episcleral circle formed by anterior ciliary branches; an intramuscular circle formed through the anastomosis between anterior ciliary arteries and long posterior ciliary artery branches; and the major arterial circle formed primarily, if not exclusively, by paralimbal branches of the long posterior ciliary arteries. The major arterial circle is the immediate vascular supply of the iris and ciliary processes [8,9].

1.4. Ciliary epithelia

The inner surfaces of the ciliary processes and the pars plana are lined by two layers of epithelium. (figure 3)

The outer layer is the pigmented epithelium, which is composed of low cuboidal cells and is adjacent to the stroma and continuous with the retinal pigmented epithelium.

The inner layer is formed by the nonpigmented epithelium, a columnar epithelium, adjacent to the aqueous humor in the posterior chamber and continuous with the retina.

These two layers of the epithelium are appositioned in their apical surfaces.

1.5. Innervation

The major innervation is provided by ciliary nerve branches (third cranial nerve-oculomotor), forming a rich parasympathetic plexus. There are also sympathetic fibers originating from the superior cervical ganglion which keep pace with arteries and their branches.

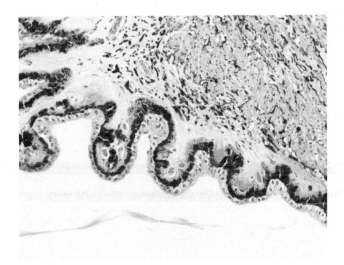

Figure 3. Histology of human ciliary epithelia

2. Ultrastructure of the ciliary processes

Each ciliary process is composed of a central stroma and capillaries, covered by a double layer of epithelium. (FIGURE 3)

The ciliary process capillaries occupy the center of each process [10]. The capillary endothelium is thin and fenestrated, representing areas with fused plasma membranes and no cytoplasm, which may have an increased permeability. A basement membrane surrounds the endothelium and contains mural cells or pericytes.

The stroma is very thin and surrounds the vascular tissues, separating them from the epithelial layers. The stroma is composed of ground substance (mucopolysaccharides, proteins and plasma of low molecular size), collagen connective tissue (especially collagen type III) and cells of connective tissue and the blood [11].

Ciliary process epithelia consist of two layers, with the apical surfaces in apposition to each other.

The pigmented epithelium is the outer layer, and the cuboidal cells contain numerous melanin granules in their cytoplasm. This layer is separated from the stroma by an atypical basement membrane, a continuation of Bruch`s membrane which contains collagen and elastic fibers [15].

The nonpigmented epithelium is composed of columnar cells with numerous mitochondria, well-developed endoplasmic reticulum seen in the cytoplasm, extensive infoldings of the membranes and tight junctions between the apical cell membranes. The basement membrane faces the aqueous humor, is composed of fibrils in a glycoprotein with laminin and collagens I, III and IV [16]. The apical cells of this membrane are connected by tight junctions (zonulae occludentae), creating a permeability barrier, which is an important component of the blood-aqueous barrier called the internal limiting membrane.

Adjacent cells within each epithelial layer and between the apical cells of the two layers are connected by gap junctions, tight junctions and desmosomes. The apical membranes of the nonpigmented epithelium are also joined by tight junctions [12,13,14]

These tight junctions are permeable only to low-molecular-weight solutes.

The anterior portion of the nonpigmented ciliary epithelium has the morphologic features of a tissue involved in active fluid transport, i.e., evidence of abundant sodium-potassium adenosine triphosphatase (Na+ K+ ATPase), glycolytic enzymes activity, and incorporation of labeled sulfate into glycolipids and glycoproteins [17]. There are many indications that the aqueous humor is produced in the anterior portion of the nonpigmented epithelia of ciliary processes [17,18,19].

There is a potential space between the two epithelial layers, called "ciliary channels". The aqueous humor may be secreted into this space after beta-adrenergic agonist stimulation, but this notion requires additional studies [20].

3. Anterior chamber angle

The iris inserts into the anterior side of the ciliary body and separates the aqueous compartment into a posterior and anterior chamber. The angle formed by the iris and the cornea is the anterior chamber angle[6].

The aqueous humor is formed by the ciliary process, passes from posterior chamber to the anterior chamber through the pupil, and leaves the eye at the anterior chamber angle. Most of the aqueous humor exits the eye through the trabecular meshwork, which is called the conventional or canalicular system, and accounts for 83 to 96% of aqueous outflow of normal human eyes [21,22].

The other 5-15% of the aqueous humor leaves the eye through the uveoscleral and uveovortex systems (unconventional systems), including anterior ciliary muscle and iris to reach supra-ciliary and suprachoroidal spaces [22,23,24].

3.1. Anatomy of anterior chamber angle (conventional outflow system)

a.   Schwalbe`s line

This line or zone represents the transition from the trabecular to corneal endothelium, the termination of Descemet`s membrane, and the trabecular insertion into the corneal stroma.

Schwalbe`s line is just anterior to the apical portion of the trabecular meshwork, is composed of collagen and elastic tissue and has a width that varies 50-150 µm; it has been called Zone S [25].

b.   Scleral spur

The posterior wall of the scleral sulcus is formed by a group of fibers, parallel to the limbus that project inward like a fibrous ring, called the scleral spur. These fibers are composed of 80% collagen (collagen type I and III) and 5% elastic fibers. The spur is attached anteriorly to the trabecular meshwork and posteriorly to the sclera and the longitudinal portion of the ciliary muscle [26].

When the ciliary muscle contracts, it pulls the scleral spur posteriorly, it increases the width of the intertrabecular spaces and prevents Schlemm`s canal from collapsing [27].

c.   Ciliary body band

This is structure that is located posterior to scleral spur.

When the iris inserts into the anterior side of the ciliary body, it leaves a variable width of the latter structure visible between the iris and scleral spur, corresponding to the ciliary body band. Gonioscopically, it appears as a brownish band.

d.   Trabecular meshwork

The aqueous humor leaves the eye at the anterior chamber angle through the conventional system consisting of the trabecular meshwork, Schlemm's canal, intrascleral channels, and episcleral and conjunctival veins.

The trabecular meshwork consists of connective tissue surrounded by endothelium. In a meridional section, it has a triangular shape, with the apex at Schwalbe's line and the base at the scleral spur.

The meshwork consists of a stack of flattened, interconnected, perforated sheets, which run from Schwalbe's line to the scleral spur. This tissue may be divided into three portions: a) uveal meshwork, b) corneoscleral meshwork and c) juxtacanalicular tissue[6]. By gonioscopy, the trabecular meshwork can be separated into two portions: an anterior (named non-pigmented) and a posterior (pigmented).

The inner layers of the trabecular meshwork can be observed in the anterior chamber angle and are referred to as the uveal meshwork. This portion is adjacent to the aqueous humor, is arranged in bands or rope-like trabeculae, and extends from the iris root and ciliary body to the peripheral cornea. These strands are a normal variant and are called by a variety names such as iris process, pectinated fibers, uveal trabeculae, ciliary fibers, and uveocorneal fibers. The deeper layers of the uveoscleral meshwork are more flattened sheets with wide perforations.

The outer layers, the corneoscleral meshwork, consist of 8 to 15 perforated sheets. The corneoscleral trabecular sheets insert into the scleral sulcus and spur. These sheets are not visible gonioscopically.

The perforations are elliptical and become progressively smaller from the uveal meshwork to the deep layers of the corneoscleral meshwork [28]. The aqueous humor leaves the trabecular in a tortuous route until reaching Schlemm's canal, because the perforations are not aligned.

The ultrastructure of the trabecular, uveal and corneoscleral meshworks is similar. Each sheet is composed of four concentric layers. The trabecular beams have a central core of connective tissue of collagen fiber types I and III and elastin. There is a layer composed of elastic fibers that provides flexibility to the trabeculae. The core is surrounded by a glass membrane, which is composed of fibronectin, laminin, heparin, proteoglycan and collagen type III, IV and V. The endothelial layer is a continuous layer and covers all the trabeculae. The endothelial cells are larger, more irregular than corneal endothelial cells. They are joined by gap junctions and tight junctions and have microfilaments, including actin filaments and intermediate filaments (vimentin and desmin) [30].

3.2. Gonioscopy of the normal anterior chamber angle

On gonioscopy, starting at the cornea and moving posteriorly toward the root of the iris, the first anatomic structure encountered is Schwalbe's line. (FIGURE 4)

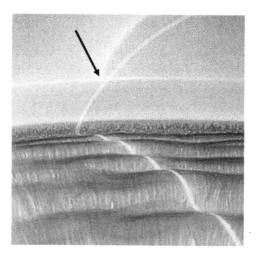

Figure 4. Normal gonioscopic vision of Schwalbe's line (black arrow)

Schwalbe's line corresponds to the termination of Descemet's membrane and marks the most anterior extension of the trabecular meshwork.

It can be seen, by slit-lamp examination, as a fine white ridge, just anterior to the meshwork, and with an indirect contact gonioscopic lens, it is identified at the point where the anterior and posterior beams of the cornea converge (parallelepiped method to identify the transition between the cornea and the meshwork).

The trabecular meshwork lies between Schwalbe's line and the scleral spur, and it may be considered as two separate portions: (a) anterior part, which is composed of corneoscleral sheets and is not pigmented, meaning it is not visible gonioscopically; (b) posterior part, which is the primary site of aqueous outflow and is the pigmented trabecular meshwork composed of a syncytium of fibers. Gonioscopically, it has an irregular roughened pigmented surface. The amount and distribution of the pigment deposition varies considerably with age and race. At birth, it has no pigment, and develops color with age from light to dark brown, depending on the degree of pigment dispersion in the anterior chamber angle.

The scleral spur is just posterior to the pigmented trabecular band, and it is the most anterior projection of the sclera internally. Gonioscopically, it is seen as a prominent white line between the ciliary body band and pigmented trabecular. It can be obscured by excessive pigment dispersion, and is not visible at variable degrees of narrow or occluded angles.

The iris processes, thickenings of the posterior uveal meshwork, may be frequently seen crossing the scleral spur. They have the appearance of a variable number of fine and pigmented strands.

The ciliary body band is the portion of ciliary body that is visible in the anterior chamber. The width of the band depends on the point of the iris insertion on the ciliary body. Gonioscopically, it appears as a densely pigmented band, gray or dark-brown, posterior to the scleral spur and anterior to the root of the iris.

4. Juxtacanalicular tissue

The corneoscleral meshwork is separated from the endothelium of Schlemm's canal by a thin tissue, the juxtacanalicular tissue [29].

The juxtacanalicular tissue is the outermost portion of the meshwork in contact with the inner wall of Schlemm's canal. This tissue consists of a layer of connective tissue (types III, IV and V collagen, fibronectin) and ground substance (glycosaminoglycans and glycoproteins), and it is lined on either side by endothelium [31,32]. There is evidence that the juxtacanalicular tissue contains elastic fibers that provide support for Schlemm's canal and that these fibers are attached to the tendons of the ciliary muscle.

5. Schlemm's canal

Schlemm's canal is a 360-degree endothelial-lined channel that runs circumferentially around the globe. Generally, it has a single lumen, but occasionally it is like a plexus with multiple branches.

The outer wall of Schlemm's canal is a single layer of endothelium, without pores but with numerous large outlet channels and series of giant vacuoles, which form projections into the lumen of Schlemm's canal, possibly serving as a pathway for fluid moviment [33].

6. Collector channels

Schlemm's canal drains into the episcleral and conjunctival veins by a complex system of vessels (collector channels or outflow channels). This system is composed of innumerous intrascleral aqueous vessels and aqueous veins of Ascher, which arise from the outer wall of Schlemm's canal up to the episcleral and conjunctival veins. These collector vessels can run like a direct system, draining directly into the episcleral venous system or like an indirect system of more numerous, fine channels, forming an intrascleral plexus before draining into the episcleral venous system [34,35].

7. Episcleral and conjunctival veins

The aqueous humor reaches the episcleral venous system by several routes [36]. Most aqueous vessels run posteriorly draining into episcleral and conjunctival veins. Some aqueous vessels run parallel to the limbus before heading posteriorly toward the conjunctival veins.

The episcleral veins drain into the cavernous sinus by the anterior ciliary and superior ophthalmic veins.

The conjunctival veins drain into superior ophthalmic or facial veins via the angular or palpebral veins [37].

Author details

Adriana Silva Borges- Giampani and Jair Giampani Junior

Federal University of Mato Grosso, Brazil

References

[1] Stamper, R. L, Lieberman, M. F, & Drake, M. V. Aqueous Humor Formation and Outflow. In Diagnosis and Therapy of the glaucomas. Becker-Shaffer's. Mosby, Seventh edition,(1999). , 20-64.

[2] Hogan, M. F, Alvarado, J. A, & Weddell, J. E. Histology of the Human Eye. Philadelphia, WB Saunders,269; (1971).

[3] Smelser GK; Electron microscopy of a typical epithelial cell and of the normal human ciliary processTrans Am Acad Ophthalmol Otolaryngol 70: 738,(1966).

[4] Brubaker, R. F. and cols; The effect of age on aqueous humor formation in man, Ophthalmology 88: 283, (1981).

[5]   Aiello, A. L, & Tran, V. T. Rao NA: Postnatal development of the ciliary body and pars plana. A morphometric study in childhood. Arch Ophthalmol 110:802, (1992).

[6]   Bruce Shields MAqueous humor dynamics: Anatomy and Physiology. In Textbook of glaucoma. Williams & Wilkins, Fourth edition,(1997). , 5-31.

[7]   Morrison, J. C. Van Burskirk EM: Anterior collateral circulation in the primate eye. Ophthalmology 90:707,(1983).

[8]   Funk, R. Rohen JW: Scanning electron microscopy study on the vasculature of the human anterior eye segment, specially with respect to the ciliary processses. Exp Eye Res 51:651, (1990).

[9]   Woodlief NF: Initial observations on the ocular circulations in manI. The anterior segment and extraocular muscles.Arch Ophthalmol 98:1268, (1980).

[10] Smelser GK: Electron microscopy of a typical epithelial cell and of the normal human ciliary processesTrans Am Acad Ophthalmol Otolaringol 70:738, (1966).

[11] Kitada, S, Shapourifar-tehrani, S, & Smyth, R. J. Lee DA: Characterization of human and rabbit pigmented and nonpigmented ciliary body epithelium. Eye Res 10:409, (1991).

[12] Hara, K. and cols: Structural differences between regions of the ciliary body of primates. Invest Ophthalmol Vis Sci 16:912, (1977).

[13] Ober, M. Rohen JW: Regional differences in the fine structure of the ciliary epithelium related to accommodation. Invest Ophthalmol vis Sci 18:655,(1979).

[14] Raviola, G. Raviola E: Intercellular injections in the ciliary epithelium, Invet Ophthalmol Vis Sci 17:958, (1978).

[15] Eichhorn, M, & Flügel, C. Lütgen-Drecoll E: Regional differences in the distribution of cytoskeletal filaments in the human and bovine ciliary epithelium. Grafe's Arch Ophthalmol 230:385, (1992).

[16] Marshall, G. E. Konstas AGP, Abrahan S, Lee WR : Extracellular matrix in aged humar ciliary body: an immunoelectron microscope study. Invest Ophthalmol Vis Sci 33:2546, (1992).

[17] Russmann W : levels of glycolytic enzyme activity in the ciliary epithelium prepared from bovine eyesOphthalmic Res 2:205,(1971).

[18] Mizuni, K. Asoka M: Cycloscopy and fluorescein cycloscopy. Invest Ophthalmol 15: 561, (1976).

[19] Feeney, L. Mixon R: Localization of 35 sulfated macromolecules at the site of active transport in the ciliary processes. Invest Ophthalmol 13:882,(1974).

[20] Fujita, H, & Konko, K. Sears M: Eine neue funktion der nicht pigmentierten epithels der ziliarkorperfortsatze bei der kammerwasserproduktion, Klin Mbl Augenheilk 185:28, (1984)

[21] Jocson, V. L. Sears ML: Experimental aqueous perfusion in enucleated human eyes. Arch Ophthalmol 86:65, (1971).

[22] Bill, A. Phillips CI: Uveoscleral drainage of aqueous humor in human eye. Exp Eye Res 12:275,(1971).

[23] Pederson, J. E, & Gaasterland, D. E. MacLellan HM: Uveoscleral aqueous outflow in the rhesus monkey: importance of uveal reabsorption. Invest Ophthalmol Vis Sci 16:1008,(1977).

[24] Sherman, S. H, & Green, K. Laties AM: The Fate of anterior chamber fluorescein inthe monkey eye. I. The anterior chamber outflow pathways. Exp Eye Res 27:159,(1978).

[25] Neufeld, A. H, & Jampol, L. M. Sears ML: Aspirin prevents the disruption of the blood aqueous barrier in the rabbit eye. Nature 238:158,(1972).

[26] Moses, R. A, & Grodzki, W. J Jr, Starcher BC, Galione MJ: Elastin content of the scleral spur, trabecular mesh and sclera. Invest Ophthalmol Vis Sci 17:817, (1978).

[27] Moses, R. A, & Grodzki, W. J Jr: The scleral spur and scleral roll. Invest Ophthalmol Vis Sci 16:925, (1977).

[28] Flocks M: The anatomy of the trabecular meshwork as seen in tangencial sectionArch Ophthalmol 56:708,(1957).

[29] Fine BS: Observations on the drainage angle in man and rhesus monkey: A concept of the pathogenesis of chronic simple glaucomaA light and electron microscopic study. Invest Ophthalmol 3:609,(1964).

[30] Ashton N: The exit pathway of the aqueousTrans Ophthalmol Soc UK 80:397,(1960).

[31] Bairati, A. Orzalesi N: The ultrastructure of the epithelium of the ciliary body: a study of the function complexes and of the changes associated with the production of plasmoid aqueous humor. Z Zellforsch Mikrosk Anat 69: 635, (1966).

[32] Cole DF : location of ouabain-sensitive adenosinetriphosp'fatase in ciliary epitheliu-mExp Eye Res 3: 72,(1964).

[33] Vegge T : An epithelial blood-aqueous barrier to horseradish peroxidase in the processes of the vervet monkey Ceropithecus aethipsZ Zellforsch Mikrosk Anat 114: 309, (1971).

[34] Hoffman, F. Dumitrescu L: Schlemm's canal under the scanning electron microscope. Ophthal Res 2:37, (1971).

[35] Rohen, J. W. Rentsch FJ: Electronmicroscopic studies on the structure of the outer wall of Schlemm's canal, its outflow channels and age changes. Grafe's Arch Ophthalmol 177:1,(1969).

[36] Ascher KW: The aqueous veinsBiomicroscopic study of the aqueous humor elimination. Springfield IL,Charles C Thomas,(1961).

[37] Last RJ: Wolff's anatomy of the eye and orbitPhiladelphia, Fifth edition, WB Saunders, (1961).

Chapter 4

Modern Aspects of Glaucoma Pathogenesis Local Factors for Development of Primary Open-Angle Glaucoma Associated with Impairment of Secretory Functions of the Eye Membranes

A.A. Zilfyan

Additional information is available at the end of the chapter

1. Introduction

The term "Glaucoma" integrates a wide range of eye diseases characterized by a diversity of clinical forms: mainly by the chronic course and rather unfavourable prognosis. Sufficient to mention that in developed countries the frequency of vision loss due to glaucoma is steadily at the level of 15-20% of the total number of all blind subjects [*Nesterov A.P., 2008*].

It is considered long-established that among various clinical-and-anatomical manifestations of the glaucomatous process the anterior open-angle glaucoma is the most frequently diagnosed form.

The severity of course of anterior open-angle glaucoma and especially the unfavourable outcomes of the disease are mainly connected with those unsolvable problems faced by ophthalmologists at the study of pathogenesis of primary and secondary glaucomas. Precisely this circumstance is the "insurmountable" obstacle in pathogenetic therapy, thus limiting the entire complex of medical interventions within the early symptomatic therapy with underlying local application of hypotensive means aimed to decrease intraocular pressure.

To a known extent, the interpretation of aspects of pathogenesis in case of anterior open-angle glaucoma is connected to the fact that this type of glaucoma is rather frequently associated with the cataract and pseudoexfoliative syndrome.

At present the etiopathogenetic links engaged in induction and the course of anterior open-angle glaucoma are conditionally divided into general and local ones.

Heredity, general type changes in specific integrative systems of the organism (CNS, endocrine, immune and cardiovascular) are among the general factors bringing forth disorders of the hematoophthalmic barrier and the increase of intraocular pressure.

Amongst the local factors relatively persistent elevation of intraocular pressure, primary dystrophic and atrophic changes, including age-related shifts in the cornea, ciliary body and the trabecular meshwork, which cause the infringement of hydrodynamic and hydrostatic properties of the aqueous humour, are considered.

As mentioned by A.P. Nesterov (2008) chronologically occurring processes, which might be conditionally subdivided into 2 stages, are engaged in the pathogenesis of glaucomas in anterior and posterior chambers of an eye. At the first stage mechanisms bringing forth the increase of intraocular pressure are triggered in the anterior chamber of an eye. At the second stage mechanisms localized in the posterior part of the eye chamber are initiated and in the long run become the cause of atrophy of the visual nerve. At that, the "glaucomatous process" firstly originates in the anterior chamber of an eye, while the dystrophic and atrophic processes in the visual nerve are resulting from the exposure to high intraocular pressure.

During the last years, rather informative evidences were obtained to discuss the role of biologically active substances produced *in situ*, i.e. in specific eye membranes, in mechanisms of anterior open-angle glaucoma origination using the clinical and experimental material.

We did not set the problem to analyze the current state of the art on the role of general pathogenetic factors engaged in induction and the course of anterior open-angle glaucoma.

The currently available data of scientific publications and results of our own investigations devoted to the role of *in situ* produced biologically active substances of cytokine, mediatory and hormonal origin in mechanisms of a stable increase of the intraocular pressure in case of anterior open-angle glaucoma will be analyzed in this work.

2. Secretory-mediatory hormone-dependent functions of eye membranes in the mechanisms of glaucoma development

2.1. The role of transforming growth factor β-2 (TgF$_{β-2}$), insulin-like growth factor-1 (IgF-1) and E$_2$ prostaglandins (PgE$_2$) in pathogenesis of primary open-angle glaucoma

Nowadays the role of TGF$_β$ produced in post-barrier membranes of an eye is considered to be of no less importance for realization of processes ensuring the drainage function of the eye anterior chamber-associated immune deviation (ACAID) [*Mansfield K. et al., 2004; Banh A. et al., 2006; Kim Y.S. et al., 2008; Dawes L.J. et al., 2009*]. According to scientific publications, TGF$_{β-2}$ produced in the post-barrier membrane of an eye (in cornea, ciliary body, retina) at some eye diseases takes an active part in the increase of intraocular pressure [*de Iongh R.U. et al., 2005; Stefan C. et al., 2008; Dawes L.J. et al., 2009; Hindman H.B. et al., 2010; Pattabiraman P.P, Rao P.V., 2010*].

To our mind, during the last years rather informative data signifying in favour of pleotropic potencies of $TGF_{\beta-2}$ produced in post-barrier membranes of the eye.

In particular, in a post-surgery period in patients operated for complicated and senile cataracts *in situ* produced $TGF_{\beta-2}$ induces trans-differentiation of epithelial cells of crystalline lens capsule into fibroblasts; this latter was manifested as opacity of lens with all the subsequent after-effects [*Dawes L.J. et al., 2009*]. The modulatory effect of $TGF_{\beta-1}$ towards the processes of activation of cells of fibroblastic line in the cornea was also established. Thus, the authors [*Karamichos D. et al., 2010*] under conditions of cultivating cells of cornea using $TGF_{\beta-1}$ dose-dependent mode activated *in situ* synthetic processes in fibroblasts, thus bringing forth intensification of collagen(ous) fibrilles synthesis and eventually to regional overgrowth of immature connective tissue with the resulting fibrosis.

$TGF_{\beta-2}$ high level was also revealed in cells of the trabecular meshwork of patients with open-angle glaucoma [*Stefan C. et al., 2008*]. The authors consider that at the mentioned disease $TGF_{\beta-2}$ stimulates fibronectin synthesis in trabecular cells, thus predefining "profibrotic" effects of $TGF_{\beta-2}$ in post-barrier membranes of the eye.

Literature data is available [*Ochiai Y., Ochiai H., 2002*], according to which in patients with anterior open-angle glaucoma, diabetes complicated by anterior open-angle glaucoma the level of $TGF_{\beta-2}$ in aqueous / intraocular humor is markedly increased. As a control, the authors studied aqueous humour of patients with cataracts.

Processes reflecting the specific precise stages of $TGF_{\beta-2}$ and IGF-1 activity in post-barrier membranes of the eye are the subject of a wide discussion. Furthermore, the study on mechanisms of their direct and/or mediated interaction in processes ensuring the drainage function of an eye is mainly emphasized.

In the organism of mammals, the post-barrier membranes of an eye also serve as a source of both cytocines. IGF-1 and its receptors, IGF-IR, were found in epitheliocytes of lens and cornea, epitheliocytes of retina meshwork, Muller's cells [*Shaw L.C. et al., 2006; Ko J.A. et al., 2009*]. $TGF_{\beta-2}$ is produced in post-barrier membranes of an eye and, first of all, in fibroblasts of cornea [*Streilein J. et al., 1992; Wilkbanks G. et al., 1992; Hollborn M. et al., 2000; Fleenor D. et al., 2006*].

According to C. Stefan et al. (2008), cells of the trabecular meshwork of the anterior angle of the eye chamber might serve as the source of $TGF_{\beta-2}$ synthesis.

S.H. Chung and associates used human lens epithelial cells (HLE B-3) to reveal the role of IGF-1 in processes of $TGF_{\beta-2}$ mediated fibronectin accumulation in lens cells [*Chung S.H. et al., 2007*]. Based on analysis performed by the authors (reverse polymerase transcriptase chain reaction, immune-fluorescent studies) mentioned researchers draw a conclusion that IGF-1 counteracts $TGF_{\beta-2}$ induced fibronectin accumulation in lens epitheliocytes.

J.A. Ko et al. (2009) studied the role of IGF-1 in intrercellular regulation in cultured fibroblasts and human corneal epitheliocytes. According to authors, the presence of epitheliocytes in the culture medium enhanced N-cadherin expression in fibroblasts. Similar effect of corneal epitheliocytes was also simulated by IGF-1, but not fibroblasts growth factor or epidermal growth factor. The authors conclude that IGF-1 produced in epitheliocytes regulates N-cadherin positive expression in corneal fibroblasts.

There is an opinion that IGF-1 and IGF-2 regulate the processes of proliferation and apoptosis in corneal epitheliocytes [*Yanai R. et al., 2006*]. According to K. Izumi and co-workers (2006), TGF_β produces an influence to corneal fibroblasts differentiation into myofibroblasts. Moreover, IGF-1 is engaged in this mechanism. Thus, treatment with $TGF_{\beta-2}$ caused expression of IGF-1, mRNA, IGF BP-3 and IGF BR-3 protein in human corneal. According to N. Yamada et al. (2005), IGF-1, alongside with fibronectin, IL-6 and substance P, actively participate in stimulation of fibroblastic processes in cornea.

The analysis of above mentioned scientific publications signifies to the important role of *in situ* produced $TGF_{\beta-2}$ and IGF-1 in mechanisms of fibroblastic processes formation and their cellular metaplasia in specific eye membranes: in post-barrier eye membranes in ACAID mechanisms and withdrawal. One cannot exclude that locally produced cytokines possess short-distant range of activity; moreover, their realization might occur according to either the principles of intercellular interaction, i.e. through the paracrine mechanism, or on the basis of intercellular autocrine regulation. Apparently, both mechanisms have an important part in infringement of drainage function of an eye at different types of glaucoma.

As known, prostaglandins play an important role in integrative activity of the mammalian organism, in particular, in regulation of immunogenesis, hemostasis, non-specific resistance at the organism level [*Kuznik B. et al., 1989*].

However, until present the probability of prostaglandins synthesis in post-barrier membranes of an eye seems still disputable.

There are only sporadic communications related to the mentioned aspect; an attempt was made to reveal E_1, E_2 and $F_{2\alpha}$ prostaglandins in post-barrier membranes of an eye and in the aqueous humour.

It is considered established that prostaglandins increase intraocular pressure and infringe the function of hematoophthalmic barrier [*Podos S.M. et al., 1972 a; b; Podos S.M., 1976a ; b; c*]. Moreover, the drainage function of an eye is simultaneously realized by prostaglandins in the aqueous humour.

According to C.B. Toris and associates, numerous prostaglandin-dependent effects in post-barrier membranes of an eye are realized according to the receptor mechanism associated at the level of mRNAs [*Toris C.B. et al., 2008*]. Similar receptors were revealed in the trabecular meshwork, celiar muscle, and sclera.

Prostaglandin-dependent receptors in post-barrier eye membranes were revealed not only in humans, but also in rats, mice, rabbits, pigs and monkeys. Considering the vasoactive properties of prostaglandins, as well as their role in sustaining the drainage function of an eye, the sysnthetic analogs of prostaglandins are widely applied in ophthalmological practice for treatment of glaucoma [*Bucci F.A., Waterbury L.D., 2008; Toris C.B. et al., 2008*].

Therefore, it is no excluded that E_2 prostaglandins might participate in maintenance of the drainage function and, appropriately, the intraocular pressure as well; similar mechanisms of prostaglandins functioning in post-barrier membranes of the eye are realized exceptionally according to the receptor mechanism.

Taking into account the abovementioned, an assumption might be proposed according to which *in situ* produced E_2 prostaglandins are engaged into the pathological process observed at the area of post-barrier membranes of an eye at primary open-angle glaucoma.

2.2. The role of fibronectin in pathogenesis of primary open-angle glaucoma

Fibronectins are a group of cold-insoluble glycoproteids with the molecular mass 400.000–450.000 D localized both on the surface of connective tissue cells and in the extracellular matrix. The following functionally active domains were revealed in fibronectin structure: NH2 terminal domain includes sites of fibrin binding; then collagen and heparin binding domains and domain ensuring cells adhesion are localized; at COOOH-cone there is one more heparin binding domain [*Kuznik B. et al., 1989*]. Fibronectins have an important part in cells proliferation and differentiation, morphogenesis and embryogenesis of tissues. In particular, tissue fibronectin of fibroblastic genesis actively participates in collagen formation both at norm (at the stage-by-stage process of the connective tissue maturation), and in pathology state (different distrophic and inflammatory processes occurring at the site of the connective tissue. Thus, in particular, an important role is assigned to fibronectin in reparative processes, influence on cells migration, growth and proliferation. Fibronectin produced by cells of the connective tissue (fibroblasts, endotheliocytes, smooth-muscle cells of arterioles, etc.) in its turn actively participates in formation of the extra-cellular matrix, especially at early stages of the connective tissue formation. The following cells of different genesis serve as the main source of fibronectin synthesis: endothelium, hepatocytes, fibroblasts, smooth myocytes, Schwann's cells, alveolar and peritoneal macrophages, epitheliocytes, and thrombocytes [*Kuznik B. et al., 1989*].

Currently the sources of fibronectin synthesis in the post-barrier membranes of an eye are disputable as well. According to H.B. Hindman et al. (2010), corneal keratocytes might be considered as probable sources of fibronectin synthesis. This fact was revealed under cultivation of keratocytes localized in the anterior and posterior parts of cornea. Furthermore, in the process of cultivating corneal cells of fibroblastic line the authors established $TGF_{\beta-1}$-dependent activation of keratocytes, in which a marked activation of fibronectin synthesis occurred. Simultaneously, Thy-1 secretion increases in the same keratocytes. According to D. Karamichos et al. (2010), *in situ* (in post-barrier membranes of an eye) produced $TGF_{\beta-2}$, under conditions of pathology might serve as a provoking factor binging forth fibrosis of the cornea. Therefore, we cannot exclude that realization of this $TGF_{\beta-2}$ related effect is mediated due to the activation of fibronectin in the same keratocytes.

C. Stefan et al. (2008) use the immune enzyme assay to determine $TGF_{\beta-2}$ and fibronectin concentration in aqueous humour of patients with anterior open-angle glaucoma. The authors revealed a significant increase of $TGF_{\beta-2}$ concentration in this cohort of patients and draw a conclusion that $TGF_{\beta-2}$ produced in post-barrier membranes of the eye should be considered as a "special" cytokine that increases fibronectin concentration in the trabecular meshwork; moreover, it might be considered as a local pro-fibrotic factor.

Sporadic, though rather informative, evidences are available according to which the trabecular meshwork localized in the angle of an anterior chamber of the eye serves as the possible source of fibronectin synthesis. In particular, R.J. Wordinger et al. (2007) studied the probable mechanisms of synthesis of the biologically active substances by trabecular meshwork cells. As known, the cells of trabecular meshwork synthesize and excrete "bone morphogenic protein" – BMP-4. The authors, under conditions of trabecular cells cultivation studied the synthetic potencies thereof at addition of BMP-4 and $TGF_{\beta-2}$ to the culture media. The study results demonstrated that $TGF_{\beta-2}$ treated cells of the trabecular meshwork launched an intense synthesisn of fibronectin, while BMP-4, if additionally introduced to $TGF_{\beta-2}$ containing media, blocked this induction of fibronectin.

Mentioned authors studied the expression of BMP-4 family gens in normal and glaucomatous cells of the trabecular meshwork. Under the influence of these receptors the levels of $TGF_{\beta-2}$ and BMP antagonist, protein gremlin, significantly increased. The authors succeeded to establish that gremlin blocked the negative impact of BMP-4 towards $TGF_{\beta-2}$ induction of fibronectin.

Another result obtained by the same authors is of no less importance: gremlin introduced in the medium *ex vivo*, caused the prototype of increased intraocular pressure glaucoma. Research findings of these authors reflect the main statements of the hypothesis according to which in case of the anterior open-angle glaucoma the enhanced expression of gremlin by trabecular meshwork cells inhibits BMP-4 antagonism to $TGF_{\beta-2}$, eventually, might bring forth the increase in deposition of the extracellular matrix and intraocular pressure.

The analysis of rather informative data obtained by mentioned authors allows to draw a conclusion, according to which the trabecular meshwork of an angle of anterior chamber of the eyes should not considered as an object that passively ensures the drainage function thus sustaining optimally stable levels of the intraocular pressure.

To our mind, the drainage function of trabecular meshwork is an active process and the leading role here belongs to "secretory" cells of the meshwork predominantly functioning according to the autocrine mechanism. At dysfunctions of trabecular meshwork cells, especially in case of open-angle glaucoma, the synchronous activity of these cells is infringed; this latter might enhance their specific medatory function – in view of the increased synthesis of fibronectin. Precisely, fibronectin depositions and the subsequent intensification of fibroblastic processes *in situ* might bring to disorders in drainage function of the trabecular meshwork of the angle of anterior chamber of the eye and, finally to the stable increase of intraocular pressure.

According to D. Fleenor et al. (2006), $TGF_{\beta-2}$ treatment of segments of trabecular meshwork cells of the angle of anterior chamber of the eye resulted in modulation of multiple gens regulating the structure of extracellular matrix. In the trabecular meshwork cells $TGF_{\beta-2}$ brings forth an increased secretion of fibronectin. $TGF_{\beta-2}$ action to cells of the trabecular meshwork was blocked by inhibitors of receptor type 1 TGF_{β}. In perfusion anterior segments of human eyes $TGF_{\beta-2}$ treatment increased the intraocular pressure and elution of fibronectin. In our opinion the authors come to the rather reasonable conclusion: $TGF_{\beta-2}$ influence on intraocular pressure might be "leveled" by $TGF_{\beta-2}$ -mediated receptors type 1 through prevention of $TGF_{\beta-2}$ stimulating effect to cells of the extracellular matrix.

According to mentioned authors, understanding these inter-mediatory and receptor interactions, which occur at the site of trabecular meshwork of an angle of anterior chamber of the eye, would then allow to develop new efficient approaches for treatment of glaucoma.

There is an opinion [*Gonzales J.M. et al., 1998*], according to which it is merely domain of heparin II (Hep II) in the structure of fibronectin that regulates the ability outflow (excretory system) in cultured anterior segments through the effects produced to the cytoskeleton in transformed cells of the trabecular meshwork of the angle of the anterior chamber of an eye. The mentioned authors cultivated cells of the trabecular meshwork under conditions of Hep II domain and revealed an active site of this domain that regulates the ability of aqueous humor efflux. According to researchers, precisely this site of a domain is responsible in case of disorders in actinic cytoskeleton of the trabecular meshwork at glaucomas.

Fibronectin concentration in aqueous (intraocular) humour of patients with cataracts and glaucomas, according to K.S. Kim et al. (1992), widely varies from 5 *ng/ml* to 100 *ng/ml* (data of immune enzyme assay – ELISA). Authors separated the aqueous humor by aspiration from the eyes of patients with cataract and glaucoma using a special puncture needle introduced through the limbal zone before the limbal incision in the anterior chamber of the eye, that is before the surgical intervention. Due to the performed immune enzyme assay the researchers managed to establish that at glaucomas the level of fibronectin significantly increases compared to its level in aqueous humour of patients with cataracts. At the same time, fibronectin levels in aqueous humor patients with cataract and glaucoma had no dependence on either age or gender of patients under preoperative study.

The aspects related to fibronectin sources in post-barrier membranes of the eye are also discussed. An assumption was made that at primary glaucomas relatively high concentrations of fibronectin accumulate in the anterior chamber of an eye, as it cannot escape the drainage pathways. There are quite opposite data, according to which in patients with the open-angle glaucoma fibrinogen concentration in the aqueous humor significantly did not differ from that of aqueous humor of patients with cataracts [*Vesaluoma M. et al., 1998*]. At the same time, upon comparison of obtained results of immune enzyme analysis for fibrinogen content on the one hand, in aqueous humor of patients with cataracts and primary glaucomas, and, on the other hand, in patients with exfoliative glaucoma, the level of fibronectin in aqueous humor significantly increased in the latter case. The authors consider that significantly higher concentration of fibronectin in patients with the pseudoexfoliative glaucoma might result from infringement of the hematoophthalmic barrier. There is evidence [*Tripathi B.J. et al., 2004*] that the growth factor ($TGF_{\beta-2}$) under conditions *in vivo* modulates fibronectin and stromelysin-1 (MMP-3) in trabecular cells of the anterior chamber of an eye. Mentioned authors studied expression of RNA and fibronectin protein at presence of growth factors in primary and secondary humour of the anterior chamber (taken in pre- and post-operative period, appropriately). In particular, under conditions of incubation of trabecular cells of the anterior chamber of the eye, growth factor containing aqueous humors taken from patients with glaucoma prior to and post the surgery were added to the culture medium. Compare to control, fibronectin mRNA expression by trabecular cells increased by 50 and 100% after incubation in primary samples of aqueous humor during 48 hours or 7 days, as well as by 50 and 160% after incubation in secondary samples of the aqueous humor. MMP-1 mRNA expression decreased by 25 and 50% after incubation in samples of primary aqueous humor during 48 hours or 7 days, as well as by 80 and 85% after incubation during 48 hours or 7 days in secondary samples of aqueous humor. The level of fibronectin increased 3.5 times and 6-fold after incubation during 48 hours with primary and secondary samples of aqueous humor.

Study results obtained by the abovementioned authors allow to draw a conclusion that induction of MMP-3 in the trabecular meshwork of glaucomatous eyes might decrease fibronectin formation in aqueous humor excretion pathways, thus decreasing the resistance of liquid outflow into the anterior chamber of an eye.

The analysis of publications relevant to the role of *in situ* produced fibronectin in post-barrier membrane of an eye allows to come the following conclusions.

Firstly, the role of *in situ* produced fibronectin in mechanisms on sustaining the local homeostasis remains debatable.

Secondly, the available scientific literature indicates to the fact that under conditions of norm fibronectin produced by cells of the trabecular meshwork performs the drainage function in outflow of the aqueous humor.

Thirdly, at some eye diseases and especially at primary open-angle glaucoma and pseudoexfoliative syndrome, the excessive synthesis of fibronectin by cells of the trabecular meshwork might bring forth a disorder of the drainage function that eventually in its turn is fraught with the increase of intraocular pressure.

Fourthly, it is not excluded that in post-barrier membranes of the eye there are engaged fibronectin-dependent mechanisms, which function according to both principles of intercellular interactions and the autocrine mechanism.

2.3. The role of cortisol in pathogenesis of anterior open-angle glaucoma

At present, aspects related to studies on "endocrine homeostasis" in post-barrier membrane of an eye at both norm and pathology are the subject of a wide discussion in ophthalmology. The available publications are not numerous; furthermore, they are of a rather statement-of-the-fact character [*Southren A. et al., 1976; Floman N., Zor U., 1977; Kasavina B. et al., 1977; Weinstein B. et al., 1983; Stone R., Wilson C., 1984; Stojek A. et al., 1991; Chiquet C., Denis P., 2004; Burch J. et al., 2005; Pleyer U. et al., 2005; Schwartz B. et al., 2005; Vessey K. et al., 2005*]. In particular, there are reports discussing the possibility of cortisol local synthesis in eye membranes.

The autopsy material (vitreous body and blood serum of healthy subjects with fatal injury) was subject to immune enzyme assay for determination of progesterone, estradiol, thyroxine, triiodothyronine, thyrotropic hormone, luteinizing hormone, follitropin, cortisol and prolactin [*Chong A., Aw S., 1986*]. The thyroid-stimulating hormone, luteinizing hormone, follitropin, cortisol and prolactin were revealed in the vitreous humour. As to other hormones, progesterone, estradiol, triiodothyronine and thyroxine, the results of immune enzyme assay were negative even despite their high solubility and relatively small size of their molecules. According to A. Steiger (2003), the role of somatotropin, somatostatin and adrenocorticotropic hormone (ACTH) in the genesis of a wide range of eye diseases with both inflammatory and degenerative genesis is also disputable.

The results obtained by mentioned authors testify in favour of the local synthesis of certain hormones in eye membranes and tissues.

It should be specially noted that regional neuroendocrine mechanisms underlying the induction of primary open-angle glaucoma have not been sufficiently studied yet. In this aspect the role of *in situ* produced cortisol in mechanisms of impaired ion exchange is exceptionally connected with disbalance of sodium ions transport between the cells and liquid media of an eye and the impaired catecholamines exchange.

As known, in peripheral "epithelial" tissues sodium and water transport are regulated by corticosteroids, 11-β-hydroxysteroid-dehydrogenase (11-β-HSD), its isoform (11-β-HSD1), due to which there occurs formation of cortisol molecule from cortisone. Considering this latter, some researchers [*Rauz S. et al., 2003*] determined levels of cortisol, cortisone, 11-β-HSD and 11-β-HSD1 in ciliary body of actually healthy volunteers. The study was aimed to reveal the role of cortisol and 11-β-HSD in regulation of intraocular pressure that is sustained due to balance of aqueous humour (intraocular liquid) depending on the sodium transport through the ciliated epithelium and drainage via the trabecular meshwork. In both study groups cortisol concentrations were higher than cortisone levels. In both groups oral application of carbenoxolone, 11-β-HSD inhibitor, was accompanied by a marked decrease of intraocular pressure. To our mind, data obtained by mentioned authors, on the one hand, signify in favour of the above-mentioned cascade of reactions for maintenance of intraocular pressure, on the other hand, in favour of cortisol local synthesis in post-barrier membranes of the eye.

There is an opinion, according to which merely 11-β-HSD1 ensures receptor Nf-dependent mechanisms through the ciliated epithelium, thus regulating the level of intraocular pressure [*Rauz S. et al., 2001*]. Mentioned authors revealed the fine mechanisms, which provide the level of glucocorticoids mediated intraocular pressure. However, the potentiating role of cortico-steroids in regulation of intraocular pressure was revealed much earlier [*Jacob E. et al., 1996*]. As known, the rate of aqueous humour production is stimulated by adrenalin. The authors studied the joint and isolated effects of adrenalin and hydrocortisone to the rate of aqueous humor production in 20 volunteers. As demonstrated by study results, joint oral application of adrenaline and hydrocortisone significantly (by 42%) enhanced production of aqueous humour compared to placebo. The authors consider that both factors simultaneously function within the post-barrier membranes of the eye (ciliary body), thus ensuring the rate of aqueous humour production.

Molecular mechanisms underlying the biological action of glucocorticosteroids in eye membranes were also studied. Specifically, in the experiment, under conditions of cornea transplantation the influence of glucocorticosteroids (SEGRA) was studied to the labeled synthesis of anti- and pro-inflammatory cytokines. The application of glucocorticosteroids brought forth more efficient engraftment. Moreover, the terms of engraftment correlated with the low expression of cytokines, especially IL-I [*Pleyer U. et al., 2005*].

A. Southren et al. (1979) performed experiments in rabbits and revealed endoplasmatic reception of glucocorticoids in corneal cells and the ciliary body. Translocation of cortisol from the surface of the cell nucleus occurred within 30 minutes after injection. As to authors, this mechanism is a stereotype for glucocorticoids towards other sensitive tissues.

It is important to note the following phenomenon as well. Similar translocation was not observed when experimental animals were administered testosterone, estradiol and progesterone. At the same time, different membranes and liquid media of the eye possess different ability of affinity to glucocorticoids and their realization (accumulation and excretion).

In 1977, B. Kasavina et al. (1977) studied cortisol distribution in sclera, ciliary body, cornea, iris, lens capsule, vitreous body and the aqueous humour. Radionuclide methods of investigation allowed to reveal that tissues and media of the eye have different intensity of cortisol absorption and excretion. According to authors, the sclera, ciliary body, and lens capsule served as target tissues for cortisol.

3. Regional mediatory hormonal mechanisms of impaired eye drainage function at primary open-angle and pseudoexfoliative glaucomas (Results of own research investigation)

It is rather difficult to interpret issues relevant to pathogenesis of primary open-angle glaucoma, as this type malady is frequently associated with cataract and pseudoexfoliative syndrome.

In particular, according to D.S. Krol (1968; 1970), among the randomly selected contingent the pseudoexfoliative syndrome was observed in 6.2% subjects above 50, in 24% patients with senile cataract and in 47% patients with open-angle glaucoma. P.P. Frolova and G.Kh. Khamitova (1984) provided similar data, according to which pseudoexfoliative syndrome was diagnosed in 5.8% examined persons above 40. Furthermore, the higher the age, the more frequent was pseudoexfoliative syndrome encountered: at the age of 40-48 years old in 1% patients, at 50-59 – in 6.4%, at 60-69 – in 12.5%, above 70 – in 36.8%. It is especially important that among persons with pseudoexfoliative syndrome glaucoma was diagnosed in 35% cases, while cataracts made 69%.

According to clinical observations of A.P. Nesterov (2008) in persons with the pseudoexfoliative syndrome glaucoma originates 20 time more often than in the general population of the same age group. According to the author, approximately in 50% patients with open-angle glaucoma symptoms of pseudoexfoliative syndrome are revealed. The type of glaucoma associated with the pseudoexfoliative syndrome is called "pseudoexfoliative glaucoma".

Nowadays, amongst the mechanisms of cataract induction and course, an importance is attributed to local immunepathological disorders, which all in all are defined as "anterior chamber associated immune deviation (ACAID) [*Wilbanks G., Streilein J., 1990; Streilein J. et al., 1992; Abrahamian A. et al., 1995; Muhaya M. et al., 1999; Fleenor D. et al., 2006*].

In pathogenesis of the primary open-angle glaucoma the specific gravity of regional immunepathological disorders, which are pathognomonic for cataracts, are open for a special discussion, because data of available scientific publications are scarce, fragmentary, sometimes contradictory and inconsistent.

At the same time, to our mind, it is rather expedient to perform studies at which in case of complicated cataracts associated with glaucoma and pseudoexfoliative syndrome the subject matter would be the entire specter of biologically active substances produced in eye membranes, which were earlier considered by us as pathogenetic factors of open-angle glaucoma. Such scientific and methodical approach is rather substantiated, as it will allow to answer the question: to what extent the processes of impaired synthesis of fibronectin, IGF-1, PgE_2 and cortisol in eye membranes are engaged in mechanisms of primary open-angle glaucoma, namely: in pathogenesis of impaired drainage function and increase of intraocular pressure.

Under our observation there were 960 patients with the senile and complicated cataracts operated at "Shengavit" Medical Center within a period of 2008-2012. The degree of lens opacity was assessed according to Emery colorimetric classification and generally accepted classification of cataracts proposed by Buratto. Undoubtedly, the state of lens capsule, folding, presence of elements of fibrous filaments, pseudoexfoliative deposits on the anterior surface of the capsule, lens subluxation to some degree, were taken into consideration together with classification of phakodonesis suggested by Pashtaev. Actual expressiveness of the pseudoexfoliative syndrome was considered based on the classification proposed by Yeroshevskaya.

All operated patents were divided into three groups.

The studied groups of patients involved civil contingent: residents of Yerevan and different provinces (marzes) of Armenia; age range was from 40 to 82 years.

The first group included patients with senile cataract. The second group was made up of patients with the complicated cataract on the background of existing anterior open-angle glaucoma, with initial and developed stages of the glaucomatous process. The third group involved patients with complicated cataract on the background of existing pseudoexfoliative glaucoma and pseudoexfoliative syndrome.

The analyses were performed using the main clinical laboratory methods accepted in ophthalmology.

Irrespective of the cataract degree and stage, all patients underwent microaxial Phacoemulsification – Microincision Cataract Surgery (MICS) through 2.2 *mm* incision with implantation of posterior chamber intraocular lens. Intra-chamber administration of antibiotics was not applied in these groups.

The methodical procedure of extracting aqueous humour was used intra-operatively under conditions of sterility. The corneocentis was done by insulin syringe through the limb; 0.1-0.2 *ml* aqueous humour was extracted. The fluid remained in a syringe until laboratory research was performed immediately after delivery of the material to the Scientific-Research Center of the Yerevan State Medical University after M. Heratsi.

All the operated patients were under intense observation and got the appropriate post-operative treatment and medical rehabilitation. We observed the patients in the early post-operative period.

Unfortunately, rather low amounts of isolated aqueous humour (0.1-0.2 *ml*) for immune enzyme assays and ion-selective analyses due to objective reasons, do not allow us simulta-neously (in one and the same sample) determine two parameters of studied biological active compounds. Inclusion of a relatively high number of operated patients (by 320 persons) in each study group is connected with the mentioned circumstance. Thereby, in all the three study groups by 40 samples of aqueous humour and blood serum were allocated for each test.

The content of fibronectin, IGF-1, PgE_2 and cortisol in aqueous humour was determined with the use of appropriate kits (DRG-International Inc., USA). The immune enzyme assay was performed on the automatic spectrophotometer "Stat-Fax 3200" (USA) in the absorbance wavelength range 420-450 *nm*.

Determination of potassium, sodium and calcium ions was done according to ion-selective method of analysis with use of Kone-microlyte analyzer (Finland).

The obtained results were exposed to statistical analysis using Student's criteria and applica-tion of SPSS-13 programme (one Sample T-Test and Paired Sample T-Test).

The results of immune enzyme assay for fibronectin, IGF-1, and PgE_2 in aqueous humour of patients with the senile and complicated cataracts are presented in Table 1.

Study groups of patients	Studied indices		
	Fibronectin (ng/ml)	IGF-1 (ng/ml)	PgE_2 (pg/ml)
I	11.26±0.99	1.10±0.18	43.05±4.13
II	20.71±2.37	2.50±0.46	66.11±7.40
	$p_1 < 0.0005$	$0.0005 < p_1 < 0.005$	$0.0005 < p_1 < 0.005$
III	33.83±5.97	2.60±0.39	76.64±7.78
	$p_1 < 0.0005$	$0.0005 < p_1 < 0.005$	$p_1 < 0.0005$
	$0.025 < p_2 < 0.05$	$p_2" / > 0.4$	$0.10 < p_2 < 0.25$

Notes: p_1 –indices of groups II and III compared to indices of the study group I; p_2 – indices of group II compared to indices of the study group III.

Table 1. Fibronectin, IGF-1, and PgE_2 content in aqueous humour of patients with the senile and complicated cataracts

As obvious from the Table, in patients with cataracts on the background of primary open-0an-gle glaucoma (study group II) the level of fibronectin in aqueous humour 1.8 times exceeded analogous level in aqueous humour of patients with senile cataracts. In those cases when cataract was observed on the background of pseudoexfoliative glaucoma (study group III) the highest indices of fibronectin were determined in the aqueous humour; these indices were 3.0 and 1.6 times higher compared to those in patients of groups I and II, appropriately.

A similar regularity was traced upon revealing shifts in PgE_2 and IGF-1 content in aqueous humour of patients in study groups I and II. Thus, the level of PgE_2 in aqueous humour of the study group II patients 1.5 times exceeded PgE_2 level in aqueous humour of the study group I patients. In study group III PgE_2 high levels were also determined (compared to the study group I), being similar to those revealed in aqueous humour of the study group II patients. As obvious from the Table, in the aqueous humour of patients in study groups II and III we recorded approximately the same IGF-1 indices, which exceeded similar values in aqueous humour of study group I patients 2.27 and 2.36 times, correspondingly.

Table 2 presents the results of immune enzyme assay for determination of cortisol in the aqueous humour of patients with senile and complicated cataracts.

Study groups of patients	Studied indices	
	Aqueous humour	Blood serum
I	12.90±0.64	56.90±4.15
II	23.38±1.46	64.84±7.28
	p<0.0005	0.1<p<0.25
III	30.4±1.56	50.70±6.91
	p<0.0005	0.1<p<0.25

Note: p – indices of complicated cataracts as related to indices of senile cataracts.

Table 2. Cortisol content in blood serum and aqueous humour of patients with the senile and complicated cataracts

As obvious from Table 2, in patients of study group II the level of cortisol in aqueous humour markedly increased (as compared to hormone levels determined in aqueous humour of patients with the senile cataract – control group). Thus, the level of cortisol in aqueous humour of patients with cataract on the background of primary open-angle glaucoma was 1.8 times higher compared to norm. The highest indices of cortisol were observed in aqueous humour of patients of the study group III. In particular, cortisol levels in aqueous humour of patients with the senile cataract on the background of primary open-angle glaucoma and pseudoexfoliative glaucoma increased 2.3 times. The results of immune enzyme assays performed on aqueous humour were compared with cortisol levels in blood serum of the same cohort of patients. As demonstrated by the research findings, the level of cortisol in blood serum of patients of all the 3 study groups was almost similar and within the range of cortisol determined in actually healthy subjects. This latter, though indirectly, signifies in favour of the local synthesis of cortisol in the eye membranes, the cells of which apart from their main functions ensure processes of *in situ* cortisol secretion as well.

The next stage of our investigation involved biochemical analysis with the use of ion-selective method aimed to determine ions of sodium, potassium and calcium in the aqueous humour of patients with senile and complicated cataracts.

Table 3 presents results of analyses performed on the aqueous humour of patients with senile and complicated cataracts.

Study groups of patients	K⁺	Na⁺	Ca⁺⁺
I	5.00±0.21	133.3±14.4	0.99±0.06
II	2.30±0.26	177.6±17.2	1.99±0.18
	p<0.0005	0.025<p<0.05	p<0.0005
III	1.92 ±0.28	196.7±18.2	2.40±0.26
	p<0.0005	0.005<p<0.01	p<0.0005

Note: p – indices of complicated cataracts as related to indices of senile cataracts

Table 3. K⁺, Na⁺ and Ca⁺⁺ content in aqueous humour of patients with senile and complicated cataracts

As obvious from Table 3, the levels of K^+, Na^+ and Ca^{++} in aqueous humour of patients with senile cataracts were similar to those in actually healthy cohort of subjects (we compared indices of ions in aqueous humour of patients with senile cataracts with the indices indicated in monograph of A. Pirie and R. van Heyningen (1968)). In aqueous humour of patients with cataract on the background of primary open-angle glaucoma low level of potassium ions was determined, it was 2.2 times lower than the level in aqueous humour of patients from the study group I. The lowest indices of potassium ions were recorded in the study group III, i.e., at cataracts on the background of pseudoexfoliative glaucoma. Thus, the level of potassium ions in aqueous humour of this study group decreased 2.15 times.

Unlike the shifts in potassium content in the aqueous humour of patients from study groups II and III, regarding the increase of sodium and calcium ions content a diametrically opposite picture was observed in the same groups. The content of sodium ions in the study group II increased 1.3 times, in the study group III – 1.5 times, compared to corresponding indices in aqueous humour of patients with senile cataracts.

Similar tendency was also observed on calcium ions content in aqueous humour of patients from study groups II and III. Thus, the level of calcium ions in aqueous humour of patients with cataracts on the background of primary open-angle glaucoma was 2.0 times above the control (group I), while in patients with cataracts on the background of pseudoexfoliative glaucoma it was 2.4 times higher.

We considered purposeful to present interpretation of our research findings of immune enzyme assay for determination of fibronectin, IGF-1, PgE_2, and cortisol in the aqueous humour of patients with cataracts associated with primary open-angle glaucoma and pseu-doexfoliative glaucoma taking into account data of scientific publications relevant to sources for the synthesis of mentioned substances in specific eye membranes and their possible biological effects realized at the level of inter-cellular relations in different cell populations of the eye.

In line with this, first of all, we considered the essential role that is related to the biological activity of TGF_2 produced in cornea and trabecular meshwork of an eye in mechanisms of inter-cellular relations *in situ* ensuring the drainage function of the eye.

It is considered to be generally accepted that in case of senile and complicated cataracts processes of $TGF_{\beta\text{-}2}$ synthesis are markedly intensified in the cornea and trabecular meshwork [*de Iongh R.U. et al., 2005; Stefan C. et al., 2008; Dawes L.J. et al., 2009; Pattabiraman P.P., Rao P.V., 2010*]. Therefore, we cannot exclude that relatively high levels of fibronectin and IGF-1 in the aqueous humour of patients with complicated cataracts are resulting from a direct stimulating influence of $TGF_{\beta\text{-}2}$ to cell populations localized in the cornea and trabecular meshwork of the eye selectively synthesizing fibronectin and IGF-1.

The proposed statement, to a known extent, is also confirmed by the available literature data relevant to the biological activity of $TGF_{\beta\text{-}2}$ – in the aspect of its selective modulatory impact to the processes of fibronectin and PgE_2 synthesis and secretion in the eye membranes.

As known, keratocytes of the cornea and trabecular meshwork cells of the eye serve as the main sources of fibronectin synthesis *in situ*, i.e. in the eye tissues. Dose-dependent stimulant effect of $TGF_{\beta\text{-}2}$ to processes of fibronectin synthesis was established [*Wordinger R. et al., 2007; Hindman H. et al., 2010; Karamichos D. et al., 2010*] under the conditions of mentioned cells cultivation. Moreover, according to [*Stefan C. et al., 2008*], $TGF_{\beta\text{-}2}$ produced in eye membranes should be considered as a "special" cytokine that under conditions of the eye barrier functions disturbance might increase fibronectin concentration in cells of trabecular meshwork of the eye anterior chamber's angle.

The IGF-1 elevated level revealed in aqueous humour of patients with the complicated cataracts should be considered as a factor hindering drainage function of trabecular meshwork and thus facilitating the increase of intraocular pressure. It is not excluded that similar mechanism functions in association with fibronectin-dependent mechanisms underlying the disturbed drainage function of the trabecular meshwork in the senile and, moreover, in the complicated cataracts.

Literature data [*Izumi K. et al., 2006; Yanai R. et al., 2006; Ko J. et al., 2009*] signify in favour to the proposed assumption: IGF-1 produced in corneal epitheliocytes and cells of the trabecular meshwork significantly activates fibroplastic processes *in situ*. To our mind, in processes of IGF-1 enhanced synthesis in the above mentioned structures of an eye the role should be assigned to $TGF_{\beta\text{-}2}$ produced in the same eye membranes, because the latter is known to markedly activate synthesis of IGF-1 and mediators, which take an active part in stimulation of fibroplastic processes [*Yamada N. et al., 2005; Izumi K. et al., 2006; Ko J. et al., 2009*], in corneal epitheliocytes and cells of trabecular meshwork.

In the light of our own and literature data, the role of $TGF_{\beta\text{-}2}$ in mechanisms of ACAID induction and withdrawal should be considered from qualitatively new positions. No doubt, the immunomodulatory effect of $TGF_{\beta\text{-}2}$ *in situ* that is conditioned by the targeted activation of the cytotoxic lymphocytes subpopulations (T-suppressors and T-killers) is determinant in processes of forming intercellular correlation among different lymphocytic subpopulations localized in eye membranes, hence ensuring reactions underlying ACAID. However, it is not excluded that the sphere of $TGF_{\beta-2}$ activity under conditions of norm is more versatile, as *in situ* produced mentioned cytokine directly and/or indirectly (activating the synthesis of fibronectin and IGF-1 in a mediated manner) participates in processes of maintaining the drainage function of trabecular meshwork, thus ensuring the constant level of intraocular pressure. Apparently, the above-mentioned mediatory effects of $TGF_{\beta-2}$ are strictly dose-dependent, as under conditions of pathology (in the given case: at senile and, especially, at the complicated cataracts) a significant elevation of $TGF_{\beta-2}$ in eye membranes brings to trabecular meshwork dysfunction; the latter is fraught with the increase of intraocular pressure.

The analysis of our own research results in the context of available publications allows to consider the important role of $TGF_{\beta-2}$ and IGF-1, which are produced in cornea and trabecular meshwork, in mechanisms ensuring the drainage function of an eye.

The facts of detection of receptors to PgE_2 in cells of trabecular meshwork and sclera allow possibility of PgE_2 participation in processes of intraocular pressure regulation.

The high level of PgE_2 found by us in aqueous humour allows possibility of its participation in processes of the impaired drainage function and increase of intraocular pressure at cataracts proceeding on the background of primary open-angle glaucoma pseudoexfoliative glaucoma.

The following phenomenon of no less importance should specially mentioned: high levels of fibronectin IGF-1 and PgE_2 in the aqueous humour of patients under study were pathogno-monic for the course of the primary open-angle glaucoma and not for cataracts, as in this latter case all the indices studied in aqueous humour were much lower than analogous indices at senile non-complicated cataract.

Our research revealed a direct correlation dependence between the high level of cortisol, on the one hand, and the content of sodium and calcium ions, on the other hand. Based on the results obtained a conclusion might be drawn that the increase of intraocular pressure in persons with complicated cataracts on the background of glaucoma is mostly conditioned by impairment of ion transfusion between the ciliary body and aqueous humour and the proc-esses of cortisol "hyperproduction" by hormone-producing cells in post-barrier membranes of the eye.

4. Conclusion

This chapter deals with one of the urgent problems of modern ophthalmology: revealing the mechanisms underlying induction of primary open-angle and pseudoexfoliative glaucoma. Till nowadays the problem remains rather actual, as the issue is open to discussion: what are the regional mechanisms underlying the disorders in functions of the trabecular apparatus of the angle of anterior chamber of an eye and in the increase of intraocular pressure at the mentioned disease case.

One of severe complications of glaucoma is the steady persistent increase of intraocular pressure that is fraught with compression of the head of optic nerve that results in its partial or complete atrophy with the partial and/or complete sight loss. Currently, the majority of specialists engaged in clinical and experimental ophthalmology are inclined to the opinion that the increase of intraocular pressure is not the consequence of general hemodynamic disorders resulting from the permeability increase in hematoophthalmic barrier, but rather originates from pathological processes occurring in the membranes and chambers of an eye.

In line with the modern views, processes underlying the increased intraocular pressure originate in the eye structures as such: in connective-tissue, epithelial and endothelial cells of the ciliary body, cornea, retina, lens, trabecular apparatus of the angle of the anterior chamber of an eye. These cells possess selective secretory activity in the aspect of producing a number of biologically active substances exerting direct and/or indirect action to the processes regulating intraocular pressure.

Moreover, numerous pathological processes proceeding in case of primary open-angle glaucoma at the site of eye membranes are fraught with the infringement of chamber humour osmolarity; furthermore, one of mechanisms increasing the volume of aqueous humour and not infrequently hindering its outflow is the impaired K^+/Na^+ balance in favour of the accumulation of this latter in the anterior chamber of an eye.

Available literary data of the last 30 years which discuss mediatory functions realized by cells of fibroblastic, epithelial and endothelial line in a ciliary body, cornea, retina, lens, a trabecular network formed a basis for carrying out the research directed at clarification of a role of *in situ* produced fibronectin, IgF-1 and a cortisol at primary open-angle glaucoma.

The drainage function of trabecular meshwork of an angle of the anterior chamber of an eye is an active process, in which the leading role belongs to secretory cells of this network. As it was specified above, secretory cells of the trabecular meshwork develop TGF_{β}-$_2$, fibronectin and an insulin-like growth factor -1, PgE_2. It is not excluded that the mentioned substances play an important role in ensuring drainage function of a trabecular meshwork, and thus, to a certain extent, in maintenance of an optimum level of the intraocular pressure.

For this reason, high indices of fibronectin and IGF-1 found in aqueous humour of patients with primary open-angle glaucoma testify in favor of hypersecretion of mentioned cytokines by cells of a trabecular meshwork. The presence of fibronectin and insulin-like growth factor-1 high concentrations at the primary open-angle glaucoma, and also at pseudoexfoliative glaucoma, testifies to violation of drainage function of a trabecular meshwork of an angle of the anterior chamber of an eye; this latter, to a certain extent, preconditions the high level of intraocular pressure. At the same time, the specific weight of fibronectin and insulin-like of growth factor -1 in hypertension formation in the aqueous humour is far from being equivalent, as on the one hand, fibronectin level in aqueous humour of patients from investigated groups II and III 10 times exceeds concentration of insulin-like growth factor-1 in the same liquid, on the other hand, as known, the weight of soluble fibronectin makes 440.000-150.000 D, while the mass of insulin-like growth factor-1 is 7.649 D [*Panteleev M. A. et al., 2011*].

Thus, on the basis of the analysis of literary data and carried-out own research it is possible to conclude that at glaucomas the infringement of drainage function and increase of intraocular pressure is in many respects caused by high concentration of fibronectin and, partially, insulin-like growth factor-1 in the intraocular liquid.

As it was noted above, the content of PgE_2 considerably increases in aqueous humour of patients with primary open-angle glaucomas and pseudoexfoliative glaucomas.

There is scanty literature about the synthesis of prostaglandins in eye membranes. Local synthesis of prostaglandins is found out only in cells of crystalline lens that was proved by research of O. Nishi et al. (1992) in model experiments *in vitro*: at cataract the extracted lens in the course of operation was located on incubation medium. With the increase of incubation terms the content of prostaglandins E_2 in the incubation environment considerably increased. At the same time, in a number of eye membranes, the ciliary body, sclera and the trabecular meshwork of an angle of the anterior chamber of an eye receptors to prostaglandins E_2 were found [*Toris C.B. et al., 2008*].

It is not excluded that the high content of PgE_2 in aqueous humour is fraught with an increase of intraocular pressure at glaucomatous patients, as according to [*Podos S.M. et al., 1972 a; b; Podos S.M., 1976 a; b; c*], PgE_2 takes an active part in maintenance of drainage function of an eye.

It is known that ionic balance in liquid media of an organism (blood, spinal, gingival, synovial and intraocular liquids) is a necessary condition for maintenance of the osmotic pressure.

The anterior and posterior chambers of an eye are main depots; water makes about 93% and a very insignificant share make proteins. It is considered established that the delay of outflow of aqueous humour or its intensive more "production" promotes considerable elevation of pressure inside an eye.

Thus, one of the factors leading to increase of intraocular pressure at glaucomas is the increase of osmolarity of intraocular liquid.

It is considered to be established long ago that at anterior open-angle glaucoma in aqueous humour there are serious impairments in its ionic structure that was shown by disorders in functioning of sodium – potassium pomp, with the superfluous accumulation of sodium ions.

In our research as demonstrated by the results of ion-selective analysis, at primary open-angle glaucomas and pseudoexfoliative glaucomas rather high indices of ions of sodium and calcium and low indices of potassium were determined in aqueous humour, as compared with the indices defined in aqueous humour of patients with senile not complicated cataracts.

The similar imbalance, being shown as superfluous accumulation of sodium and calcium in aqueous humour, complicates normal outflow of aqueous humour from the anterior chamber of an eye that, in its turn, is fraught with the increase of intraocular pressure.

Without considering the questions connected with mechanisms of shifts found by us regarding electrolytes content in aqueous humour (that was not an actual problem of the present research), nevertheless we consider expedient to discuss some aspects connected with the fact established by us on impaired ionic balance between eye membranes and the intraocular liquid.

Firstly, the increase of Na^+ and Ca^{++} levels observed by us in aqueous humour should be considered from positions of the broken ionic balance between specific membranes of an eye and intraocular liquid, and not as a result of the general disorder of electrolytes composition in blood of experimental animals, because the level of studied electrolytes in blood serum was within the limits of control values.

Secondly, the high level of a cortisol found by us in aqueous humour can serve one of possible causes of infringement of the ionic balance. This assumption appears very reasonable, as it is known that high concentrations of cortisol in separate membranes of an eye lead to ionic imbalance in connection with enhanced inflow of ions of sodium in aqueous humour that results in an increase of intraocular pressure.

Thirdly, it is not excluded that realization of hormonal and cytokine-dependent processes conditioned by regional shifts in the content of cortisol, prolactin, fibronectin, insulin-like growth factor-1 at cataracts proceeding on the background of primary open-angle glaucoma and pseudoexfoliative glaucoma, is caused by activation of calcium-dependent reactions in secretory cells of eye membranes.

It is considered established that the pseudoexfoliative syndrome represents itself as a provoking factor for development of the open-angle glaucoma, the course of which has a progressing character and is characterized by high resistance to carried-out medicamentous therapy and an unfavourable forecast [*Prince A.J, Ritch R., 1986; Streeten B.W. et al., 1990; Tarkkanen A. et al., 2002; Takhchidi K.P. et al., 2010*].

One of severe complications at development of a pseudoexfoliative syndrome is cataract as well [*Küchle M. et al., 1997; Puska P., Tarkkanen A., 2001*].

The impairment of immunological tolerance (of immunological privileges of an eye – ACAID) acts as an initiating factor for development of pseudoexfoliative syndrome [*Takhchidi K.P. et. al., 2010*].

It is not excluded that in pathogenesis of pseudoexfoliative syndrome emergence are also involved the local hormonal-mediatory mechanisms connected not with the operational intervention, but rather with infringement of processes of synthesis and secretion of such cytokines as $TgF_{\beta-2}$, IGF-1 and, first of all, fibronectin in cornea, ciliary body and trabecular meshwork of synthesis.

At a pseudoexfoliative syndrome essential physical and chemical changes occur in aqueous humour: the concentration of proteins considerably raises, including fibronectin as well [*Takhchidi K.P. et al., 2010*]. At the same time, shifts found by us in aqueous humour of patients with cataract on the background of pseudoexfoliative glaucoma, in many respects depend on the character of disease course: not so much of cataract, as glaucoma and the pseudoexfoliative syndrome. It is not excluded that in this studied group the high level of fibronectin in aqueous humour in many respects depends on features of pseudoexfoliative syndrome development.

On the basis of the analysis of literary data, it is possible to come to conclusion, according to which $TGF_{\beta-2}$ developed in eye membranes plays far not the last role in pathogenesis of primary open-angle glaucoma, including pseudoexfoliative glaucoma as well. So, at glaucomas of $TGF_{\beta-2}$ stimulates synthesis of such cytokines as insulin-like growth factor-1 and fibronectin in cornea, ciliary body and a trabecular meshwork of an angle of the anterior chamber of an eye. Their high levels found by us in aqueous humour testify to possible violation of drainage function of the trabecular meshwork that is fraught with an increase of intraocular pressure.

In conclusion, in the form of generalized schemes 1 and 2 the possible pathogenetic links engaged in the induction and a course of primary open-angle glaucoma, including pseudoexfoliative glaucoma as well, are presented to attention of ophthalmologists. The specific subject matter is regional disorder that is fraught with impairment of secretory activity of the polypotent cells localized in various eye membranes, which besides the main functions produce a number of biologically active substances of the cytokine, hormonal and mediatory nature.

At anterior open-angle glaucoma (see schemes 1 and 2) the synthesis of fibronectin in cells of the trabecular meshwork is considerably activated which is caused by the stimulating influence of fibroblasts transforming growth factor ($TGF_{\beta-2}$). Realization of this effect, to a certain extent, is caused by blocking of inhibitory effect of a bone morfogenic protein (BMP-4) towards the activity of $TGF_{\beta-2}$ due to which the stimulating effect of the latter on processes of fibronectin intra-cellular synthesis is realized. It is not excluded that at the same time there occurs blocking of inhibitory effect of $TGF_{\beta-1}$ on domain of heparin (Hep-2) responsible for synthesis of fibronectin in a cell.

Further, as a result of fibronectin "hyper production", there is a deposition of fibronectin in extracellular matrix (EM) owing to which, as a result of drainage function impairment in trabecular meshwork, there proceeds an increase of intraocular pressure.

It is not excluded that in the conditions of physiological activity of trabecular meshwork cells the processes of intra-cellular synthesis of fibronectin are regulated according to cytokine mechanisms in realization of which, on the one hand, $TGF_{\beta-2}$ serves as a stimulating factor, on the other hand, this stimulating effect is adjusted due to gremin (G) and BMP-4 produced in trabecular meshwork cells. It is precisely the coordinated activity of aforementioned cytokines, $TGF_{\beta-2}$, G and BMP-4, that strictly supervises the balanced synthesis of fibronectin cells by trabecular network cells in the conditions of norm.

The specified Scheme 1 was constructed by us upon the analysis of the modern data concerning a role fibronectin, which is produced in keratocytes and cells of a trabecular meshwork, in violation of the drainage function of an eye at glaucomas and complicated cataracts [*Gonzales J.M. et al., 1998; Fleenor D. et al., 2006; Wordinger R.J. et al., 2007; Stefan C. et al., 2008; Zilfyan A., 2009; 2012; Hindman H.B. et al., 2010*].

In addition, due to analysis of the modern scientific data in the aspect of our own research findings we propose a summary scheme (Scheme 2) that presents the role of *in situ* produced biologically active compounds, which under conditions of disorders in synchronous activity of secretory cells localized in various membranes of the eye might bring to impairment of the drainage function and development of a symptom complex that is characteristic for primary open-angle and pseudoexfoliative glaucoma.

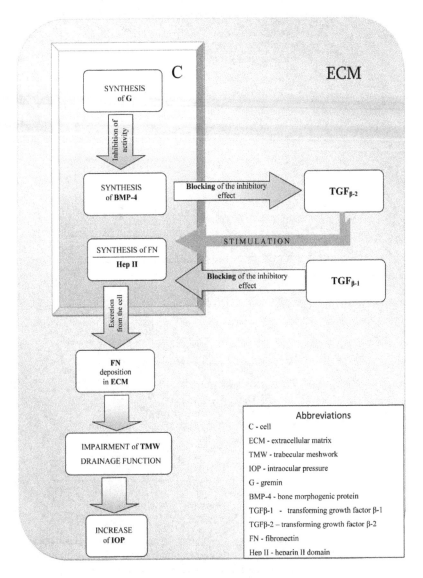

Scheme 1. The role of trabecular meshwork cells of the anterior chamber angle of an eye in mechanisms of fibronectin-dependent drainage function impairment and the increase of intraocular pressure at anterior open-angle glaucoma

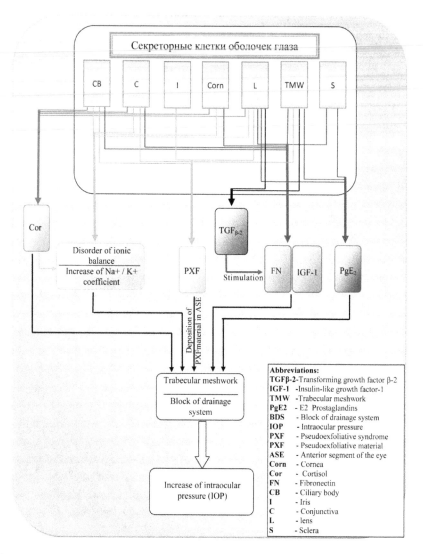

Scheme 2. The role of mediators and hormones in mechanisms of intraocular pressure increase at complicated cataracts: cataracts on the background of primary open-angle glaucoma and pseudoexfoliative glaucoma

As obvious from Scheme 2, regional factors engaged in mechanisms of drainage function impairment and intraocular pressure increase might be conditionally divided into 2 categories. Secretory processes associated with dysfunction of cornea and trabecular meshwork cells (in the aspect of their targeted synthesis of $TGF_{\beta\text{-}2}$ should be related to category 1. Category 2 should embrace hormonal disorders, impairment of the regional ionic homeostasis and destructive processes, mechanisms of which are not sufficiently studied until present. In the given scheme we consider only 1 point of application that is affected by the influence of all the above mentioned factors: as a "target" here serves the trabecular meshwork of the anterior chamber of an eye with impaired drainage function that eventually rings to an increase of intraocular pressure. As evident from Scheme 2, in case of anterior open-angle glaucoma the regional $TGF_{\beta-2}$ dependent mechanisms are engaged, being conditioned by its stimulating influence to secretory cells of some eye membranes: in the aspect of their "excessive" synthesis of fibronectin and $IGF_{\beta-2}$, which cumulate both in stroma of the trabecular meshwork and in the aqueous humour finally resulting in block of drainage system and an increase of intraocular pressure. The hyperproduction of PgE_2 in secretory cells of trabecular meshwork, sclera and, probably, the lens, also brings forth impairment of the drainage function. In impairment of drainage network functions a definite role is also devoted to *in situ* produced cortisol and processes resulting in disorders of ionic balance between the membranes and liquid media of an eye (first of all: between the cells of the ciliary body, cornea, trabecular meshwork and the aqueous humour). In the mechanism of impaired ionic balance that at the primary open-angle glaucoma is characterized by excessive accumulation of sodium ions in aqueous humour a certain part belongs also to cortisol produced in eye membranes. In cases of pseudoexfoliative glaucoma deposition of pseudoexfoliative matter in the anterior segment of an eye might cause blocking of the drainage system.

Author details

A.A. Zilfyan[1,2*]

Address all correspondence to: namj@ysmu.am, zilf.art@mail.ru

1 Scientific-Research Center, Yerevan State Medical University, Yerevan, Armenia

2 "Shengavit" Medical Center, Yerevan, Armenia

References

[1] Abrahamian, A, Xi, M, Donnelly, J, & Rockey, J. Effect of interferon-gamma on the expression of transforming growth factor-beta by human corneal fibroblasts: role in corneal immunoseclusion. J. Interferon Cytokine Res. (1995). , 15(4), 323-330.

[2] Banh, A, Deschamps, P. A, Gauldie, J, Overbeek, P. A, Sivak, J. G, & West-mays, J. A. Lens-specific expression of TGF-beta induces anterior subcapsular cataract formation in the absence of Smad3. Invest. Ophthalmol. Vis. Sci. (2006). Aug; , 47(8), 3450-3460.

[3]   Bucci, F. A. Jr., Waterbury L.D. Comparison of ketorolac 0.4% and bromfenac 0.09% at trough dosing: aqueous drug absorption and prostaglandin E2 levels. J. Cataract Refract. Surg. (2008). Sep; , 34(9), 1509-1512.

[4]   Burch, J, Mair, D, Meny, G, Moroff, G, Ching, S, Naidoff, M, Steuer, E, Loftus, S, Armstrong, J, Clemons, T, & Klein, B. The risk of posterior subcapsular cataracts in granulocyte donors. Transfusion. (2005). , 45(11), 1701-1708.

[5]   Chiquet, C, & Denis, P. The neuroanatomical and physiological bases of variations in intraocular pressure. J. Fr. Ophthalmol. (2004). , 27(2), 2511-2518.

[6]   Chong, A, & Aw, S. Postmortem endocrine levels in the vitreous humor. Ann. Acad. Med. Singapore. (1986). , 15(4), 606-609.

[7]   Chung, S. H, Jung, S. A, Cho, Y. J, Lee, J. H, & Kim, E. K. IGF-1 counteracts TGF-beta-mediated enhancement of fibronectin for in vitro human lens epithelial cells. Yonsei. Med. J. (2007). Dec 31; , 48(6), 949-954.

[8]   Cinatl, J, Blaheta, R, Bittoova, M, Scholz, M, Margraf, S, Vogel, J, Cinatl, J, & Deorr, H. Decreased neutrophil adhesion to human cytomegalovirus-infected retinal pigment epithelial cells is mediated by virus-induced up-regulation of Fas ligand independent of neutrophil apoptosis. J. Immunol. (2000). , 165(8), 4405-4413.

[9]   Dawes, L. J, Sleeman, M. A, Anderson, I. K, Reddan, J. R, & Wormstone, I. M. TGFbeta/Smad4-dependent and-independent regulation of human lens epithelial cells. Invest. Ophthalmol. Vis. Sci. (2009). Nov; Epub 2009 Jun 10., 50(11), 5318-27.

[10] De Iongh, R. U, Wederell, E, Lovicu, F. J, & Mcavoy, J. W. Transforming Growth Factor-β-Induced Epithelial-Mesenchymal Transition in the Lens: A Model for Cataract Formation. Cells Tissues Organs. (2005).

[11] Fleenor, D, Shepard, A, Hellberg, P, Jacobson, N, Pang, I, & Clark, A. TGFbeta2- induced changes in human trabecular meshwork: implications for intraocular pressure. Invest. Ophthalmol. Vis. Sci. (2006). , 47(1), 226-234.

[12] Floman, N, & Zor, U. Mechanism of steroid action in ocular inflammation: Inhibition of prostaglandin production. Invest. Ophthalmol. Vis. Sci. (1977). , 16(1), 69-73.

[13] Frolova, P. P, & Khamitova, G. Kh. [On the frequency of pseudoexfoliative syndrome at dispensary medical examination of population][published in Russian]. Vestn. Ophthalm. (1984). (4), 8-9.

[14] Gonzales, J. M. Jr, Hu Y., Gabelt B.T., Kaufman P.L., Peters D.M. Identification of the active site in the heparin II domain of fibronectin that increases outflow facility in cultured monkey anterior segments. Eye (Lond) (1998). Pt 5): 886-890.

[15] Hindman, H. B, Swanton, J. N, Phipps, R. P, Sime, P. J, & Huxlin, K. R. Differences in the TGF-{beta}1-induced profibrotic response of anterior and posterior corneal kera-

tocytes in vitro. Invest. Ophthalmol. Vis. Sci. (2010). Apr; Epub 2009 Nov 11., 51(4), 1935-1942.

[16] Hollborn, M, Enzman, V, Barth, W, Wiedemann, P, & Kohen, L. Changes in the mRNA expression of cytokines and chemokines by stimulated RPE cells in vitro. Curr. Eye Res. (2000). , 20(6), 488-495.

[17] Izumi, K, Kurosaka, D, Iwata, T, Oguchi, Y, Tanaka, Y, Mashima, Y, & Tsubota, K. Involvement of insulin-like growth factor-I and insulin-like growth factor binding protein-3 in corneal fibroblasts during corneal wound healing. Invest. Ophthalmol. Vis. Sci. (2006). Feb; , 47(2), 591-598.

[18] Jacob, E. FitzSimon J., Brubaker R. Combined corticosteroid and catecholamine stimulation of aqueous humor flow. Ophthalmology. (1996). , 103(8), 1303-1308.

[19] Karamichos, D, Guo, X. Q, Hutcheon, A. E, & Zieske, J. D. Human corneal fibrosis: an in vitro model. Invest. Ophthalmol. Vis. Sci. (2010). Mar; Epub 2009 Oct 29., 51(3), 1382-1388.

[20] Kasavina, B, Ukhina, T, & Churakova, T. Distribution of labeled cortisol in the tissues and media of the eye. Bull. Exp. Biol. Med. (1977). , 83(4), 401-402.

[21] Kim, K. S, Lee, B. H, & Kim, I. S. The measurement of fibronectin concentrations in human aqueous humor. Korean J. Ophthalmol. (1992). Jun; , 6(1), 1-5.

[22] Kim, Y. S, Kim, N. H, Jung, D. H, Jang, D. S, Lee, Y. M, Kim, J. M, & Kim, J. S. Genistein inhibits aldose reductase activity and high glucose-induced TGF-beta2 expression in human lens epithelial cells. Eur. J. Pharmacol. (2008). Oct 10; 594(1-3): 18-25. Epub 2008 Jul 25.

[23] Ko, J. A, Yanai, R, & Nishida, T. IGF-1 released by corneal epithelial cells induces up-regulation of N-cadherin in corneal fibroblasts. J. Cell. Physiol. (2009). Oct; , 221(1), 254-261.

[24] Kroll, D. S. Pseudoexfoliative syndrome and exfoliative glaucoma][published in Russian]. Author's Thesis of Doctoral Dissertation (Med. Sci.). (1970). p.

[25] Kroll DS [Pseudoexfoliative syndrome and its role in pathogenesis of glaucoma] [published in Russian]. Vestnik Ophthalm. (1968). , 1, 9-15.

[26] Küchle, M, Amberg, A, Martus, P, et al. Pseudoexfoliation syndrome and secondary cataract. Br. J. Ophthalmol. (1997). , 81, 862-866.

[27] Kuznik, B, Vasiliev, N, & Zybikov, N. Immunogenesis, homeostasis and non-specific resistance of the organism][published in Russian]. Moscow. "Medicine". (1989). p.

[28] Mansfield, K. J, Cerra, A, & Chamberlain, C. G. FGF-2 counteracts loss of TGF beta affected cells from rat lens explants: implications for PCO (after cataract). Mol. Vis. (2004). Jul 22; , 10, 521-532.

[29] Nesterov, A. P. Glaucoma][published in Russian]. Moscow. "Medical Information Agency" LLC. (2008). p.

[30] Nishi, O, Nishi, K, & Imanishi, M. Synthesis of interleukin-1 and prostaglandin E2 by lens epithelial cells of human cataracts. Br. J. Ophthalmol. (1992). Jun; , 76(6), 338-341.

[31] Ochiai, Y, & Ochiai, H. Higher concentration of transforming growth factor-beta in aqueous humor of glaucomatous eyes and diabetic eyes. Jpn J. Ophthalmol. (2002). May-Jun; , 46(3), 249-253.

[32] Orge, Y, & Gungor, S. Immunological etiopathogenesis of senile and complicated cataract. Microbiol. Bull. (1984). , 18(3), 145-153.

[33] Panteleev, M. A, Vasiliev, S. A, Sinauridze, E. I, Vorobiev, A. I, & Atallakhanov, F. I. Practical coagulology] [published in Russian]. Moscow. "Practical Medicine". (2011). p.

[34] Pattabiraman, P. P, & Rao, P. V. Mechanistic basis of Rho GTPase-induced extracellular matrix synthesis in trabecular meshwork cells. Am. J. Physiol. Cell Physiol. (2010). Mar; 298(3): CEpub 2009 Nov 25., 749-63.

[35] Pirie, A, & Van Heyningen, R. Biochemistry of the eye. Blackwell Scientific Publications. Oxford. Russian edition: Moscow. Meditsina (Medicine Publishers). (1968). p.

[36] Pleyer, U, Yang, J, Knapp, S, Schacke, H, Schmees, N, Orlic, N, Otasevic, L, De Ruijter, M, Ritter, T, & Keipert, S. Effects of a selective glucocorticoid receptor agonist on experimental keratoplasty. Graefes Arch. Clin. Exp. Ophthalmol. (2005). , 243(5), 450-455.

[37] Podos, S. M. Animal models of human glaucoma. Trans. Sect. Ophthalmol. Am. Acad. Ophthalmol. Otolaryngol. (1976). a Jul-Aug; 81(4 Pt 1): OP, 632-635.

[38] Podos, S. M. Prostaglandins, nonsteroidal anti-inflammatory agents and eye disease. Trans. Am. Ophthalmol. Soc. (1976 b). , 74, 637-660.

[39] Podos, S. M. The effect of cation ionophores on intraocular pressure. Invest. Ophthalmol. (1976). c Oct; , 15(10), 851-854.

[40] Podos, S. M, Becker, B, Beaty, C, & Cooper, D. G. Diphenylhydantoin and cortisol metabolism in glaucoma. Am. J. Ophthalmol. (1972 a). Sep; , 74(3), 498-500.

[41] Podos, S. M, Jaffe, B. M, & Becker, B. Prostaglandins and glaucoma. Br. Med. J. (1972). b Oct 28; 4(5834): 232.

[42] Prince, A. J, & Ritch, R. Clinical signs of the pseudoexfoliation syndrome. Ophthalmology. (1986). , 93, 803-807.

[43] Puska, P, & Tarkkanen, A. Exfoliation syndrome as a risk factor for cataract development: five year follow-up of lens opacities in exfoliation syndrome. J. Cataract Refract. Surg. (2001). Dec.; , 27(12), 1992-1998.

[44] Rauz, S, Cheung, C, Wood, P, Coca-prados, M, Walker, E, Murray, P, & Stewart, P. Inhibition of 11β-hydroxysteroid dehydrogenase type 1 lowers intraocular pressure in patients with ocular hypertension. QJM. (2003). , 96(7), 481-490.

[45] Rauz, S, Walker, E, Shackleton, C, Hewison, M, Murray, P, & Stewart, P. Expression and putative role of 11 beta-hydroxysteroid dehydrogenase isozymes within the human eye. Invest. Ophthalmol. Vis. Sci. (2001). , 42(9), 2037-2042.

[46] Schwartz, B, Wysocki, A, & Qi, Y. Decreased response of plasma cortisol to intravenous metyrapone in ocular hypertension and primary open-angle glaucoma. J. Glaucoma. (2005). , 14(6), 474-481.

[47] Shaw, L. C, Pan, H, Afzal, A, Calzi, S. L, Spoerri, P. E, Sullivan, S. M, & Grant, M. B. Proliferating endothelial cell-specific expression of IGF-I receptor ribozyme inhibits retinal neovascularization. Gene Ther. (2006). May; , 13(9), 752-760.

[48] Southren, A, Altman, K, Vittek, J, Boniuk, V, & Gordon, G. Steroid metabolism in ocular tissues of the rabbit. Invest. Ophthalmol. (1976). , 15(3), 222-228.

[49] Southren, A, Gordon, G, Yeh, H, Dunn, M, & Weinstein, B. Nuclear translocation of the cytoplasmic glucocorticoid receptor in the iris-ciliary body of the rabbit. Invest. Ophthalmol. Vis. Sci. (1979). , 18(5), 517-521.

[50] Stefan, C, Dragomir, L, Dumitrica, D. M, Ursaciuc, C, Dobre, M, & Surcel, M. TGF-beta2 involvements in open angle glaucoma][published in Romanian]. Oftalmologia. (2008). , 52(3), 110-112.

[51] Steiger, A. Sleep and endocrinology. J. Intern. Med. (2003). l): , 13-22.

[52] Stojek, A, Kasprzak, B, & Slabikowski, A. Intraocular pressure and prolactin measures in seasonal affective disorder. Psychiatr. Pol. (1991).

[53] Stone, R, & Wilson, C. Steroid effects on uveal transport. Ophthalmic Res. (1984). , 16(6), 297-301.

[54] Streeten, B. W, Dark, A. J, Wallace, R. N, Li, Z. Y, & Hoepner, J. A. Pseudoexfoliative Fibrillopathy in the Skin of Patients with Ocular Pseudoexfoliation. Am. J. Ophthalmol. (1990). , 5, 490-499.

[55] Streilein, J, Wilbanks, G, Taylor, A, & Cousins, S. Eye-derived cytokines and the immunosuppressive intraocular microenvironment: a review. Curr. Eye Res. (1992). Suppl.): , 41-47.

[56] Takhchidi, K. P, Barinov, Z, Agafonova, F, Frankovska-gerlak, V. V, Sulaeva, M, & In, O. N. Pathology of an eye at pseudoexfoliative syndrome"][published in Russian]. Moscow. "Ophthalmologia" Publishers. (2010). p.

[57] Tarkkanen, A, Kivela, T, & John, G. Lindberg and the discovery of exfoliation syndrome. Acta Ophthalmol. Scan. (2002). , 80(12), 151-154.

[58] Toris, C. B, Gabelt, B. T, & Kaufman, P. L. Update on the mechanism of action of topical prostaglandins for intraocular pressure reduction. Surv. Ophthalmol. (2008). Nov; 53 (Suppl. 1): S, 107-120.

[59] Tripathi, B. J, Tripathi, R. C, Chen, J, Gotsis, S, & Li, J. Trabecular cell expression of fibronectin and MMP-3 is modulated by aqueous humor growth factors. Exp. Eye Res. (2004). Mar; , 78(3), 653-660.

[60] Vesaluoma, M, Mertaniemi, P, Mannonen, S, Lehto, I, Uusitalo, R, Sarna, S, Tarkkanen, A, & Tervo, T. Cellular and plasma fibronectin in the aqueous humour of primary open-angle glaucoma, exfoliative glaucoma and cataract patients. Eye (Lond). (1998). Pt 5): 886-890.

[61] Vessey, K, Lencses, K, Rushforth, D, Hruby, V, & Stell, W. Glucagon receptor agonists and antagonists affect the growth of the chick eye: a role for glucagonergic regulation of emmetropization? Invest. Ophthalmol. Vis. Sci. (2005). , 46(11), 3922-3931.

[62] Weinstein, B, Gordon, G, & Southren, A. Potentiation of glucocorticoid activity by 5 beta-dihydrocortisol: its role in glaucoma. Science. (1983). , 222(4620), 172-173.

[63] Wilbanks, G, Mammoli, M, & Streilen, J. Studies on the induction of anterior chamber-associated immune deviation (ACAID). III. Induction of ACAID depends upon intraocular transforming growth factor-beta. Eur. J. Immunol. (1992). , 22(1), 165-173.

[64] Wordinger, R. J, Fleenor, D. L, Hellberg, P. E, Pang, I. H, Tovar, T. O, Zode, G. S, Fuller, J. A, & Clark, A. F. Effects of TGF-beta2, BMP-4, and gremlin in the trabecular meshwork: implications for glaucoma. Invest. Ophthalmol. Vis. Sci. (2007). Mar; , 48(3), 1191-1200.

[65] Yamada, N, Yanai, R, Inui, M, & Nishida, T. Sensitizing effect of substance P on corneal epithelial migration induced by IGF-1, fibronectin, or interleukin-6. Invest. Ophthalmol. Vis. Sci. (2005). Mar; , 46(3), 833-839.

[66] Yanai, R, Yamada, N, Inui, M, & Nishida, T. Correlation of proliferative and anti-apoptotic effects of HGF, insulin, IGF-1, IGF-2, and EGF in SV40-transformed human corneal epithelial cells. Exp. Eye Res. (2006). Jul; Epub 2006 Mar 10., 83(1), 76-83.

[67] Zilfyan, A. A. Shifts in content of fibronectin, insulin-like growth factor-1 and E_2 prostaglandins in aqueous humour in case of senile and complicated cataracts. The New Armenian Medical Journal. (2012). , 6(3), 34-41.

[68] Zilfyan, A. A. The role of cortisol, prolactin, CD_4 and CD_8 in induction of anterior chamber associated immune deviation (ACAID) in case of cataracts. The New Armenian Medical Journal. (2009). , 3(1), 59-67.

Chapter 5

Emerging Concept of Genetic and Epigenetic Contribution to the Manifestation of Glaucoma

Barkur S. Shastry

Additional information is available at the end of the chapter

1. Introduction

In recent years many mutations in genes that are responsible for several Mendelian eye diseases have been identified and characterized. Genome-wide association studies also advanced our knowledge of complex diseases [1-4]. However, for many diseases, variation in phenotype with a single genotype, disease susceptibility among individuals, discordance in monozygotic twins, progressive nature of the disorder and age-related onset cannot be explained by accumulating mutations alone [5-6]. Therefore, there must be another layer of information. This missing link could be epigenetic factors. The term epigenetics refers to the mitotically heritable changes in the pattern of gene expression without any changes in the DNA sequence and the term epigenomics denotes the study of epigenetics on a genome wide basis. Epigenetics is an emerging field in ophthalmology and is involved in the regulation of gene expression during normal eye development. It has also a role in the etiology and progression of several common human diseases [7]. Epigenetic regulation through environmental factors such as diet, smoking and pollution may result in changes in gene expression that may lead to an increase in disease susceptibility, variation in phenotype and progressive nature of many common diseases such as age-related macular degeneration and glaucoma. These epigenetic changes may be age-related and cell or tissue specific. They may also persist throughout the lifetime of an individual. An understanding of the role of epigenetics is important to the success of the stem cell-based therapies [8]. Although epigenetic studies on glaucoma are limited at present [9], in this short article, an attempt has been made to summarize this emerging concept of genetic and epigenetic contribution to the manifestation of glaucoma.

2. Genetic contribution to glaucoma: Classification and pathophysiology

Glaucoma is a group of complex, genetically and clinically heterogeneous condition and affects all age groups throughout the world [10]. Approximately 70 million people worldwide are affected and it is one of the leading causes of bilateral blindness in humans [11]. The glaucomas are classified into primary and secondary glaucomas and within these two groups the disorder is divided into primary open-angle (POAG; the trabecular mesh work seems to be open and unobstructed by the iris), primary closed angle (PCAG; partial or complete anterior chamber angle closure) and primary congenital glaucoma (PCG; which mainly affects children). The disorder is characterized by the progressive degeneration of the retinal ganglion cells (RGCs) and is frequently associated with elevated intraocular pressure (IOP) [12]. A host of genetic and environmental factors contribute to the glaucoma phenotypes. For instance in certain population, older age, history of thyroid diseases, higher IOP and high myopia have been reported to be significant risk factors for POAG [13-16]. Similarly, drinking coffee, antioxidant intake and post menopausal hormone use may influence the development of POAG. These environmental risk factors exert their effects on IOP (by decreasing or increasing) and/or the rate of retinal ganglion cell apoptosis. In advanced glaucoma, the cone photoreceptors were also affected suggesting that photoreceptors may also be sequentially damaged in the disorder [17].

Epidemiological studies suggest that POAG is the most common type of glaucoma in most populations and is consistently associated with elevated IOP [18-19]. However, patients with POAG can also have IOP within the normal range and they are classified as having normal tension glaucoma (NTG) – most likely an independent entity [20]. In NTG, the optic nerve head is just susceptible to normal IOP. This may be due to the difference in the ultra structure of the optic nerve head or due to micro-level of biochemical agents. It is only a limited subset of patients with elevated IOP will develop POAG. This is consistent with the finding that, a significant number of glaucoma patients although respond well to therapies to lower the eye pressure, continue to lose vision [21-22]. Many individuals have IOP elevation without optic nerve damage (they are considered as having ocular hypertension) and some individuals develop optic nerve degeneration without elevated IOP [10]. Therefore, it has been proposed that elevation in IOP is neither necessary nor sufficient for the onset of the progression of the disorder or optic nerve damage [10, 23-24]. Recent research suggests that transforming growth factor - beta (TGF - beta) and tumor necrosis factor - alpha (TNF - alpha) signaling pathways may contribute to the optic nerve disease in glaucoma [10].

3. Primary open-angle glaucoma (POAG)

The genetic basis of glaucoma is not fully understood. However, familial aggregation, occurrence of bilateral PCG in monozygotic twins and environmental factors such as advanced age, race, vascular risk factors, diabetes and hypertension suggest a multifactorial contribution to the etiology of the disease [12, 25-26]. Although details about the inheritance of the disease remain unclear, candidate gene, genome-wide association and traditional linkage studies have identified at least 14 chromosomal loci that are influencing POAG [27-29]. However, glaucoma-causing genes have been identified in only three of these loci including myocilin (MYOC; also called GLC1A), optineurin (OPTN) and WDR 36 (tryptophan and aspartic acid repeat domain 36). Subsequent studies have demonstrated that mutations in MYOC and OPTN genes are associated with POAG accounting for less than 5% of all POAG cases [29-30]. The WDR 36 gene may be a minor disease-causing gene in adult onset POAG [31] at least in German population. This suggests that more than 90% of the genetic contribution of POAG cases is unknown. Additionally, association studies have identified at least another 27 genes (Table 1) that are reported to be involved in glaucoma. However, these results are either not replicated in other populations or contradictory and hence their role in glaucoma is not still understood. Recently, genome wide association studies have also identified Si RNA binding domain 1 (SRBD1) and fatty acid elongase 5 (ELOVL5) genes as new susceptibility genes for NTG [32] as well as POAG but their significance remains to be established.

4. Biology of mutant genes

Although the exact role of MYOC and OPTN genes in the pathogenesis of glaucoma is unknown, it was suggested that myocilin might be involved in the trabecular meshwork (TM) homeostasis. Interestingly, MYOC mutations Y437H and I477N were shown to sensitize cells to oxidative stress induced apoptosis. Similarly, invitro transfection experiments suggested that mutations in MYOC might also cause mitochondrial defects that may lead to TM cell death. Additionally, biological and cell biological studies demonstrated that mutant MYOC was misfolded and accumulated in the endoplasmic reticulum (ER). This leads to ER stress and activates the unfolded protein response that may cause cellular toxicity and death. However, MYOC gene overexpression is not a cause or effect of elevated IOP. Similarly, OPTN may have a role in reducing the susceptibility of RGCs to hydrogen peroxide-induced cell death. Mutations in OPTN gene may also cause oxytosis and apoptosis. For instance, OPTN gene regulates endocytic trafficking of transferin receptor that is important for maintaining homeostasis. The E50K mutation of OPTN was shown to impair with trafficking and this may have implications for the pathogenesis. The TM is the target tissue in the anterior chamber. The development and progression of glaucoma was reported to cause the oxidative damage to the tissue. These changes can be minimized by the use of anti-oxidants and IOP lowering substances. Therefore, it is possible to reduce the progression of POAG by preventing the oxidative stress exposure to the TM tissue. The WDR gene on the other hand, encodes a member of the WD (tryptophan and aspartic acid) repeat protein family and the members of this family are involved in a variety of cellular processes such as apoptosis and signal transduction. Mutations in the gene may interfere in its normal functions. Despite strong genetic influence in POAG pathogenesis, only a small part of the disease can be explained in terms of genetic mutations.

Gene	Chromosomal location	Gene	Chromosomal location
ANP	1p36.2	TNF	6p21.3
MTHFR	1p36.3	NOS-3	7q36
GSTM1	1p13.3	PON1	7q21.3
IL-1beta	2q14	TLR4	9q32-q33
NCK2	2q12	IGF2	11p15.5
OPA1	3q28-q29	CDH1	16q21.1
PARL	3q27	TP53	17p13.1
EDNRA	4q31.2	APOE	19q13.2
CDKN1A	6p21.2	NTF4	19q13.3
HSPA1A	6p21.3	AGTR2	Xq22-q23

ANP = Atrial natriuretic peptide; MTHFR = methylenetetrahydrofolate reductase; IL-1beta = interleukin 1-beta; NCK = adapter protein 2; OPA1 = optic atrophy-1; PARL = presenilin associated rhomboid-like; EDNRA = endothelin receptor type A; CDKN1A = cyclin dependent kinase inhibitor 1A; HSPA1A = heat-shock 70 kD protein 1A; TNF = Tumor necrosis factor; NOS-3 = nitric oxide synthetase –3; PON1 = paraoxonase –1; TLR4 = toll-like receptor 4; IGF2 = insulin-like growth factor 2;CDH-1 = E-cadherin; TP53 = tumor protein p53; APOE = apolipoprotein E; NTF-4 = neurotrophin 4; AGTR2 = angiotensin II receptor type 2; GSTM1 = glutathione S-transferase mu 1; Asterisk (*) = detailed references can be found in ref. # 18.

Table 1. A partial list of genes that are reported to be associated with POAG and NTG *

5. Primary angle-closure glaucoma (PACG)

PACG also involves progressive and irreversible degeneration of the optic nerve with gradual visual field loss. It is estimated that in Saudi Arabia 40% of glaucoma patients belong to PACG. Although hereditary component for PACG exists, causative genes have not been identified except occasional differences in the frequency of polymorphisms in some genes. For instance, variations in Best disease (BEST1), hepatocyte growth factor (HGF), matrix metalloproteinase - 9 (MMP-9) and methylenetetrahydrofolate reductase (MTHFR) genes have been reported [28]. However, some of these results were not extended to other populations.

6. Primary congenital glaucoma (PCG)

In children, PCG is an important cause of visual loss and diagnosed during the neonatal period. It is a heterogeneous group of disorder and is characterized by an elevated IOP due to an abnormal development of the aqueous outflow system. The majority of PCG cases are sporadic but there are some familial cases. The familial condition is inherited as an autosomal recessive trait with variable expression and penetrance. Recently three PCG loci (2p21, 1p36 and 14q24.3-q31.3) corresponding to GLC3A, GLC3B and GLC 3C genes respectively, have been mapped. More than 60 different mutations in CYP1B1 (or GLC3A) – a member of the cyto-chrome P450 superfamily enzyme-encoding gene - have been reported in several PCG fami-lies [33-38]. Mutations in CYP1B1 were associated with wide range of phenotypes and the alterations of this gene could impair the morphogenesis of the outflow angle because it has been suggested that CYP1B1 gene participates in iridocorneal angle development [39]. In short, the current concept of glaucoma pathogenesis (Fig. 1) suggests that it is a group of het-erogeneous optic neuropathies caused by genetic, epigenetic and environmental factor [40].

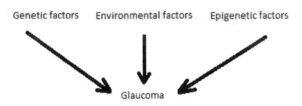

Figure 1. A complex glaucoma pathogenesis may include interplay among several factors such as genetic, epigenetic and environmental factors.

7. Inherited glaucoma in animals

Inherited glaucoma also occurs in several breeds of dogs including beagles. Primary glauco-ma in beagles is inherited as an autosomal recessive trait and appears when the animals are 9 to 18 months old. The pathogenesis, clinical signs and pharmacological responses of glau-coma in beagles have been investigated and reported previously [41-43]. Glaucoma in bea-gles however, does not involve mutations in MYOC and CYP1B1 genes [44-45]. Similarly, mutations in MYOC gene are unlikely to play a role in the pathogenesis of PCAG in Shiba Inu dogs [46]. Recently, a candidate gene for the beagle model has been isolated [47] and the mutant protein is suggested to be altering the processing of the extracellular matrix that may affect the aqueous humor outflow thereby contributing to the elevated IOP. However, the mechanism underlying RGCs death is not well understood. Interestingly, it was reported that impaired neurotrophin signaling or compromised trophic support as well as p53 medi-ated apoptosis may not be the underlying mechanism of RGCs death in a beagle model of glaucoma [48]. Recently, there has been some success in stem cell therapy in animal models [49]. Transplantation of induced pluripotent stem (iPS) cells restored retinal structure and function in degenerative animals. Therefore, these animal models are very useful in further understanding of the pathogenesis as well as drug development in glaucoma.

8. Pigmentary dispersion syndrome, pigmentary glaucoma and Axenfeld-Rieger syndrome

A number of ocular conditions such as pigment dispersion syndrome (PDS), Axenfeld-Rieger syndrome (ARS) can lead to secondary open-angle glaucoma. PDS affects the young people and is characterized by the presence of TM pigmentation, iris-transillumination defects, Krukenberg spindle and backward bowing of the iris [50]. It is transmitted in a direct linear manner from parent to sibling [51]. Genetic analysis revealed a homozygous mutation (C677T) in methylenetetrahydrofolate reductase gene (MTHFR) in a patient [52] and the higher level of plasma homocysteine was suggested to be associated with pigmentary glaucoma. Additionally, a gene responsible for the PDS has been mapped to chromosome 7q35-q36 [53]. Regarding pigmentary glaucoma, the risk of developing it from PDS is about 10% at 5 years. Young myopic men are most likely to develop the disorder [54]. Interestingly, PDS and pigmentary glaucoma are not associated with mutations in lysyl oxidase like-1 (LOXL1) and tyrosinase related protein-1 (TYRP1) genes [55-56]. Another anterior segment disease with the risk of developing congenital glaucoma is called ARS. It is a rare autosomal dominant disorder with genetic heterogeneity and exhibits a range of congenital malformations of the anterior segment of the eye. In addition, patients with ARS may present systemic malformations such as mild tooth abnormalities, craniofacial dysmorphism, sensory hearing loss and congenital heart defect. It is caused by mutations in paired-like homeodomain 2 (PITX2) and forkhead box C1 (FOXC1) genes [57-61]. In the United States, it has been estimated that mutations in PITX2 and FOXC1 genes are associated with 25% - 30% cases of ARS [62]. In severely affected patients, digenic inheritance of mutations in PITX2 and FOXC1 has also been reported [63].

9. Epigenetics: Three major types of epigenetic modifications

A vast spectrum of epigenetic changes has been described. The most common epigenetic variations involve DNA methylation, various modifications of histones, microRNA (miRNA) and small non-coding RNA expression. All these factors can modulate the expression of genes that in turn may affect phenotypes and response to drugs. DNA methylation may be tissue specific [64] and disrupts the transcriptional activity of genes by affecting the accessibility of transcription factors. A large number of CpG residues are concentrated in a region of DNA sequence (CpG island). Methylation of cytosine may reduce or prevent the binding of sequence specific transcription factors. This results in changes in gene expression. The CpG region methylation also regulates the expression of a large number of miRNA. On the other hand, genomic hypomethylation may lead to genome instability. This kind of epigenetic abnormality can be influenced by environmental factors such as tobacco smoking, dioxin and nutrition [65] and can lead to complex disorders. Studies including monozygotic twins also suggest that non-Mendelian and complex diseases (including neurological and psychiatric disorders) are likely to be caused by the combination of genetic and epigenetic factors [66]. DNA methylation and its maintenance may depend upon chromatin-associated factors and histone modifications but it is not clear how DNA demethylation process is achieved [67-68].

The other epigenetic marks are posttranslational modifications such as acetylation, methylation and phosphorylation of N-terminal tails of histone proteins. They may also regulate gene activity [66] because they affect the chromatin structure. For instance, acetylation of histone H3 and H4 leads to the formation of euchromatin and deacetylation leads to heterochromatin (tightly packed) formation (see below). These can also be influenced by environmental factors such as diet. Similarly, miRNAs regulate (down regulation) the translation of mRNAs by binding to their complementary sequence in the 3'untranslated region [69] and small RNAs are involved in gene silencing at the transcriptional level [70].

10. The potential role of epigenetics in glaucoma

The eye is a model organ for epigenetic studies because external ocular tissues are exposed to the outside environment and may be sensitive to epigenetic effects. Although the epigenetics is well known in diseases such as cancer [71], and hereditary and environmental determinants have been long suspected for eye disorders [72], epigenetic studies on eye disorders are slowly progressing [9; 73-74]. For instance, retinal and lens differentiation involves specific changes in DNA methylation, expression of non-coding RNA and nucleolar organization [73]. In addition, cell-specific DNA methylation may play an important role in modulating eye specific genes [64]. Similarly, histone modifications were involved in the pathologic course of retinal ganglion cells [75] and site-specific DNA hypomethylation permits the expression of interphotoreceptor retinoid binding protein (IRBP) gene [76]. Overexpression of mutant OPTN (E50K) is also found to induce RGC apoptosis [77-78]. Recently, it was also shown that histone deacetylase 4 (HDAC4) was involved in the survival of retinal neurons by preventing apoptosis of rod photoreceptor and bipolar cells [79-80]. Additionally, histone acetyltransferase p300 was found to promote intrinsic axonal regeneration [81]. Similarly, in an animal model (rat/mice), it has been observed that there was a regional gene expression changes including pro-survival, pro-death and acute stress genes [82-84]. Moreover, miRNAs can act as either oncogenes or tumor suppressor genes and can influence the growth of uveal melanoma [85]. Similarly, smoking and nutritional factors were involved in the etiology of age-related macular degeneration (AMD) in addition to genetic susceptibility [65].

Another example to illustrate the epigenetic effect is the pseudoexfoliation syndrome (XFS), which is one of the most common subtypes of POAG. It is the major risk factor for secondary POAG. The condition is characterized by a pathological accumulation of the whitish material in the anterior segment of the eye, predisposing to glaucomatous optic neuropathy [86]. The disorder is frequent among Icelanders, increases with age and rarely identified in people below the age of 50. Mutations in the LOXL1 gene were found to be associated with XFS in the Caucasian Australian population. [87]. However, this does not account for the large difference in disease prevalence between different populations. This raises the possibility of unidentified genetic, racial and environmental modulators [88]. In support of this is the finding that XFS may be associated with geographic and climatic factors such as sun exposure and ambient temperature [89]. The mechanisms involved are not known at present. Retinal cell death, the most common pathophysiology of all forms of glaucoma involves many factors such as oxidative stress, mitochondrial dysfunction, excitotoxic damage, axonal transport failure, deprivation of neurotrophic factors and activation of intrinsic and extrinsic apoptotic signals [90-91]. Some of these could be modulated by epigenetic changes. In support of this is the finding that heavy smoking, exposure to pesticides and nutrient intake was significantly associated with POAG [92-94]. This suggests that the interaction between gene and environmental factors may play a role in the pathogenesis of glaucoma. Intrauterine exposure (obesity and diabetes), variable DNA methylation and environmental factors may also have profound influence on adult epigenetic status. Thus in general, epigenetic may provide an additional layer of important information on inherited as well as age-related eye disorders including glaucoma.

11. Pharmacogenetics and pharmacoepigenetics in glaucoma

Adverse drug reactions (ADRs) and individual variations in drug response were well known in medicine. There are many systemic and other drugs that produce adverse effects in eye care [95-96]. For instance, many steroid drugs induce glaucoma in some patients [97]. Therefore, efficacy and safety are important aspects of initiation of any medication. Presently, there are no biochemical markers (proteins or genes) to predict which group of patients develops ADR and which group does not. Physicians in all medical branches have to make a guessing game to find out, which medication will work best for a given patient. This trial-and error method is often inefficient. Now because of the advancement in genetics, physicians will have better opportunities to treat individual patients based on their genotype (Fig. 2). In order to understand the relationship between genes and inter-individual variations in drug response, two related fields namely pharmacogenetics and pharmacogenomics have been developed. They have taken massive studies on genetic personalization of drug response [98]. Some of the pharmacogenetic studies that are related to eye disorders including glaucoma have been discussed previously [99-100]. For instance, heterozygosity in N363S mutation in glucocorticoid receptor gene has been found to be associated with steroid induced ocular hypertension in Hungarian population although it may not be the major risk factor in the pathogenesis of elevated IOP. Similarly, a beta-adrenergic antagonist timolol has been used for the treatment of glaucoma. However, a topically administered eye drop may cause adverse cardiovascular and respiratory effects. Recent investigation of a single nucleotide polymorphism (SNP) in beta-adrenergic receptor suggests that this polymorphism may be associated with positive clinical response to topical beta-blockers. In addition, R296C polymorphism in CYP 2D6 (cytochrome P450) gene may confer susceptibility to timolol induced bradycardia. Patients with CC genotype were unlikely to suffer from timolol induced bradycardia and those with TT genotype were found to suffer. Many studies address the pharmacology of several glaucoma medications but it is still not possible to explain the variable IOP response to glaucoma drugs between patients [101] using their genotype alone. This missing link could be due to several factors including environmental factors such as chemicals, alcohol, tobacco, diet and other drugs. In addition, age and gender may contribute to the physiological and biochemical status of the targeted cells (with respect to gene expression). Therefore, it is not simply genetics or environment but it is the interplay between them that is important in pharmacology and medicine.

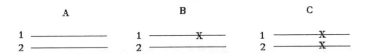

Figure 2. A schematic illustration of the relationship between genotype and drug response of an individual. Two horizontal lines 1 and 2 (panels A to C) denote a pair of homologous genes encoding a drug-metabolizing enzyme. In panel A, genes are normal and hence the individual is a fast responder and metabolizes the drug more efficiently. Therefore high doses are needed to treat. In panel B, the individual is heterozygous for the mutation and metabolizes the drug slowly. Therefore, lower doses are needed to avoid side effect or toxicity. In panel C, the individual is homozygous for the mutation and metabolizes the drug very poorly. Therefore, it may have fatal effect. The X mark denotes mutation.

12. Concluding remarks

Epigenetic is an emerging field in ophthalmology. One benefit of understanding epigenetic changes is at the level of treatment. Epigenetic modifications are reversible. For instance, disease associated DNA methylation can be reversed by inhibitors such as adenosine or deoxycytidine. However, these reagents might become cytotoxic and may lead to a wide spread DNA hypomethylation that may be resulting in and causing destabilization of genome. We need to develop less toxic inhibitors of DNA mythyltransferases. Similarly, inhibitors of histone deacetylase (HDAC) may have some therapeutic applications. For instance, HDAC inhibitors have been found to have protective effects in animal model of ischemia and optic nerve damage in the retina [71, 102-103]. At present IOP is the only modifiable risk factor for the prevention or progression of glaucoma and low IOP is associated with reduced progression of visual field defect [104-105]. Recent development on stem-cell therapy may be interesting. The initial results of clinical trials in patients using stem-cell therapy showed some visual benefits with no sign of tumorigenicity [106-111]. Therefore, stem-cell therapy may be a promising approach to treat patients with retinal disease in the future. However, further research will be needed and an understanding of the role of epigenetics is also important to the success of the stem cell-based therapies [8]. In the future, studies will uncover the epigenetic mechanism contributing to glaucoma. A strong emphasis must be placed on epigenetics in the analysis of complex phenotypic variation. It may be necessary to develop a human methylation map to understand the difference in transcript expression. Epigenetic mechanisms in ophthalmology are truly exciting areas of research.

Glossary

Apoptosis: genetically programmed cell death

Chromatin : a complex of nucleic acids and proteins

Euchromatin: a less condensed, mostly transcriptionally active chromatin

Heterochromatin: a highly condensed chromatin

Histones: small DNA binding proteins

miRNA: short regulatory non-coding RNAs

Author details

Barkur S. Shastry

Department of Biological Sciences, Oakland University, Rochester, MI, USA

References

[1] Hysi PG, Young TL, MacKey DA, Andrew T, Fernandez-Medarde A, Solonki AM, Hewitt AW, Macgregor S, Vingerling JR, Li YJ, Ikram MK, Fai LY, Sham PC, Manyes L, Porteros A, Lopes MC, Carbonaro F, Fahy SJ, Martin NG, Van Duijn CM, Spector TD, Rahi JS, Santos E, Klaver CC, Hammond CJ. A genome-wide association study for myopia and refractive error identifies a susceptibility locus at 15q25. Nat Genet 2010; 42: 902-905.

[2] Solonki AM, Verhoeven VJ, Van Duijn CM, Verkerk AJ, Ikram MK, Hysi PG, Despriet DD, Van Koolwijk LM, Ho L, Ramdas WD, Czudowska M, Kuijpers RW, Amin N, Struchalin M, Aulchenko YS, Van Rij G. et al. A genome-wide association studies identifies a susceptibility locus for refractive error and myopia at 15q14. Nat Genet 2010; 42: 897-901.

[3] Thorleifsson G, Walters GB, Hewitt AW et al. Common variants near CAV1 and CAV2 are associated with primary open-angle glaucoma. Nat Genet 2010; 42: 906-909.

[4] Burdon KP, Macgregor S, Hewitt AW, Sharma S, Chidlow G, Mills RA, Danoy P, Casson R, Viswanathan AC, Liu ZZ, Landers J, Henders AK, Wood J, Souzeau E, Crawford A, Leo P, Wang JJ, Rochtchina E, Nyholt DR, Martin NG, Montgomery GW, Mitchell P, Brown MA, Mackey DA, Craig JE. Genome-wide association study identifies susceptibility loci for open-angle at TMCO1 and CDKN2B-AS1. Nat Genet 2011; 43: 574-578.

[5] Manolino TA, Collins FS, Cox NJ, Goldstein DB, Hondorff LA, Hunter DJ, McCarthy MI, Ramos EM, Cardon LR, Chakravarti A, Cho JH, Guttmacher AE, Kong A, Kruglyak L, Mardis E, Rotimi CN, Slatkin M, Valle D, Whittemore AS, Boehnke M, Clark AG, Eichler EE, Gibson G, Haines JL, Mackay TF, McCarroll SA, Visscher PM. Finding the missing heretability of complex diseases. Nature 2009; 461: 747-753.

[6] Petronis A. Epigenetics as a unifying principle in the etiology of complex traits and diseases. Nature 2010; 465: 721-727.

[7] Bjornsson HT, Fallin MD, Feinberg AP. An integrated epigenetic approach to common human disease. Trends Genet 2004; 20: 350-358.

[8] Lister R, Pelizzola M, Dowen RH, Hawkins RD, Hong G, Tonti-Filippini J, Nery JR, Lee L, Ye Z, Ngo QM, Edsall L, Antosiewicz-Bourget J, Stewart R, Routti V, Millar AH, Thomson JA, Ren B, Ecker JR. Human DNA methylomes at base resolution show wide spread epigenetic differences. Nature 2009; 462: 315-322.

[9] Hewitt AW, Wang JJ, Liang H, Craig JE. Epigenetics effects on eye diseases. Expert Rev Ophthalmology 2012; 7: 127-134.

[10] Wiggs JL. The cell and molecular biology of complex forms of glaucoma: updates on genetic, environmental, and epigenetic risk factors. Invest Ophthalmol Vis Sci 2012; 53: 2467-2469.

[11] Quigley H. Number of people with glaucoma worldwide. Br J Ophthalmol 1996; 80: 389-393.

[12] Raymond V (1997) Molecular genetics of glaucomas: mapping of the first five GLC loci. Am J Hum Genet 1997; 60: 272-277.

[13] Kim M, Kim TW, Parker KH, Kim JM. Risk factors for primary open-angle glaucoma in South Korea. Jpn J Ophthalmol 2012; 56: 324-329.

[14] Suzuki Y, Iwase A, Araie M, Yamamoto T, Abe H, Shirato S, Kuwayama Y, Mishima HK, Shimizu H, Tomita G, Inoue Y, Kitazawa Y. Risk factors for open-angle glaucoma in a Japanese population: the Tijimi study. Ophthalmol 2006; 113: 1613-1617.

[15] Marcus MW, deVries MM, Montolio JFG, Jansonius NM. Myopia as a risk factors for open-angle glaucoma: a systematic review and meta-analysis. Ophthalmol 2011; 118: 1989-1994 e2.

[16] Xu L, Wang Y, Wang S, Wang Y, Jonas JB. High myopia and glaucoma susceptibility: the Beijing eye study. Ophthalmol 2007; 114: 216-220.

[17] Vincent A, Shetty R, Devi SA, Kurian MK, Balu R, Shetty B. Functional involvement of cone photoreceptors in advanced glaucoma: a multifocal electroretinogram study. Doc Ophthalmol 2010; 121: 21-27.

[18] Fuse N. Genetic basis of glaucoma. Tohoku J Exp Med 2010; 221: 1-10.

[19] Quigley H. Open-angle glaucoma. New Engl J Med 1993; 328: 1097-1106.

[20] Werner E. Normal tension glaucoma. In The Glaucoma, Ritch R, Shields BM, Krupin T. ed Mosby St. Louis 1996; 2: 769-797.

[21] Friedman DS, Wilson MR, Liebmann JM, Fechtner RD, Weinreb RN. An evidence based assessment of risk factors for the progression of ocular hypertension and glaucoma. Am J Ophthalmol 2004; 138: 19-31.

[22] Caprioli J. Neuroprotection for the optic nerve in glaucoma. Acta Ophthalmol Scand 1997; 75: 364-367.

[23] Drance SM. Glaucoma: a look beyond intraocular pressure. Am J Ophthalmol 1997; 123: 817-819.

[24] Pascale A, Drago F, Govoni S. Protecting the retinal neurons from glaucoma: lowering ocular pressure is not enough. Pharmacol Res 2012; 66: 19-32.

[25] Wiggs JL. Genetic etiologies of glaucoma. Arch Ophthalmol 2007; 125: 30-37.

[26] Ben-Zion I, Bogale A, Moore DB, Helveston EM. Bilateral primary congenital glaucoma in monozygotic twins. J Pediatr Ophthalmol Strabismus 2010; 47: 124-126.

[27] Shastry BS. Genetic risk factors in glaucoma. In Advances in Medicine and Biology. Berhardt LV ed, Nova Science Publishers, Inc. NY 2011; 26: 71-87.

[28] Liu Y, Allingham RR. Molecular genetics in glaucoma. Exp Eye Res 2011; 93: 331-339.

[29] Fingert JH. Primary open-angle glaucoma genes. Eye 2011; 25: 587-595.

[30] Fingeret JH, Stone EM, Sheffield VC, Alward WL. Myocilin glaucoma. Surv Ophthalmol 2002; 47: 547-561.

[31] Pasutto F, Mardin CY, Michels-Rautenstrauss K, Weber BHF, Sticht H, Chavarria-Soley G, Rautenstrauss B, Kruse F, Reis A. Profiling of WDR 36 missense variants in German patients with glaucoma. Invest Ophthalmol Vis Sci 2008; 49: 270-274.

[32] Megnro A, Inoko H, Ota M, Muzukin N, Bahram S and the normal tension glaucoma genetic study group of Japan glaucoma society. Genome wide association study of normal tension glaucoma: common variants in SRBD1 and ELOVL5 contribute to disease susceptibility. Ophthalmol 2010; 117: 1331-1338 e5.

[33] Bejjani BA, Lewis RA, Tomey KF, Anderson KL, Dueker DK, Jabak M, Astele WF, Otterud B, Leppert M, Lupski JR. Mutations in CYP1B1, the gene for cytochrome P450 1B1, are the predominant cause of primary congenital glaucoma in Saudi Arabia. Am J Hum Genet 1998; 62: 325-333.

[34] Bagiyeva S, Marfany G, Gonzalez-Duarte R. Mutational screening of CYP1B1 in Turkish PCG families and functional analyses of newly detected mutations. Mol Vis 2007; 13: 1458-1468.

[35] Demasi DP, Hewitt AW, Straga T, Pater J, MacKinnon JR, Elder JE, Casey T, Mackey DA, Craig JE. Prevalence of CYP1B1mutations in Australian patients with primary congenital glaucoma. Clin Genet 2007; 72: 255-260.

[36] Mashima Y, Suzuki Y, Sergeev Y, Ohtake Y, Tanino T, Kimura I, Miyata H, Aihara M, Tanihara H, Inatani M, Azuma N, Iwata T, Araie M. Novel cytochrome P450 1B1 (CYP1B1) gene mutations in Japanese patients with primary congenital glaucoma. Invest Ophthalmol Vis Sci 2001; 42: 2211-2216.

[37] Stoilov IR, Costa VP, Vasconcellos JP, Melo MB, Betinjane AJ, Carani JC, Oltrogge EV Sarfarazi M. Molecular genetics of primary congenital glaucoma in Brazil. Invest Ophthalmol Vis Sci 2002; 43: 1820-1827.

[38] Colomb E, Kaplan J, Gaechon HJ. Novel cytochrome P450 1B1(CYP1B1) mutations in patients with primary congenital glaucoma in France. Hum Mutat 2003; 22: 496.

[39] Libby RT, Smith RS, Savimova OV, Zableta A, Martin JE, Gonzalez FJ, John SW. Mutations of ocular defects in mouse developmental glaucoma models by tyrosinase. Science 2003; 299: 1578-1581.

[40] Ray K, Mookherjee S. Molecular complexities of primary open-angle glaucoma: current concepts. J Genet 2009; 88: 451-467.

[41] Gelatt KN, Gum GG. Inheritance of primary glaucoma in beagles. Am J Vet Res 1981; 42: 1691-1693.

[42] Samuelson DA, Gum GG, Gelatt KN. Ultrastructural changes in the aqueous outflow apparatus in the beagles with inherited glaucoma. Invest Ophthalmol Vis Sci 1989; 30: 550-561.

[43] Gelatt KN, Gum GG, Gwin RN, Bromberg NM, Merideth RE, Samuelson DA. Inherited primary open-angle glaucoma in the beagles. Am J Pathol 1981; 102: 292-295.

[44] Kato K, Sasaki N, Gelatt KN, MacKay EO, Shastry BS. Autosomal recessive primary open-angle glaucoma (POAG) in beagles is not associated with myocilin (MYOC) gene. Graefes Arch Clin Exp Ophthalmol 2009; 247: 1435-1436.

[45] Kato K, Kamida A, Sasaki N, Shastry BS. Evaluation of the CYPB1 gene as a candidate gene in beagles with primary open-angle glaucoma (POAG). Mol Vis 2009; 15: 2470-2474.

[46] Kato K, Sasaki N, Matsunaga S, Nishimura R, Ogawa H. Cloning of canine myocilin cDNA and molecular analysis of the myocilin gene in Shiba Inu dogs. Vet Ophthalmol 2007; 10: 53-62.

[47] Kuchtey J, Olson LM, Rinkoski T, MacKay EO, Iverson TM, Gelatt KN, Haines JL, Kuchtey RW. Mapping of the disease locus and identification of ADANTS locus candidate gene in a canine model of primary open-angle glaucoma. PLoS Genetics 2011; 7: e1001306.

[48] Kato K, Sasaki N, Shastry BS. Retinal ganglion cell (RGS) death in glaucomatous beagles is not associated with mutations in p53 and NTF4 genes. Vet Ophthalmol 2012; 15: 8-12..

[49] Ong JM, da Cruz L. A review and update on the current status of stem-cell therapy and retina. Br Med Bull 2012; 102: 133-146.

[50] Niyadurupola N, Broad DC. Pigent dispersion syndrome and pigementary glaucoma – a major review. Clin Exp Ophthalmol 2008; 36: 868-882.

[51] Mandelkorn RM, Hoffman ME, Olander KW, Zimmerman TJ, Harsha D. Inheritance and the pigmentary dispersion syndrome. Ophthalmic Pediatr Genet 1985; 6: 325-331.

[52] Jaksic V, Markovic V, Milenkovic S, Stefanovic I JakovicN, Knezevic M. MTHFR C677T homozygous mutation in patient with pigmentary glaucoma and central retinal vein occlusion. Ophthalmic Res 2010; 43: 193-196.

[53] Andersen JS, Pralea AM, DeBono EA, Haines JL, Gorin MB, Schuman JS, Mattox CG, Wiggs JL. A gene responsible for the pigment dispersion syndrome maps to chromosome 7q35-36. Arch Ophthalmol 1997; 115: 384-388.

[54] Siddiqui Y, Ten Hulzen RD, Cameron JD, Hodge DO, Johnson DH. What is the risk of developing pigmentary glaucoma from pigment dispersion syndrome? Am J Ophthalmol 2003; 135: 794-797.

[55] Rao KN, Ritch R, Dorairaj SK, Kaur I, Liebmann JM, Thomas R, Chakrabarti S. Exfoliation syndrome and exfoliation glaucoma associated LOXL1 variations are not involved in pigment dispersion syndrome and pigmentary glaucoma. Mol Vis 2008; 14: 1254-1262.

[56] Lynch S, Yanagi G, DelBono E, Wiggs JL. DNA sequence variants in the tyrosinase related protein 1 (TYRP1) gene are not associated with human pigmentary glaucoma. Mol Vis 2002; 8: 127-129.

[57] Semina EV, Ferrell RE, Mintz-Hittner HA, Bitoun P, Alward WL, Reiter RS, Funkhauser C, Daack-Hirsch S, Murray JC. A novel homeobox gene PITX3 is mutated in families with autosomal dominant cataract and ASMD. Nat Genet 1998; 19: 167-170.

[58] Nishimura DY, Swiderski RE, Alward WL, Searby CC, Patil SR, Bennet SR, Kanis AB, Gastier JM, Stone EM, Sheffield VC. The forkhead transcription factor gene FKHL7 is responsible for glaucoma phenotypes which maps to 6p25. Nat Genet 1998; 19: 140-147.

[59] Mears AJ, Jordan T, Mirzayans F, Dubois S, Kume T, Parlee M, Ritch R, Koop B, Kuo WL, Collins C, Marshall J, Gould DB, Pearce W, Carlsson W, Enerback S, Morissette J, Bhattacharya S, Hogan B, Raymond V, Walter MA. Mutations of the forkhead/wingled helix gene FKHLK7 in patients with Axenfeld-Rieger anomaly. Am J Hum Genet 1998; 63: 1316-1328.

[60] Reis LM, Tyler RC, Volkmann KBA, Schilter KF, Levin AV, Lowry RB, Zwijnenburg PJ, Stroh E, Broeckel U, Murray JC, Semina EV. PITX2 and FOXC1 spectrum of mutations in ocular syndrome. Eur J Hum Genet (in press).

[61] Tumer Z, Bach-Holm D. Axenfeld-Rieger syndrome and spectrum of PITX2 and FOXC1 mutations. Eur J Hum Genet 2009; 17: 1527-1539.

[62] Alward WL. Axenfeld-Rieger syndrome in the age of molecular genetics. Am J Ophthalmol 2000; 130: 107-115.

[63] Kelberman D, Islam L, Holder SE, Jaques TS, Calvas P, Hennekam RC, Nischal KK, Sowden JC. Digenic inheritance of mutations in FOXC1 and PITX2: correlating transcription factor function and Axenfeld-Rieger disease severity. Hum Mutat 2011; 32: 1144-1152.

[64] Merbs SL, Khan MA, Heckler L Jr, Oliver VF, Wan J, Qian J, Zack DJ. Cell-specific DNA methylation patterns of retina-specific genes. PLoS One 2012; 7: e32602.

[65] Seddon JM, Reynolds R, Shah HR, Rosner B. Smoking, dietary betaine, methionine and vitamin D, in monozygotic twins with discordant macular degeneration: epigenetic implications. Ophthalmol 2011; 118: 1386-1394.

[66] Fraga MF, Ballestar E, Paz MF, Ropero S, Setien F, Ballestar ML, Heine-Suner D, Cigudosa JC, Urioste M, Benitez J, Boix-Chornet M, Sanchez-Aguilera A, Ling C, Carlsson E, Poulsen P, Vaag A, Stephan Z, Spector TD, Wu YZ, Plass C, Esteller M. Epigenetic differences arise during lifetime of monozygotic twins. Proc Natl Acad Sci. USA 2005; 102: 10604-10609.

[67] Chen Z-X, Riggs AD. DNA methylation and demethylation in mammals. J Biol Chem 2011; 286: 18347-18353.

[68] Zaidi SK, Young DW, Montecino M, van Wijnen AJ, Stein JL, Lian JB, Stein GS. Book marking the genome: maintenance of epigenetic information. J Biol Chem 2011; 286: 18355-18361.

[69] Shomron N. MicroRNAs and pharmacogenomics. Pharmacogenomics 2010; 11: 629-632.

[70] Zhang X, Rossi JJ. Phylogenetic comparison of small RNA-triggered transcriptional gene silencing. J Biol Chem 2011; 286: 29443-29448.

[71]]. Berdasco M, Esteller M. Aberrant epigenetic landscape in cancer: how cellular identity goes awry. Dev Cell 2010; 19: 698-711.

[72] Schwartz JT. Twin studies in ophthalmology: hereditary and environmental determinants of eye disease. Am J Ophthalmol 1968; 66: 323-327.

[73] Cvekl A, Mitton KP. Epigenetic regulatory mechanisms in vertebrate eye development and disease. Heredity 2010; 105: 135-151.

[74] Nickells RW, Merbs SL. The potential role of epigenetics in ocular diseases. Arch Ophthalmol 2012; 130: 508-509.

[75] Pelzel HR, Schlamp CL, Nickells RW. Histone H4 deacetylation plays a critical role in early gene silencing during neuronal apoptosis. BMC Neurosci 2010; 11: 62.

[76] Boatright JH, Nickerson JM, Borst DE. Site specific DNA methylation permits expression of the IRBP gene. Brain Res 2000; 887: 211-221.

[77] Meng Q, Lu J, Ge H, Zhang L, Xue F, Zhu Y, Liu P. Overexpressed mutant optineurin (E50K) induces retinal ganglion cells apoptosis via the mitochondrial pathway. Mol Biol Rep 2012; 39: 5867-5873.

[78] Chi ZL, Akahori M, Obazawa M, Minami M, Noda T, Nakaya N, Tomarev S, Kawase K, Yamamoto T, Noda S, Sasaoka M, Shimazaki A, Takada Y, Iwata T. Overexpression of optineurin E50K disrupts Rab 8 interaction and leads to a progressive retinal degeneration in mice. Hum Mol Genet 2010; 19: 2606-2615.

[79] Chen B, Cepko CL. Requirement of histone deacetylase activity for the expression of critical photoreceptor gene. BMC Dev Biol 2007; 7: 78.

[80] Chen B, Cepko CL. HDAC4 regulated neuronal survival in normal and diseased retinas. Science 2009; 323: 256-259.

[81] Gaub P, Joshi Y, Wuttke A, Naumann U, Schnichels S, Heiduschka P, Di Giovanni S. The histone acetyltransferase p300 promotes intrinsic axonal regeneration. Brain 2011; 134: 2134-2148.

[82] Panagis L, Zhao X, Ge Y, Ren L, Mittag TW, Danias J. Gene expression changes of in areas of focal loss of retinal ganglion cells in the retina of DBA/2J mice. Invest Ophthalmol Vis Sci 2010; 51: 2024-2034.

[83] Wang D, Ray A, Rodgers K, Ergorul C, Hyman BT, Huang W, Crosskreutz CL. Global gene expression changes in rat retinal ganglion cells in experimental glaucoma. Invest Ophthalmol Vis Sci 2010; 51: 4084-4095.

[84] Fan BJ, Liu K, Wang D, Tham CC, Tam PO, Lam DS, Pang CP. Association of polymorphisms of tumor necrosis factorand tumor protein p53 with primary open-angle glaucoma: a replication study of ten genes in a Chinese population. Invest Ophthalmol Vis Sci 2010; 51: 4110-4116.

[85] Chen X, Wang J, Shen H, Lu J, Li C, Hu DN, Dong XD, Yan D, Tu L. Epigenetics, microRNAs and carcinogenesis: functional role of microRNA-137 in uveal melanoma. Invest Ophthalmol Vis Sci 2011; 52: 1193-1199.

[86] Schlotzer-Schrehardt U. Genetics and genomics of pseudoexfoliation syndrome/glaucoma. Middle East Afr J Ophthalmol 2011; 18: 30-36.

[87] Rautenbach RM, Bardien S, Harvey J, Ziskind A. An investigation into LOXL1 variants in black South African individuals with exfoliation syndrome. Arch Ophthalmol 2011; 129: 206-210.

[88] Hewitt AW, Sharma S, Burdon KP, Wang JJ, Baird PN, Damasi DP, Mackey DA, Mitchell P, Craig JE. Ancestral LOXL1 variants are associated with pseudoexfoliation in Caucasian Australian but with markedly lower penetrance than in Nordic people. Hum Mol Genet 2008; 17: 710-716.

[89] Stein JD, Pasquale LR, Talwar N, Kim DS, Reed DM, Nan B, Kang JH, Wiggs JL, Richards JE. Geographic and climatic factors associated with exfoliation syndrome. Arch Ophthalmol 2011; 129: 1053-1060.

[90] Almasieh M, Wilson AW, Morquette B, Cueva Vergas JL, Di Polo A. The molecular basis of retinal ganglion cell death in glaucoma. Prog Retn Eye Res 2012; 31: 152-181.

[91] Nickells RW. The cell and molecular biology of glaucoma: mechanisms of retinal ganglion cell death. Invest Ophthalmol Vis Sci 2012; 53: 2476-2481.

[92] Renard JP, Rouland JF, Bron A, Sellem E, Nordmann JP, Baudouin C, Denis P, Villain M, Chaine G, Collin J, de Pouvourville G, Pinchinat S, Moore N, Estephan M, Delcourt C. Nutritional, life style and environmental factors in ocular hypertension and primary open-angle glaucoma: an exploratory case control study. Acta Ophthalmol 2012; (in press)

[93] Ramdas WD, Wolfs RC, Kiefte-de Jong JC, Hofman A, de Jong PT, Vingerling JR, Jansonius NM. Nutrient intake and risk of open-angle glaucoma: the Rotterdam study. Eur J Epidemiol 2012; 27: 385-393.

[94] Wise LA, Rosenberg L, Radin RG, Mattox C, Yang EB, Palmer JR, Seddon JM. A prospective study of diabetes, lifestyle factors and glaucoma among African-American women. Ann Epidemiol 2011; 21: 430-439.

[95] Li J, Tripathi RC, Tripathy BJ. Drug induced ocular disorders. Drug Saf 2008; 31: 127-141.

[96] Santaella RM, Fraunfelder FW. Ocular adverse effects associated with systemic medications: recognition and management. Drugs 2007; 67: 75-93.

[97] Razeghinejad MR, Pro MJ, Katz LJ. Non-steroid drug induced glaucoma. Eye 2011; 25: 971-980.

[98] McLeod HL, Evans WE. Pharmacogenomics: unlocking the human genome for better drug therapy. Ann Rev Pharmacol Toxicol 2001; 41: 101-121.

[99] BS. Genetic diversity and medicinal drug response in eye care. Graefes Arch Clin Exp Ophthalmol 2010; 248: 1057-1061.

[100] Shastry BS. Pharmacogenomics in ophthalmology. Discov Med 2011; 12: 159-167.

[101] McLaren NC, Moroi SE. Clinical implications of pharmacogenetics for glaucoma therapeutics. Pharmacogenomics J 2003; 3: 197-201.

[102] Biermann J, Grieshaber P, Goebel U, Martin G, Thanos S, Givonni S, Lagreze WA. Valproic acid mediated neuroprotective and regeneration in injured retinal ganglion cells. Invest Ophthalmol Vis Sci 2010; 51: 526-534.

[103] Crosson CE, Mani SK, Husain S, Alsarraf O, Menick DR. Inhibition of histone deacetylase protects the retina from ischemic injury. Invest Ophthalmol Vis Sci 2010; 51: 3639-3645.

[104] The AGIS investigators. The advanced glaucoma intervention study (AGIS): 7. The relationship between control of intraocular pressure and visual field deterioration. Am J Ophthalmol 2000; 130: 429-440.

[105] Heijl A, Leske MC, Bengtsson B. Hyman L, Bengtsson B, Hussein M, early manifest glaucoma trial group. Reduction of intraocular pressure and glaucoma progression: results from the early manifest glaucoma trial. Arch Ophthalmol 2002; 120: 1268-1279.

[106] Baker PS, Brown GC. Stem-cell therapy in retinal disease. Curr Opin Ophthalmol 2009; 20: 175-181.

[107] Tibbetts MD, Samuel MA, Chang TS. Ho AC. Stem-cell therapy for retinal disease. Curr Opin Ophthalmol 2012; 23: 226-234.

[108] Schwartz SD, Hubschman JP, Heilwell G. Franco-Cardenas V, Pan CK, Ostrick RM, Mickunas E, Gay R, Klimanskaya I, Lanza R. Embryonic stem-cell trials for macular degeneration: a preliminary report. Lancet 2012; 379: 713-720.

[109] Boucherie C, Sowden JC, Ali RR. Induced pluripotent stem cell technology for generating photoreceptors. Regen Med 2011; 6: 469-479.

[110] Tucker BA, Park IH, Qi SD. Klassen HJ, Jiang C, Yao J, Redenti S, Daley GQ, Young MJ. Transplantation of adult mouse iPS cell derived photoreceptor precursors restores retinal structure and function in degenerative mice. PLoS One 2011; 6: e18992.

[111] Zhou L, Wang W, Liu Y. Fenandez de Castro J, Ezashi T, Telugu BP, Roberts RM, Kaplan HJ, dean DC. Differentiation of induced pluripotent stem cells of swine into rod photoreceptors and their integration into the retina. Stem Cells 2011; 29: 972-980.

Chapter 6

Functional Defects Caused by Glaucoma – Associated Mutations in Optineurin

Ghanshyam Swarup, Vipul Vaibhava and
Ananthamurthy Nagabhushana

Additional information is available at the end of the chapter

1. Introduction

Glaucomas are a heterogeneous group of optic neuropathies characterized by progressive loss of retinal ganglion cells (RGCs) leading to visual field defects. The distinctive pattern of optic nerve degeneration results in glaucomatous cupping. The atrophy of optic nerve cells initially leads to loss of peripheral vision and visual field loss increases with increased damage to optic nerve. Worldwide glaucoma is the second leading cause of blindness affecting more than 70 million people [1, 2]. Traditionally elevated intraocular pressure (IOP) is considered as a major risk factor for glaucomatous neuropathy. In addition to increased IOP, other risk factors include age, genetic and environmental factors, myopia, primary vascular dysregulation and hypertension [3, 4].

Glaucoma has been classified into different types based on various criteria. One of the widely used classifications depends on the nature of iridio-corneal angle [5]. Primary open angle glaucomas (POAGs) are the most common and clinically well defined subsets of glaucomas among Caucasians [6]. As its name suggests, in POAG there is no anatomical hindrance to the flow of aqueous humor as the angle structures remain 'open'. However, the drainage of humor is still inefficient resulting in an increase in IOP. Based on the age of onset, POAG can be juvenile (5-35 years) or adult onset (onset after 45 years) [6]. POAGs are usually chronic and largely asymptomatic, with gradual elevation of IOP and consequent visual field loss. In a significant fraction of POAG, glaucoma occurs even in the absence of elevation of IOP. These are recognized as normal tension glaucomas (NTG) [7].

Angle closure glaucomas (ACGs) are relatively rare among Caucasians and usually are acute. It is the most common form of glaucoma in Asian population [8, 9]. In ACGs, the iridiocorneal angle is closed, blocking the drainage of aqueous humor and resulting in elevation of IOP. People with shallower anterior chamber, with hypermetropia and hence narrower angles, are more susceptible to ACGs. Unlike POAG, ACG can be associated with symptoms like eye pain, blurred vision, headache, nausea, and hence is usually detected earlier [10].

In developmental or congenital glaucoma, developmental anomalies in tissues like trabecular meshwork and Schlemm's canal cause optic neuropathies [5].

2. Genetic basis of glaucoma

Glaucomas are genetically heterogeneous. Very few cases of glaucoma exhibit typical Mendelian inheritance, though familial history increases the risk factor [11, 12]. Majority of glaucoma cases appear to be multifactorial that are affected by multiple genetic and (or) environmental factors. In certain cases, mutations in some genes may cause glaucoma only when present in a susceptible genetic background. These and other complexities confound genotype-phenotype associations, making it difficult to identify genes that actually cause the disease. As a result, only a small fraction of glaucomas are associated with mutations in specific genes. Genetic studies have led to the identification of over 20 chromosomal loci that have been linked to glaucoma: GLC1A-1N, GLC3A-3C [5]. However, only five genes have so far been linked to glaucoma. While four genes – Myocilin/TIGR (trabecular meshwork inducible glucocorticoid response), Optineurin, NTF4 (neurotrophin 4) and WDR36 (WD repeat 36), have been shown to be associated with POAGs, CYP1B1 (cytochrome p450-1B1) has been linked to congenital glaucoma [5, 6, 11, 13, 14]. But mutations in CYP1B1 have been shown to be associated with POAG also [15, 16]. A better understanding of the genetic basis of the disease, with the genes involved, is critical for early detection of the disease and development of therapeutic agents that can target specific pathways.

Mutations in the gene OPTN, which encodes the protein optineurin (optic neuropathy inducing), cause NTG and amyotrophic lateral sclerosis (ALS) [17, 18]. Both of these are neurodegenerative diseases. Like glaucoma, ALS is also a progressive disease, which involves degeneration of motor neurons in the primary cortex, brainstem and spinal cord [19]. Optineurin is also seen in pathological structures present in some other neurodegenerative diseases, such as Alzheimer's disease and Parkinson's disease [20]. Despite its association with glaucoma almost a decade ago, the cellular functions of optineurin, and how its mutations alter these functions, are beginning to be understood only now. This review focuses on the recent advances in cellular functions of optineurin and defective molecular events because of optineurin mutations.

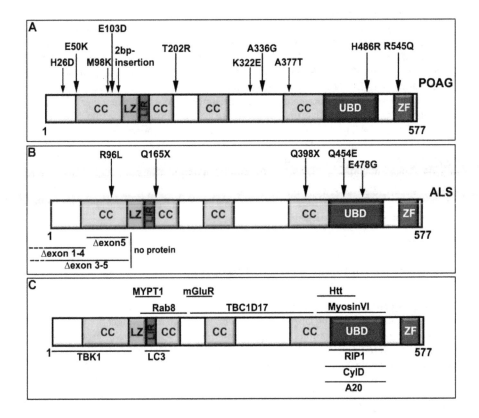

Figure 1. Disease associated mutations in optineurin. Schematic of optineurin, showing its various domains. CC-coiled coil, UBD- ubiquitin binding domain, LZ- leucine zipper, LIR- LC3 interacting region, ZF- zinc finger. A. Various glaucoma causing mutations identified in the optineurin. Of these, R545Q and M98K are polymorphisms. B. Amyotrophic Lateral Sclerosis (ALS) associated mutations in optineurin. Deletion of some of the exons have been found in ALS patients but not in glaucoma patients. C. Schematic shows regions of optineurin interacting with various proteins. Htt-Huntingtin, a protein found to be mutated in Huntington's disease; mGluR- metabotropic glutamate receptor; MYPT1- myosin phosphatase targeting subunit 1; TBK1- TANK binding kinase 1; RIP1- receptor interacting protein 1.

3. Glaucoma-associated mutations in optineurin

Rezaie et al. (2002) showed that certain mutations in the coding region of the gene *OPTN* are associated with 16.7% of the families with NTG, the only gene to be implicated in this sub-type of POAG. One of the mutations, in which glutamic acid at 50th position is replaced by lysine (E50K), segregates with the disease in a large family affected with NTG [18]. This provided strong evidence for the conclusion that this mutation in optineurin causes glaucoma. Such strong evidence is not available for other mutations of optineurin but some of the mutations have not been found in normal population. The E50K mutation was found in 13.5% of affected families [18]. Subsequent studies have identified several other mutations in optineurin that are associated with adult onset NTG and in rare cases of juvenile onset glaucoma. However, the frequency of optineurin mutation in sporadic cases is low, generally less than 1%. A polymorphism in optineurin, M98K, is associated with glaucoma in some South Asian populations but not in Caucasians [21, 22]. Most of these optineurin mutations are missense mutations (mutation which leads to replacement of the pre-existing amino acid with another). One of the rare mutations is an insertion in exon5, which would lead to production of a truncated protein due to frameshift [18] (Figure 1A). Certain point mutations that do not cause a change in amino acid sequence, for example, V148V, have also been reported [23]. Recently, certain mutations in optineurin have been shown to cause ALS [17, 24-26]. These mutations are mostly different from those that cause glaucoma (Figure. 1B). Almost all the glaucoma-associated mutations of optineurin are single copy alterations, indicating therefore, that these are likely to be dominant. An alternate possibility is that these point mutations cause a loss of function and the resulting haploinsufficiency may cause the disease.

4. Interaction of optineurin with cellular proteins

Optineurin is predominantly a coiled coil protein of 577 amino acids [27] (Figure 1). It has a well defined ubiquitin-binding UBAN domain (UBD) [28], and a zinc finger domain, which is also believed to bind to ubiquitin [29]. Optineurin interacts with a diverse array of cellular proteins through multiple interaction domains [28, 30-45] (Figure 1C). Over 20 proteins are known to interact with optineurin but functional significance of only some of these interactions is known. Emerging evidences suggest that optineurin is an adaptor protein with no known enzymatic or catalytic activity. Therefore, its functions are likely to be mediated by interaction with other proteins [46, 47].

5. Functions of optineurin

Optineurin is a multifunctional protein involved in regulating various cellular functions such as signal transduction, membrane vesicle trafficking, autophagy, NF-κB signalling, and cell survival [46, 47] (Figure 2). These functions are mediated through interaction with a wide variety of proteins.

5.1. Role of optineurin in vesicular trafficking

Vesicular trafficking is one of the most fundamental processes of eukaryotic cells. As the name suggests, it is the process of movement of cargo packaged in the vesicles or cell organelles across the cytosol inside the cell. It ensures supply of nutrients and signals to various compartments of the cell, crosstalk between the various organelles inside the cell, secretion and exocytosis [48, 49]. In a typical vesicular trafficking event, four basic steps are involved -

selection of cargo and budding of a vesiculo-tubular transport intermediate, movement of this vesicle on a cytoskeletal track, tethering or docking with an appropriate target compartment and finally fusion of the vesicle with the target membrane [50]. Several proteins like small GTPases, motor proteins, SNAREs (Soluble *N*-ethylmaleimide sensitive-factor-Attachment Protein Receptors), tethers, etc. mediate different steps of vesicular trafficking. One family of proteins, which mediates virtually all these steps in vesicular trafficking, is a class of Ras superfamily of small GTPases, the Rab GTPases (Ras-like GTPases in brain) [51, 52]. Rab GTPases confer identity to certain vesicular intermediates and organelles inside the cell, e.g. Rab5 associates with early endosome or sorting endosome and acts as a marker for it. Apart from imparting vesicle identity to some organelles, these Rab GTPases act as master regulators of trafficking events controlling vesicle budding, vesicle fusion, signal transduction and motility [53]. Rab GTPases function as molecular switches in the cell as they exist in two different forms, a GTP-bound active form that is membrane associated, and a GDP-bound inactive form that is cytoplasmic.

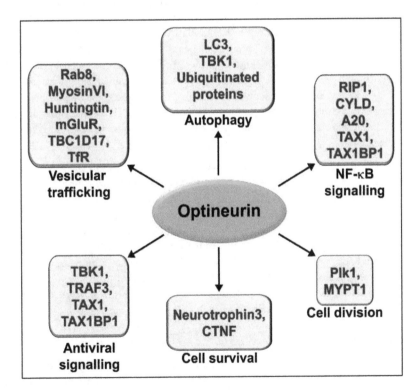

Figure 2. Functions of optineurin. Optineurin is involved in several cellular pathways. Schematic shows various functions performed by optineurin inside the cell. Proteins shown in the boxes are the ones involved in these pathways. Most of these proteins are involved in direct interaction with optineurin.

Rab GTPases mediate their functions mainly through effector proteins. By definition, effectors are the proteins, which preferentially bind to the membrane associated activated form of Rabs [54]. Given the importance of trafficking in normal cellular functions, it is not surprising that defects in trafficking have been implicated in many diseases, including glaucoma [3, 55-57].

Since optineurin interacts with multiple proteins like Rab8, huntingtin, myosinVI, transferrin receptor (TfR), TBC1D17 etc. that are involved in various intra-cellular trafficking pathways, its role in vesicular trafficking is evident [30, 34, 36, 43, 45]. But the exact mechanisms by which optineurin performs its functions in trafficking are being uncovered only recently. Rab8 is a GTPase involved in exocytosis, trafficking at recycling endosome, insulin dependent GLUT4 trafficking at plasma membrane, transferrin receptor recycling etc [30, 58-63]. Optineurin preferentially interacts with activated (GTP-bound) form of Rab8; therefore, it is an effector of some of the functions of Rab8 [34]. MyosinVI is an actin based motor protein involved in various trafficking pathways [64]. Optineurin, in conjunction with myosinVI, is required for maintenance of Golgi ribbon structure [30], polarized delivery of EGF receptor to the plasma membrane [65], sorting of AP-1B-dependent cargo to the basolateral domain in polarized cells [66] and secretory vesicle fusion at the plasma membrane [67]. Most of these processes are mediated by Rab8, also an optineurin-interacting protein. Optineurin was earlier identified as Huntingtin-interacting protein [68]. Later study showed that optineurin interacts with Rab8 through its N-terminus and recruits huntingtin to Rab8-positive vesicles [34]. Rab8 recruits optineurin to link huntingtin and myosinVI to coordinate the movement of vesicles on microtubule and actin tracks [30]. This has been reviewed in detail recently [46].

Studies from our laboratory and others have shown that optineurin interacts with TfR and mediates its trafficking [31, 32]. However, the mechanism by which optineurin regulates this, is not very clear. Recently we have shown that optineurin mediates TfR recycling by regulating the function of Rab8 through interaction with TBC1D17, a GTPase activating protein (GAP) [45] (Figure 3A). Optineurin directly interacts with TBC1D17 and also with Rab8 through adjacent but distinct binding sites. TBC1D17 does not bind directly with Rab8 and requires optineurin for this interaction. Optineurin essentially functions as an adaptor protein to recruit TBC1D17, a Rab GAP to its target Rab, Rab8, leading to inactivation of Rab8 [45]. This is a novel mechanism of regulation of Rab GTPase by its effector through a complex negative feedback mechanism.

5.2. Regulation of NF-κB by optineurin

Nuclear factor κB (NF-κB) is a family of inducible transcription factors, which is involved in regulating expression of genes involved in cell survival, immunity, inflammation, cell cycle, apoptosis etc. [69, 70] (Figure 4). Deregulation of NF-κB is associated with several human disorders including chronic inflammation, cancer, glaucoma and neurodegeneration [71].

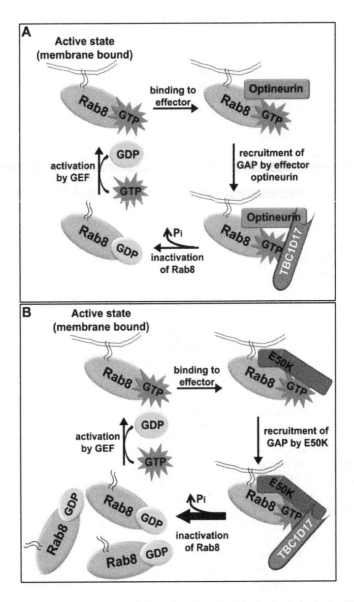

Figure 3. A model showing regulation of Rab8 by optineurin and its defective regulation by the E50K mutant.
A. GTP-bound active Rab8 performs its various functions by its interaction with effector proteins. Optineurin, an effector of Rab8, binds to the activated form of Rab8. Upon binding to activated Rab8, optineurin recruits a GAP, TBC1D17, in close proximity to Rab8. This leads to inactivation of Rab8 and thus maintenance of homeostasis. B. E50K-optineurin causes enhanced inactivation of Rab8 by recruiting TBC1D17 more efficiently.

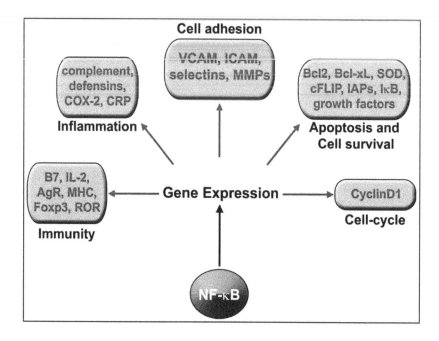

Figure 4. Schematic showing functions of transcription factor NF-κB. NF-κB is an inducible transcription factor. After its activation, it can activate transcription of various genes (shown in the boxes) and hence regulate various pathways.

It is generally kept in an inactive state in the cytoplasm through interaction with IκB (inhibitor of kappa B) inhibitory proteins. Activation of NF-κB can occur either via canonical (classical) or noncanonical (alternate) pathway. In classical pathway, upon stimulation of cells with a cytokine such as TNFα (tumor necrosis factorα), the inhibitory proteins IκBα and IκBβ are phosphorylated. This phosphorylation and consequent ubiquitination marks them for degradation by ubiquitin proteasome system. This allows NF-κB (p50-p65 complex) to move to the nucleus, where it acts as a transcriptional activator. Upon binding of TNFα to its cell surface receptor, TNFR1 (TNFα receptor 1), a signalling complex is formed in the cytoplasm, which consists of several proteins including TRADD (TNFR1-associated death domain protein), TRAF2 (TNF receptor associated factor 2) and RIP (receptor interacting protein). This leads to activation of IκB kinase (IKK), which consists of the catalytic sub-units IKKα and β, and the regulatory sub-unit NEMO / IKK-γ. Activation of IKK involves addition of polyubiquitin chains to RIP, which then binds to NEMO that leads to activation of catalytic sub-units of IKK [72]. Activated IKK phosphorylates IκB proteins leading to their degradation by ubiquitin-proteasome system (Figure 5A).

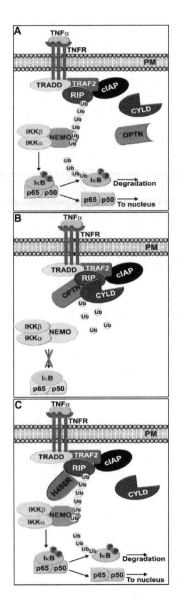

Figure 5. Schematic showing the regulation of TNFα-induced NF-κB signalling by optineurin and defective regulation caused by its H486R mutant. A. Binding of TNFα to its receptor leads to receptor trimerization, which promotes assembly of a multimolecular complex on TNF receptor in which ubiquitination of RIP takes place. Then NEMO is recruited to ubiquitinated RIP, which leads to activation of IKK. Active IKK phosphorylates IκB, which acts as a trigger for ubiquitination and degradation of IκB. This leads to the release of p50/p65 complex of NF-κB and movement to the nucleus leading to transcription activation. B. Optineurin regulates this process by acting as a competitive inhibitor of NEMO

and binds to ubiquitinated RIP by displacing NEMO. Optineurin then recruits CYLD (a deubiquitinase) to the molecular complex thus facilitating deubiquitination of polyubiquitinated RIP by CYLD leading to downregulation of downstream pathway. C. In the case of H486R mutation in optineurin, CYLD is not recruited to ubiquitinated RIP resulting in accumulation of ubiquitinated RIP. This leads to constitutive activation of NF-κB.

Role of optineurin in TNFα and NF-κB signalling was long suspected, when it was observed that it shares 53% similarity to NEMO, which led to its earlier nomenclature, NRP (NEMO related protein) [27]. It is induced by TNFα [42]. The role of optineurin in NF-κB signalling was shown by Zhu et al. [28]. Their work showed that optineurin acts as a negative regulator of TNFα–induced NF-κB signalling by binding to polyubiquitinated RIP [28]. Later, optineurin was shown to interact with CYLD, product of a tumor suppressor gene *CYLD* involved in cylindromatosis or turban tumor syndrome [36]. CYLD is a deubiquitinase which negatively regulates TNFα-induced NF-κB signalling by deubiquitinating polyubiquitinated RIP [36, 73-75]. By interacting with CYLD and also with polyubiquitinated RIP, optineurin facilitates deubiquitination of polyubiquitinated RIP by CYLD [76]. In the absence of optineurin, CYLD is unable to deubiquitinate RIP, leading to accumulation of polyubiquitinated RIP, resulting in enhanced basal NF-κB activity. Thus, in NF-κB signalling optineurin acts as an adaptor protein that brings together an enzyme (CYLD) and its substrate (polyubiquitinated RIP) together [76] (Figure 5B).

Optineurin gene expression is induced by cytokines such as TNFα and interferons [27, 77]. Human optineurin promoter has been cloned and characterized [77] and harbours, among others, NF-κB sites. TNFα induces optineurin gene expression in various cells [42, 77]. This induction is mediated by NF-κB, which binds to a site in optineurin promoter [77]. The NF-κB-binding site in optineurin promoter is located very close to the transcription start site, and is essential for TNFα mediatied induction. The activation of NF-κB is tightly regulated by complex feedback loops. Like many of its regulators, expression of optineurin, a negative regulator of NF-κB, is governed by NF-κB. Thus, there is a feedback loop in which TNFα-induced NF-κB enhances expression of optineurin, which itself negatively regulates NF-κB activation [77].

The NF-κB activity is elevated in the cells of trabecular meshwork obtained from the eyes of glaucoma patients of diverse etiology [78]. Trabecular meshwork controls aqueous outflow that regulates intraocular pressure. Elevated NF-κB activity, due to increased interleukin-1 level, protects glaucomatous trabecular meshwork cells from oxidative stress induced apoptotic cell death [78]. NF-κB p50-deficient mice show glaucoma-like pathological features such as age induced death of RGCs, hypertrophy of astrocytes with an enlargement of axons, decreased number of axons in optic nerve leading to excavation of the optic nerve head and production of autoantibodies against RGCs [79]. Therefore, it appears that NF-κB plays a cytoprotective role in various tissues of the eye. Overexpressed optineurin is known to protect NIH3T3 fibroblasts from oxidative stress-induced cell death [80]. Whether increased level of NF-κB in glaucomatous trabecular meshwork cells leads to enhanced optineurin level or optineurin-mediated cytoprotection, is yet to be investigated.

Optineurin interacts with UXT (ubiquitously expressed transcript) [36], a protein involved in the regulation of NF-κB signalling [81]. UXT is localized predominantly in the nucleus and interacts specifically with NF-κB. UXT forms a complex with NF-κB and is recruited to the NF-κB enhanceosome upon stimulation by TNFα [81]. Enhanceosome is a protein complex that binds to the "enhancer" region of a gene, which can be upstream or downstream of the promoter, or within a gene. It accelerates the gene's transcription [82, 83]. However, functional significance of optineurin-UXT interaction has not been investigated.

5.3. Role of optineurin in autophagy

Autophagy is one of the intracellular quality control mechanisms for removing and degrading defective proteins and organelles in the lysosomes [84]. During induction of autophagy, specialized membranous structures known as autophagosomes are formed, which engulf the cargo (cytoplasmic components and organelles) and deliver it to the lysosomes [85]. LC3 (microtubule-associated protein 1 light chain 3) is present in autophagosomal membranes. Overexpressed GFP conjugated LC3 or endogenous LC3 upon immunostaining is seen predominantly in autophagosomes; therefore, LC3 serves as a very useful marker for auto-phagosomes [86]. LC3 on autophagosomes interacts with autophagy receptors, which help in recruiting ubiquitinated proteins and organelles to autophagosomes. Autophagy receptors are believed to play a crucial role in the selection and recruitment of cargo to autophagosomes by simultaneously binding to LC3 and ubiquitinated cargo [85, 87, 88]. Optineurin was identified as an autophagy receptor due to its ability to bind LC3 and ubiquitin directly and simultane-ously through well defined binding sites [37]. Optineurin is involved in clearance of cytosolic Salmonella in macrophages [37]. However, so far no specific protein of Salmonella has been identified that binds to optineurin and is targeted to autophagosomes for degradation. Overexpressed normal optineurin and its E50K mutant induce formation of autophagosomes in retinal ganglion cells in culture and also in transgenic mice expressing E50K-optineurin [89].

5.4. Role of optineurin in cell survival and cell death

One of the glaucoma-associated optineurin mutations (2 bp insertion in exon 5) leads to frameshift resulting in truncation of a major part of the protein. This mutant protein is unlikely to be functional; therefore it was speculated that optineurin has a cytoprotective role in the retina that is lost by mutations [18]. Some support for this hypothesis was provided by experiments in which overexpressed optineurin protected NIH3T3 cells from oxidative stress-induced cell death whereas a glaucoma-causing mutant, E50K, did not [80]. However, this protective effect of optineurin against oxidative stress is yet to be tested in cells relevant for glaucoma or ALS. Recently, using a mouse retinal ganglion cell line, RGC-5, it was shown that knockdown of endogenous optineurin results in induction of apoptotic cell death due to reduced secretion of neurotrophin 3 (NT-3) and ciliary neurotrophic factor (CNTF) [90]. Addition of NT3 to the medium was able to suppress this cell death. The level of NT-3 or CNTF mRNA was not affected significantly upon knockdown of optineurin. Knockdown of opti-neurin resulted in breakdown of the Golgi structure [30, 90] and accumulation of NT-3 positive vesicles due to a block in vesicle trafficking in the secretory pathway [90]. Overexpression of optineurin sensitizes RGC-5 cells to TNFα-induced cell death but interestingly, in Hela cells, overexpressed optineurin does not increase TNFα-induced cell death. In fact, in Hela cells optineurin inhibits TNFα-induced cell death [91]. This is consistent with the observation that an interplay between polymorphism in TNFα and optineurin gene increases the risk of glaucoma [92]. Thus it appears that maintenance of optimum level of optineurin is important for survival of RGCs. The mechanism by which optineurin causes different effects in RGCs and in Hela cells is not known.

5.5. Regulation of mitosis by optineurin

Polo-like kinase (Plk1) is an important regulator of various events in cell division cycle such as G2/M (Gap2 of interphase to mitosis) transition, centrosome maturation, chromosome segregation and cytokinesis. The precise control of these events depends on the kinase activity of Plk1 [93-95]. During mitosis optineurin is phosphorylated by Plk1 at Ser177 that leads to its relocalization to the nucleus from the Golgi. In the nucleus optineurin enhances phosphorylation of MYPT1 (myosin phosphatase target subunit 1) by Cdk1 (cyclin dependent kinase 1) that leads to binding of MYPT1 with Plk1 and inactivation of Plk1. Knockdown of optineurin leads to defects in chromosome separation and formation of multinucleate cells [39]. Formation of multinucleate cells upon optineurin knockdown has been observed in RGC-5 cells also [90]. Thus optineurin is involved in a feedback mechanism by which Plk1 modulates localization of optineurin that in turn regulates Plk1 activity and mitosis progression [39].

5.6. Role of optineurin in antiviral signalling

Our body responds to viral infection through innate immune response and produces type I interferons (IFNα / IFNβ). These induce signalling to activate transcription of many genes to produce an antiviral state in the cells [96]. A tight regulation of this antiviral signalling is necessary to prevent unwanted tissue damage due to inflammatory response. Optineurin has emerged as one such negative regulator limiting IFNβ production in response to RNA virus infection [40]. This negative regulation of IFNβ production is mediated by interaction of optineurin with TBK1 (TANK binding kinase 1), a protein kinase involved in the activation of IRF3/7 (interferon regulatory factor 3/7) transcription factors [97]. Optineurin inhibits TBK1-mediated phosphorylation of IRF3 induced by Sendai virus or extracellular poly (I:C) [98]. But another group has suggested that optineurin is an activator of TBK1 and mediates IFNβ production in response to lipopolysaccharide or poly (I:C) [99]. UBD of optineurin plays an essential role in this process. However, a negative regulatory role for optineurin in innate immune response is supported by the observation that optineurin inhibits IRF3 activation in response to MDA5 (melanoma differentiation associated gene 5) or TRIF (TIR-domain-containing adapter-inducing interferon-β) overexpression [98].

6. Functional defects caused by optineurin mutants

Considering the importance of diverse cellular functions optineurin assists in, defects caused by its mutants are imperative. Recent work has revealed some of the normal cellular functions of optineurin. However, our understanding of functional defects due to mutations in optineurin, is only beginning to emerge. So far, functional defects caused by only two disease associated mutants are known. Here we are providing some insight into how optineurin mutants might be leading to defective cellular functions.

6.1. Defective NF-κB regulation

Aberrant NF-κB signalling has been implicated in many neurodegenerative diseases like Alzheimer's, Parkinson's and Huntington's diseases, and glaucoma [100, 101]. Recently it has been shown that a glaucoma-associated mutant of optineurin, H486R, is defective in inhibiting TNFα-induced NF-κB activation [76]. The H486R mutant is associated with JOAG and POAG patients, and this mutant has not been found in any normal individual [23, 102]. This mutation lies in the ubiquitin-binding domain (Figure 1A). The H486R mutant shows drastically reduced interaction with CYLD and also shows somewhat re-duced interaction with polyubiquitinated RIP [76]. The inability of H486R mutant to in-hibit TNFα-induced NF-κB activation is primarily due to defective interaction with CYLD although reduced interaction with RIP may also contribute to a small extent. This conclusion is supported by the finding that overexpressed CYLD was unable to deubi-quitinate RIP and inhibit TNFα-induced NF-κB activity in presence of the H486R mutant [76] (Figure 5C). Thus it is clear that the interaction of optineurin with CYLD plays a crucial role in the regulation of TNFα-induced NF-κB activation [76].

What is the mechanism of pathogenesis of glaucoma caused by the H486R mutant? In glaucoma, loss of vision occurs due to the death of retinal ganglion cells in the optic nerve head. Several mechanisms have been implicated as cause of RGC death in glaucoma such as direct effect on RGCs, activation of glial cells to secrete cytotoxic proteins like TNFα, changes in trabecular meshwork, and autoimmunity [3, 103]. However, unlike E50K mutant, the H486R mutant does not cause RGC death in cell culture or in transgenic mice [91, 104]. Therefore, it is likely that indirect effects through other cells might contribute to H486R-induced glaucoma. Increased NF-κB activity is associated with autoimmune response and also with glaucomatous trabecular meshwork [78, 79, 105]. Deregulation of NF-κB by H486R mutant provides a basis for exploring its indirect mechanisms of neurodegeneration associated with glaucoma. Since CYLD knockout mice show autoimmune defects [106], it is possible that the H486R mutant, by blocking the function of CYLD, might also cause autoimmune defects relevant for glauco-ma. Whether increased NF-κB activity associated with glaucomatous trabecular meshwork [78] is a cause or an effect of elevated IOP is not known. The relevance of NF-κB deregulation by H486R-optineurin to elevated IOP is not known but an interesting possibility is that increased NF-κB activity in trabecular meshwork might cause increased IOP by altering growth or other properties of trabecular meshwork cells.

The ALS-associated mutant E478G is unable to inhibit TNFα-induced NF-κB activation but the molecular mechanism of this defect is not known [17]. This mutant is predicted to be defective in binding to ubiquitin but this is yet to be tested. It would be of interest to know whether this mutant is defective in binding to CYLD or not. Relevance of defective NF-κB regulation by E478G mutant to disease pathogenesis is not clear.

6.2. Defective cell survival and membrane vesicle trafficking

The E50K is a dominant mutation [18], which upon overexpression induces death of RGC-5 cells in culture but not of other cell lines tested. None of the other glaucoma-associated mutants tested (H26D, H486R, R545Q) induced RGC death [91]. This suggests that the E50K mutant causes glaucoma by directly inducing death of RGCs. Transgenic mice expressing E50K mutant showed apoptotic death of RGCs suggesting, therefore, that RGC-5 cell line is a useful cell culture model to study molecular mechanisms of pathogenesis of glaucoma [104]. The E50K transgenic mice showed degeneration of entire retina resulting in reduced thickness of retina [104]. The E50K-induced death of RGCs is mediated by oxidative stress although the mechanism of induction of oxidative stress by E50K is not known. The oxidative stress is due to formation of reactive oxygen species probably produced by mitochondria because E50K-induced RGC death and production of reactive oxygen species were abolished by coexpression of mitochondrial superoxide dismutase [91]. The E50K mutant inhibits endocytic trafficking and recycling of transferrin receptor leading to accumulation of transferrin receptor in large foci/vesicular structures (recycling endosomes, autophagosomes). This defective Rab8 mediated TfR trafficking by E50K mutant is due to altered interaction of this mutant with Rab8 and transferrin receptor [31, 32]. Optineurin functions as an adaptor protein to mediate negative regulation of Rab8 by the GTPase activating protein, TBC1D17. The E50K mutant recruits TBC1D17 more efficiently to the multimolecular complex leading to enhanced inactivation of Rab8 by TBC1D17. This leads to inhibition of Rab8-mediated TfR trafficking and recycling. This hypothesis is supported by the observation showing that E50K-optineurin dependent inhibition of transferrin receptor trafficking can be prevented by knockdown of TBC1D17 or by expressing a catalytically inactive mutant of TBC1D17. A constitutively active mutant of Rab8, Q67L also reverses E50K-optineurin induced inhibition of transferrin receptor trafficking [45]. Whether E50K-induced TBC1D17-mediated Rab8 inactivation, or defective TfR trafficking, play a role in RGC death, is yet to be investigated. A blockade in axonal vesicular trafficking of brain-derived neurotrophic factor and its receptor, that are vital for RGC survival, has been considered as one of the causes for glaucomatous cell death [107, 108].

It appears that the molecular mechanism of defective TfR trafficking by the E50K mutant is somewhat complex. Optineurin forms a multimolecular complex containing Rab8 and TfR as seen by co-immunoprecipitation [31, 32]. Co-immunoprecipitation identifies protein-protein interactions, which may be direct or indirect (mediated by another protein) [109]. The E50K mutant forms a stronger complex with transferrin receptor and Rab8. Stronger colocalization of E50K mutant with Rab8 and transferrin receptor in the same structures/foci provides support for this suggestion [31]. But, direct interaction between E50K mutant and Rab8 is lost as shown in mammalian cells and also by yeast two-hybrid assay [45, 104]. Based on these observations it appears that in the multimolecular complex, direct interaction between E50K mutant and Rab8 is lost but indirect interaction (through other proteins) is increased. Therefore, it is likely that the functional positioning of these proteins in the multimolecular complex is altered in such a way that the inactivation of Rab8 by TBC1D17 is increased in E50K-expressing cells [45]. This is depicted schematically in Figure 3.

Optineurin plays a role in maintaining the structure of the Golgi complex and expression of E50K mutant results in breakdown of the Golgi [110]. However, the molecular mechanism of this effect of E50K mutant and its relevance to RGC death are not known. Whether Golgi breakdown is a contributory factor for E50K-induced defective trafficking and hence RGC death is not clear. The relationship between Rab8 inactivation and Golgi breakdown by E50K is yet to be investigated.

6.3. Defective autophagy

Formation of aggregates is one of the hallmarks of many neurodegenerative diseases like Alzheimer's, Parkinson's, Huntington's diseases and prion deseases. Accumulation of aggregates is indicative of either an inability to degrade mutant protein or an overall inhibition of the cellular trafficking and degradative machinery [111-113].

Overexpression of optineurin results in the formation of vesicular structures or foci. Some of these foci are autophagosomes and overexpression of E50K mutant results in the formation of larger autophagosomes [89]. This formation of larger autophagosomes by E50K mutant is perhaps due to a block in autophagy, which partly contributes to E50K-induced death of RGCs. This conclusion is supported by the observation that rapamycin, an inducer of autophagy, reduces E50K-induced death of RGC-5 cells [89]. However, the mechanism of increased formation of larger autophagosomes in E50K expressing cells is not known. Interaction of E50K with ubiquitinated proteins is perhaps required for autophagosome formation because inactivation of UBD by point mutation in E50K causes nearly complete loss of foci formation [31].

6.4. Other defects of optineurin mutants

RNA virus infection is sensed by components of innate immune response, including RIG-1 (retinoic acid inducible gene 1), MDA5 (melanoma differentiation associated gene 5) and Toll like receptors [114-116]. This sensing of receptors leads to activation of TBK1 and IRF3 [117]. Optineurin is a negative regulator of IRF3 activation, which is involved in IFNβ production [40]. ALS-associated mutants of optineurin, E478G and Q398X, are defective in this negative regulation [98]. Whether any of the glaucoma-associated mutants show this defect is yet to be examined.

Optineurin interacts with proteins involved in immunity, IK-cytokine and BAT4 [36]. But the functional significance of these interactions is not known.

7. Conclusions and future directions

Optineurin functions as an adaptor protein and thereby plays a crucial role in several functions including vesicle trafficking in the secretory and recycling pathways, NF-κB signalling, control of mitosis, Golgi organization, autophagy and antiviral signalling. The relationship between these different functions of optineurin is not clear. Since optineurin is an adaptor protein, mutations in it can lead to altered interactions with other proteins impairing its normal cellular functions. Identifying the functions that are affected by disease-associated mutations of optineurin is a major challenge towards understanding the molecular mechanisms of etiopathogenesis of neurodegenerative disease like glaucoma. Presently, our understanding of the molecular mechanisms of functional defects caused by E50K mutation, the best studied mutant, is far from complete. Several questions remain to be answered. How does E50K mutation cause a block in autophagy? Does E50K mutant cause inhibition of secretion of neutrophins/survival factors? Is Rab8 involved in this process? Does impaired transferrin receptor trafficking or function contribute to E50K-induced RGC death? How does H486R mutant cause glaucoma? Does it cause autoimmune defects by impairing the function of CYLD? How do other mutants of optineurin alter its function? Why some mutations cause ALS and others cause glaucoma? Are mutations of optineurin also prevalent in other neurodegenerative diseases? Is interaction of optineurin or its mutants altered with huntingtin or its mutants? If so, what is its relevance for Huntington's disease and glaucoma? Role of various mutants of optineurin in affecting known functions of optineurin needs to be examined. This would help in understanding the molecular mechanisms of pathogenesis of glaucoma and other neurodegenerative diseases. Most of the optineurin mutants do not directly induce death of RGC-5 cells upon overexpression, indicating, therefore, that these optineurin mutations might cause glaucoma by indirect mechanisms involving defects in other cells/tissues (Figure 6]. Survival of RGCs is influenced by other accessory cells like glial cells. Role of optineurin mutants in autoimmunity and glial cell activation needs to be explored.

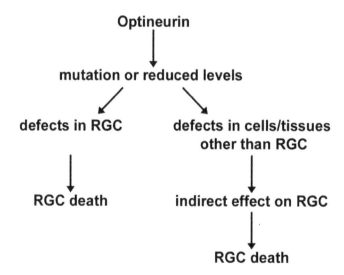

Figure 6. Overview of role of optineurin mutations in causing Glaucoma.

Functional defects caused by mutations in optineurin in cells other than RGC, especially glial cells could also be relevant for glaucoma pathogenesis. However, molecular mechanism of such effects and relevance to glaucoma needs to be established. Transgenic and knockout animal models are needed to understand the complex and diverse mechanisms involved in the pathogenesis of glaucoma and ALS caused by mutations in optineurin.

Abbreviations

RGC, Retinal ganglion cells; IOP, Intraocular pressure; POAG, Primary open angle glaucoma; JOAG, Juvenile open angle glaucoma; NTG, Normal tension glaucoma; ACG, Angle closure glaucoma; TIGR, trabecular meshwork inducible glucocorticoid response; WDR36, WD repeat 36; CYP1B1, cytochrome p4501B1; NTF3/4, neurotrophin3/4; ALS, amyotrophic lateral sclerosis; UBD, ubiquitin-binding domain; GLUT4, glucose transporter member 4; EGF, epidermal growth factor; GAP, GTPase activating protein; NF-κB, Nuclear factor κB; IκB, inhibitor of kB; TNFα, tumor necrosis factor α; TNFR1, tumor necrosis factor Receptor1; TRADD- TNFR1-associated DEATH domain protein; TRAF2, TNF receptor associated factor 2; RIP, receptor interacting protein; IKK, IκB kinase; NEMO, NF-κB essential modifier; UXT, ubiquitously-expressed transcript; LC3- microtubule-associated protein 1 light chain 3; CTNF, ciliary neurotrophic factor; Plk1, Polo-like kinase; MYPT1, myosin phosphatase target subunit 1; Cdk1, cyclin dependent kinase 1; IRF3, Interferon regulatory factor 3; TBK1, TANK binding kinase; MDA5, melanoma differentiation associated gene 5; TRIF, TIR-domain-containing adapter-inducing interferon-β; ROS, reactive oxygen species; RIG1, retinoic acid inducible gene 1.

Acknowledgements

This work was supported by a grant to GS from the Department of Biotechnology, Government of India. GS gratefully acknowledges the Department of Science and Technology, Government of India for J C Bose National Fellowship. VV is recipient of a Senior Research Fellowship from the CSIR, New Delhi, India.

Author details

Ghanshyam Swarup*, Vipul Vaibhava and Ananthamurthy Nagabhushana

*Address all correspondence to: gshyam@ccmb.res.in

Centre for Cellular and Molecular Biology, Council of Scientific and Industrial Research, Hyderabad, India

References

[1] Quigley HA. Neuronal death in glaucoma. Prog Retin Eye Res. 1999 Jan;18:39-57.

[2] Resnikoff S, Pascolini D, Etya'ale D, et al. Global data on visual impairment in the year 2002. Bull World Health Organ. 2004 Nov;82:844-51.

[3] Vrabec JP, Levin LA. The neurobiology of cell death in glaucoma. Eye (Lond). 2007 Dec;21 Suppl 1:S11-4.

[4] Weinreb RN, Khaw PT. Primary open-angle glaucoma. Lancet. 2004 May 22;363:1711-20.

[5] Vasiliou V, Gonzalez FJ. Role of CYP1B1 in glaucoma. Annu Rev Pharmacol Toxicol. 2008;48:333-58.

[6] Fan BJ, Wang DY, Lam DS, et al. Gene mapping for primary open angle glaucoma. Clin Biochem. 2006 Mar;39:249-58.

[7] Quigley HA. Glaucoma. Lancet. 2011 Apr 16;377:1367-77.

[8] He M, Foster PJ, Ge J, Huang W, Zheng Y, Friedman DS, et al. Prevalence and clinical characteristics of glaucoma in adult Chinese: a population-based study in Liwan District, Guangzhou. Invest Ophthalmol Vis Sci. 2006 Jul;47:2782-8.

[9] Friedman DS, Foster PJ, Aung T, et al. Angle closure and angle-closure glaucoma: what we are doing now and what we will be doing in the future. Clin Experiment Ophthalmol. 2012 May-Jun;40:381-7.

[10] Libby RT, Gould DB, Anderson MG, et al. Complex genetics of glaucoma susceptibility. Annu Rev Genomics Hum Genet. 2005;6:15-44.

[11] Hewitt AW, Craig JE, Mackey DA. Complex genetics of complex traits: the case of primary open-angle glaucoma. Clin Experiment Ophthalmol. 2006 Jul;34:472-84.

[12] Challa P. Glaucoma genetics. Int Ophthalmol Clin. 2008 Fall;48:73-94.

[13] Hilal L, Boutayeb S, Serrou A, et al. Screening of CYP1B1 and MYOC in Moroccan families with primary congenital glaucoma: three novel mutations in CYP1B1. Mol Vis. 2010;16:1215-26.

[14] Pasutto F, Matsumoto T, Mardin CY, et al. Heterozygous NTF4 mutations impairing neurotrophin-4 signaling in patients with primary open-angle glaucoma. Am J Hum Genet. 2009 Oct;85:447-56.

[15] Chakrabarti S, Devi KR, Komatireddy S, et al. Glaucoma-associated CYP1B1 mutations share similar haplotype backgrounds in POAG and PACG phenotypes. Invest Ophthalmol Vis Sci. 2007 Dec;48:5439-44.

[16] Melki R, Colomb E, Lefort N, et al. CYP1B1 mutations in French patients with early-onset primary open-angle glaucoma. J Med Genet. 2004 Sep;41:647-51.

[17] Maruyama H, Morino H, Ito H, et al. Mutations of optineurin in amyotrophic lateral sclerosis. Nature. 2010 May 13;465:223-6.

[18] Rezaie T, Child A, Hitchings R, et al. Adult-onset primary open-angle glaucoma caused by mutations in optineurin. Science. 2002 Feb 8;295:1077-9.

[19] Kiernan MC, Vucic S, Cheah BC, et al. Amyotrophic lateral sclerosis. Lancet. 2011 Mar 12;377:942-55.

[20] Osawa T, Mizuno Y, Fujita Y, et al. Optineurin in neurodegenerative diseases. Neuropathology. 2011 Dec;31:569-74.

[21] Alward WL, Kwon YH, Kawase K, et al. Evaluation of optineurin sequence variations in 1,048 patients with open-angle glaucoma. Am J Ophthalmol. 2003 Nov; 136:904-10.

[22] Ayala-Lugo RM, Pawar H, Reed DM, et al. Variation in optineurin (OPTN) allele frequencies between and within populations. Mol Vis. 2007;13:151-63.

[23] Leung YF, Fan BJ, Lam DS, et al. Different optineurin mutation pattern in primary open-angle glaucoma. Invest Ophthalmol Vis Sci. 2003 Sep;44:3880-4.

[24] Iida A, Hosono N, Sano M, et al. Novel deletion mutations of OPTN in amyotrophic lateral sclerosis in Japanese. Neurobiol Aging. 2012 Aug;33:1843 e19-24.

[25] Millecamps S, Boillee S, Chabrol E, et al. Screening of OPTN in French familial amyotrophic lateral sclerosis. Neurobiol Aging. 2011 Mar;32:557 e11-3.

[26] van Blitterswijk M, van Vught PW, van Es MA, et al. Novel optineurin mutations in sporadic amyotrophic lateral sclerosis patients. Neurobiol Aging. 2011 May;33:1016 e1-7.

[27] Schwamborn K, Weil R, Courtois G, et al. Phorbol esters and cytokines regulate the expression of the NEMO-related protein, a molecule involved in a NF-kappa B-independent pathway. J Biol Chem. 2000 Jul 28;275:22780-9.

[28] Zhu G, Wu CJ, Zhao Y, et al. Optineurin negatively regulates TNFalpha- induced NF-kappaB activation by competing with NEMO for ubiquitinated RIP. Curr Biol. 2007 Aug 21;17:1438-43.

[29] Laplantine E, Fontan E, Chiaravalli J, et al. NEMO specifically recognizes K63-linked poly-ubiquitin chains through a new bipartite ubiquitin-binding domain. EMBO J. 2009 Oct 7;28:2885-95.

[30] Sahlender DA, Roberts RC, Arden SD, et al. Optineurin links myosin VI to the Golgi complex and is involved in Golgi organization and exocytosis. J Cell Biol. 2005 Apr 25;169:285-95.

[31] Nagabhushana A, Chalasani ML, Jain N, et al. Regulation of endocytic trafficking of transferrin receptor by optineurin and its impairment by a glaucoma-associated mutant. BMC Cell Biol. 2010;11:4.

[32] Park B, Ying H, Shen X, et al. Impairment of protein trafficking upon overexpression and mutation of optineurin. PLoS One. 2010;5:e11547.

[33] Journo C, Filipe J, About F, et al. NRP/Optineurin Cooperates with TAX1BP1 to potentiate the activation of NF-kappaB by human T-lymphotropic virus type 1 tax protein. PLoS Pathog. 2009 Jul;5:e1000521.

[34] Hattula K, Peranen J. FIP-2, a coiled-coil protein, links Huntingtin to Rab8 and modulates cellular morphogenesis. Curr Biol. 2000 Dec 14-28;10:1603-6.

[35] Anborgh PH, Godin C, Pampillo M, et al. Inhibition of metabotropic glutamate receptor signaling by the huntingtin-binding protein optineurin. J Biol Chem. 2005 Oct 14;280:34840-8.

[36] Chalasani ML, Swarup G, Balasubramanian D. Optineurin and its mutants: molecules associated with some forms of glaucoma. Ophthalmic Res. 2009;42:176-84.

[37] Wild P, Farhan H, McEwan DG, et al. Phosphorylation of the autophagy receptor optineurin restricts Salmonella growth. Science. 2011 Jul 8;333:228-33.

[38] Morton S, Hesson L, Peggie M, et al. Enhanced binding of TBK1 by an optineurin mutant that causes a familial form of primary open angle glaucoma. FEBS Lett. 2008 Mar 19;582:997-1002.

[39] Kachaner D, Filipe J, Laplantine E, et al. Plk1-dependent phosphorylation of optineurin provides a negative feedback mechanism for mitotic progression. Mol Cell. 2012 Feb 24;45:553-66.

[40] Mankouri J, Fragkoudis R, Richards KH, et al. Optineurin negatively regulates the induction of IFNbeta in response to RNA virus infection. PLoS Pathog. 2010 Feb; 6:e1000778.

[41] Moreland RJ, Dresser ME, Rodgers JS, et al. Identification of a transcription factor IIIA-interacting protein. Nucleic Acids Res. 2000 May 1;28:1986-93.

[42] Li Y, Kang J, Horwitz MS. Interaction of an adenovirus E3 14.7-kilodalton protein with a novel tumor necrosis factor alpha-inducible cellular protein containing leucine zipper domains. Mol Cell Biol. 1998 Mar;18:1601-10.

[43] del Toro D, Alberch J, Lazaro-Dieguez F, et al. Mutant huntingtin impairs post-Golgi trafficking to lysosomes by delocalizing optineurin/Rab8 complex from the Golgi apparatus. Mol Biol Cell. 2009 Mar;20:1478-92.

[44] Harjes P, Wanker EE. The hunt for huntingtin function: interaction partners tell many different stories. Trends Biochem Sci. 2003 Aug;28:425-33.

[45] Vaibhava V, Nagabhushana A, Chalasani ML, et al. Optineurin mediates negative regulation of Rab8 function by TBC1D17, a GTPase activating protein. J Cell Sci. 2012 Aug 1.

[46] Kachaner D, Genin P, Laplantine E, et al. Toward an integrative view of Optineurin functions. Cell Cycle. 2012 Aug 1;11.

[47] Ying H, Yue BY. Cellular and molecular biology of optineurin. Int Rev Cell Mol Biol. 2012;294:223-58.

[48] Mellman I. Endocytosis and molecular sorting. Annu Rev Cell Dev Biol. 1996;12:575-625.

[49] Jahn R, Sudhof TC. Membrane fusion and exocytosis. Annu Rev Biochem. 1999;68:863-911.

[50] Zerial M, McBride H. Rab proteins as membrane organizers. Nat Rev Mol Cell Biol. 2001 Feb;2:107-17.

[51] Hutagalung AH, Novick PJ. Role of Rab GTPases in membrane traffic and cell physiology. Physiol Rev. 2011 Jan;91:119-49.

[52] Segev N. Coordination of intracellular transport steps by GTPases. Semin Cell Dev Biol. 2010 Feb;22:33-8.

[53] Stenmark H. Rab GTPases as coordinators of vesicle traffic. Nat Rev Mol Cell Biol. 2009 Aug;10:513-25.

[54] Grosshans BL, Ortiz D, Novick P. Rabs and their effectors: achieving specificity in membrane traffic. Proc Natl Acad Sci U S A. 2006 Aug 8;103:11821-7.

[55] Nixon RA. Endosome function and dysfunction in Alzheimer's disease and other neurodegenerative diseases. Neurobiol Aging. 2005 Mar;26:373-82.

[56] Laird FM, Farah MH, Ackerley S, et al. Motor neuron disease occurring in a mutant dynactin mouse model is characterized by defects in vesicular trafficking. J Neurosci. 2008 Feb 27;28:1997-2005.

[57] Schweitzer JK, Krivda JP, D'Souza-Schorey C. Neurodegeneration in Niemann-Pick Type C disease and Huntington's disease: impact of defects in membrane trafficking. Curr Drug Targets. 2009 Jul;10:653-65.

[58] Henry L, Sheff DR. Rab8 regulates basolateral secretory, but not recycling, traffic at the recycling endosome. Mol Biol Cell. 2008 May;19:2059-68.

[59] Huber LA, Pimplikar S, Parton RG, et al. Rab8, a small GTPase involved in vesicular traffic between the TGN and the basolateral plasma membrane. J Cell Biol. 1993 Oct; 123:35-45.

[60] Hattula K, Furuhjelm J, Tikkanen J, et al. Characterization of the Rab8-specific membrane traffic route linked to protrusion formation. J Cell Sci. 2006 Dec 1;119:4866-77.

[61] Ishikura S, Klip A. Muscle cells engage Rab8A and myosin Vb in insulin-dependent GLUT4 translocation. Am J Physiol Cell Physiol. 2008 Oct;295:C1016-25.

[62] Peranen J. Rab8 GTPase as a regulator of cell shape. Cytoskeleton (Hoboken). 2011 Oct;68:527-39.

[63] Rahajeng J, Giridharan SS, Cai B, et al. Important relationships between Rab and MI-CAL proteins in endocytic trafficking. World J Biol Chem. 2011 Aug 26;1:254-64.

[64] Buss F, Spudich G, Kendrick-Jones J. Myosin VI: cellular functions and motor properties. Annu Rev Cell Dev Biol. 2004;20:649-76.

[65] Chibalina MV, Poliakov A, Kendrick-Jones J, et al. Myosin VI and optineurin are required for polarized EGFR delivery and directed migration. Traffic. 2010 Oct; 11:1290-303.

[66] Au JS, Puri C, Ihrke G, et al. Myosin VI is required for sorting of AP-1B-dependent cargo to the basolateral domain in polarized MDCK cells. J Cell Biol. 2007 Apr 9;177:103-14.

[67] Bond LM, Peden AA, Kendrick-Jones J, et al. Myosin VI and its binding partner optineurin are involved in secretory vesicle fusion at the plasma membrane. Mol Biol Cell. 2010 Jan 1;22:54-65.

[68] Faber PW, Barnes GT, Srinidhi J, et al. Huntingtin interacts with a family of WW domain proteins. Hum Mol Genet. 1998 Sep;7:1463-74.

[69] Gilmore TD. Introduction to NF-kappaB: players, pathways, perspectives. Oncogene. 2006 Oct 30;25:6680-4.

[70] Schreck R, Albermann K, Baeuerle PA. Nuclear factor kappa B: an oxidative stress-responsive transcription factor of eukaryotic cells (a review). Free Radic Res Commun. 1992;17:221-37.

[71] Courtois G, Gilmore TD. Mutations in the NF-kappaB signaling pathway: implications for human disease. Oncogene. 2006 Oct 30;25:6831-43.

[72] Skaug B, Jiang X, Chen ZJ. The role of ubiquitin in NF-kappaB regulatory pathways. Annu Rev Biochem. 2009;78:769-96.

[73] Trompouki E, Hatzivassiliou E, Tsichritzis T, et al. CYLD is a deubiquitinating enzyme that negatively regulates NF-kappaB activation by TNFR family members. Nature. 2003 Aug 14;424:793-6.

[74] Kovalenko A, Chable-Bessia C, Cantarella G, et al. The tumour suppressor CYLD negatively regulates NF-kappaB signalling by deubiquitination. Nature. 2003 Aug 14;424:801-5.

[75] Sun SC. CYLD: a tumor suppressor deubiquitinase regulating NF-kappaB activation and diverse biological processes. Cell Death Differ. 2010 Jan;17:25-34.

[76] Nagabhushana A, Bansal M, Swarup G. Optineurin is required for CYLD-dependent inhibition of TNFalpha-induced NF-kappaB activation. PLoS One. 2011;6:e17477.

[77] Sudhakar C, Nagabhushana A, Jain N, et al. NF-kappaB mediates tumor necrosis factor alpha-induced expression of optineurin, a negative regulator of NF-kappaB. PLoS One. 2009;4:e5114.

[78] Wang N, Chintala SK, Fini ME, et al. Activation of a tissue-specific stress response in the aqueous outflow pathway of the eye defines the glaucoma disease phenotype. Nat Med. 2001 Mar;7:304-9.

[79] Takahashi Y, Katai N, Murata T, et al. Development of spontaneous optic neuropathy in NF-kappaBetap50-deficient mice: requirement for NF-kappaBetap50 in ganglion cell survival. Neuropathol Appl Neurobiol. 2007 Dec;33:692-705.

[80] De Marco N, Buono M, Troise F, et al. Optineurin increases cell survival and translocates to the nucleus in a Rab8-dependent manner upon an apoptotic stimulus. J Biol Chem. 2006 Jun 9;281:16147-56.

[81] Sun S, Tang Y, Lou X, et al. UXT is a novel and essential cofactor in the NF-kappaB transcriptional enhanceosome. J Cell Biol. 2007 Jul 16;178:231-44.

[82] Carey M. The enhanceosome and transcriptional synergy. Cell. 1998 Jan 9;92:5-8.

[83] Merika M, Thanos D. Enhanceosomes. Curr Opin Genet Dev. 2001 Apr;11:205-8.

[84] Son JH, Shim JH, Kim KH, et al. Neuronal autophagy and neurodegenerative diseases. Exp Mol Med. 2012 Feb 29;44:89-98.

[85] Yang Z, Klionsky DJ. An overview of the molecular mechanism of autophagy. Curr Top Microbiol Immunol. 2009;335:1-32.

[86] Tanida I, Ueno T, Kominami E. LC3 conjugation system in mammalian autophagy. Int J Biochem Cell Biol. 2004 Dec;36:2503-18.

[87] Kirkin V, McEwan DG, Novak I, et al. A role for ubiquitin in selective autophagy. Mol Cell. 2009 May 15;34:259-69.

[88] Kraft C, Peter M, Hofmann K. Selective autophagy: ubiquitin-mediated recognition and beyond. Nat Cell Biol. 2010 Sep;12:836-41.

[89] Shen X, Ying H, Qiu Y, et al. Processing of optineurin in neuronal cells. J Biol Chem. 2010 Feb 4;286:3618-29.

[90] Sippl C, Bosserhoff AK, Fischer D, et al. Depletion of optineurin in RGC-5 cells derived from retinal neurons causes apoptosis and reduces the secretion of neurotrophins. Exp Eye Res. 2011 Nov;93:669-80.

[91] Chalasani ML, Radha V, Gupta V, et al. A glaucoma-associated mutant of optineurin selectively induces death of retinal ganglion cells which is inhibited by antioxidants. Invest Ophthalmol Vis Sci. 2007 Apr;48:1607-14.

[92] Funayama T, Ishikawa K, Ohtake Y, et al. Variants in optineurin gene and their asso-
      ciation with tumor necrosis factor-alpha polymorphisms in Japanese patients with
      glaucoma. Invest Ophthalmol Vis Sci. 2004 Dec;45:4359-67.

[93] Petronczki M, Lenart P, Peters JM. Polo on the Rise-from Mitotic Entry to Cytokinesis
      with Plk1. Dev Cell. 2008 May;14:646-59.

[94] van de Weerdt BC, Medema RH. Polo-like kinases: a team in control of the division.
      Cell Cycle. 2006 Apr;5:853-64.

[95] Song B, Liu XS, Liu X. Polo-like kinase 1 (Plk1): an Unexpected Player in DNA Repli-
      cation. Cell Div. 2012;7:3.

[96] Muller U, Steinhoff U, Reis LF, et al. Functional role of type I and type II interferons
      in antiviral defense. Science. 1994 Jun 24;264:1918-21.

[97] Fitzgerald KA, McWhirter SM, Faia KL, et al. IKKepsilon and TBK1 are essential
      components of the IRF3 signaling pathway. Nat Immunol. 2003 May;4:491-6.

[98] Sakaguchi T, Irie T, Kawabata R, et al. Optineurin with amyotrophic lateral sclerosis-
      related mutations abrogates inhibition of interferon regulatory factor-3 activation.
      Neurosci Lett. 2011 Nov 21;505:279-81.

[99] Gleason CE, Ordureau A, Gourlay R, et al. Polyubiquitin binding to optineurin is re-
      quired for optimal activation of TANK-binding kinase 1 and production of interferon
      beta. J Biol Chem. 2011 Oct 14;286:35663-74.

[100] Memet S. NF-kappaB functions in the nervous system: from development to disease.
      Biochem Pharmacol. 2006 Oct 30;72:1180-95.

[101] Zhou X, Li F, Kong L, et al. Involvement of inflammation, degradation, and apopto-
      sis in a mouse model of glaucoma. J Biol Chem. 2005 Sep 2;280:31240-8.

[102] Willoughby CE, Chan LL, Herd S, et al. Defining the pathogenicity of optineurin in
      juvenile open-angle glaucoma. Invest Ophthalmol Vis Sci. 2004 Sep;45:3122-30.

[103] Wax MB, Tezel G. Neurobiology of glaucomatous optic neuropathy: diverse cellular
      events in neurodegeneration and neuroprotection. Mol Neurobiol. 2002 Aug;
      26:45-55.

[104] Chi ZL, Akahori M, Obazawa M, et al. Overexpression of optineurin E50K disrupts
      Rab8 interaction and leads to a progressive retinal degeneration in mice. Hum Mol
      Genet. 2010 Jul 1;19:2606-15.

[105] Grus FH, Joachim SC, Wuenschig D, et al. Autoimmunity and glaucoma. J Glauco-
      ma. 2008 Jan-Feb;17:79-84.

[106] Reiley WW, Jin W, Lee AJ, et al. Deubiquitinating enzyme CYLD negatively regu-
      lates the ubiquitin-dependent kinase Tak1 and prevents abnormal T cell responses. J
      Exp Med. 2007 Jun 11;204:1475-85.

[107] Pease ME, McKinnon SJ, Quigley HA, et al. Obstructed axonal transport of BDNF and its receptor TrkB in experimental glaucoma. Invest Ophthalmol Vis Sci. 2000 Mar;41:764-74.

[108] Quigley HA, McKinnon SJ, Zack DJ, et al. Retrograde axonal transport of BDNF in retinal ganglion cells is blocked by acute IOP elevation in rats. Invest Ophthalmol Vis Sci. 2000 Oct;41:3460-6.

[109] Phizicky EM, Fields S. Protein-protein interactions: methods for detection and analysis. Microbiol Rev. 1995 Mar;59:94-123.

[110] Park BC, Shen X, Samaraweera M, et al. Studies of optineurin, a glaucoma gene: Golgi fragmentation and cell death from overexpression of wild-type and mutant optineurin in two ocular cell types. Am J Pathol. 2006 Dec;169:1976-89.

[111] Xilouri M, Stefanis L. Autophagy in the central nervous system: implications for neurodegenerative disorders. CNS Neurol Disord Drug Targets. 2010 Dec;9:701-19.

[112] Harris H, Rubinsztein DC. Control of autophagy as a therapy for neurodegenerative disease. Nat Rev Neurol. 2011 Feb;8:108-17.

[113] Jellinger KA. Recent advances in our understanding of neurodegeneration. J Neural Transm. 2009 Sep;116:1111-62.

[114] Kawai T, Akira S. Toll-like receptor and RIG-I-like receptor signaling. Ann N Y Acad Sci. 2008 Nov;1143:1-20.

[115] Creagh EM, O'Neill LA. TLRs, NLRs and RLRs: a trinity of pathogen sensors that cooperate in innate immunity. Trends Immunol. 2006 Aug;27:352-7.

[116] Yoneyama M, Onomoto K, Fujita T. Cytoplasmic recognition of RNA. Adv Drug Deliv Rev. 2008 Apr 29;60:841-6.

[117] Yanai H, Savitsky D, Tamura T, et al. Regulation of the cytosolic DNA-sensing system in innate immunity: a current view. Curr Opin Immunol. 2009 Feb;21:17-22.

Chapter 7

The Role of Apolipoprotein E Gene Polymorphisms in Primary Glaucoma and Pseudoexfoliation Syndrome

Najwa Mohammed Al- Dabbagh,
Sulaiman Al-Saleh, Nourah Al-Dohayan,
Misbahul Arfin, Mohammad Tariq and
Abdulrahman Al-Asmari

Additional information is available at the end of the chapter

1. Introduction

Primary glaucoma (PG) is one of the most common eye diseases which may potentially result in bilateral blindness. Glaucoma affects 70 million people and is the second leading cause of blindness worldwide. It is estimated that by the year 2020, this number would rise to around 79.6 million [1]. The prevalence of glaucoma varies widely across the different ethnic groups [2-8] and is significantly higher in blacks (4.7%) as compared to the white (1.3%) population [9]. The prevalence of both primary open angle glaucoma (POAG) and primary angle closure glaucoma (PACG) is higher in western region of Saudi Arabia as compared to other Asian countries [10]. To date no national study has been undertaken to determine the exact prevalence of glaucoma in Saudi Arabia, though it is one of the major causes of blindness in this country.

The glaucomas are a group of relatively common optic neuropathies in which pathological loss of retinal ganglion cells cause progressive loss of sight and associated alteration in the retinal nerve fiber layer and optic nerve head. Recent studies clearly suggest that abnormalities in structure and function of retinal nerve fiber layer (RNFL) are proportional to the loss of retinal ganglion cells in glaucoma [11]. Studies on two independent patients' populations also confirmed a close association between RNFL thickness and several visual parameters [12]. The retina is a light capturing tissue consisting of more than fifty different types of cells each performing unique function that ultimately provide the visual centers in the brain the information to achieve image formation and visual perception. Photo production require the retina to have a high metabolic rate, multiple and complex membrane structures [13,14]. The photo receptor outer segments are enriched in polyunsaturated fatty acids including highly light sensitive docosahexenoic acid [15]. Recent experimental study suggests a clear role of fatty acids and cholesterol in optic nerve head blood flow and retinal nerve fibers structures. Retina has a unique mechanism for lipid uptake of low density lipoproteins which provides blood-borne lipids to all the cellular layers of retina [16,17]. Moreover, to keep its steady state lipid composition retina has the ability to synthesize cholesterol [18]. Defects in lipid metabolism in neural retina result in detrimental consequences on its structure and function. Published data clearly suggest the crucial role of lipids and lipoproteins in the pathophsiology of glaucoma [19]. Evidence from population and family studies supports heredity of glaucoma to be a complex trait. It is a genetically heterogeneous disorder attributed to the effects of individual causative mutations as well as interactions of multiple genes with a variety of environmental factors [20].

Pseudoexfoliation syndrome (PEX) is another common and clinically significant systemic condition and represents a complex, multifactorial, late-onset disease of worldwide significance with an estimated prevalence ranging from 10% to 20% of the general population [21]. It is clinically diagnosed by observation of whitish flake-like deposits of PEX material on anterior segment structures, particularly on the anterior lens surface and the pupillary border of the iris. Despite its worldwide distribution, there is a clear tendency for PEX syndrome to cluster geographically and in certain racial or ethnic subgroups. For example, there is a high prevalence of PEX syndrome in Nordic, Baltic, Mediterranean, and Arabian populations, where it affects up to 30% of individuals over age 60. The reported mean age of PEX patients ranges from 69 to 75years, and most epidemiological surveys demonstrate an increasing prevalence with increasing age. There is a significantly higher frequency and severity of optic nerve damage at the time of diagnosis, worse visual field damage, poor response to medications, more severe clinical course, and more frequent necessity for surgical intervention.

PEX is characterized by the pathological production and accumulation of an abnormal fibrillar extracellular material in the surface lining of the anterior and posterior chambers of the eye. The characteristic fibrillar PEX material is composed of microfibrillar subunits surrounded by an amorphous matrix. The material has a complex glycoprotein/proteoglycan structure composed of a protein core surrounded by glycosaminoglycan [22,23].

The fibrillar portion has been characterized as amyloid laminin, oxytalan, and various elastic tissue and basement membrane components [24-26]. Numerous studies showed positive reactions of PEX material to Congo red, showing its intense fluorescence with thioflavin T and S, and positive immunofluorescence with antiserum to amyloid, affinity for ruthenium red, positive histochemical tests for tyrosine and tryptophan [27-30]. However some other studies failed to demonstrate a positive reaction with Congo red in exfoliative deposits [24,27]. Hypothetically, amyloid might deposit in the vicinity of PEX material fibers because of the affinity they both have for elastic tissues. Moreover amyloid in the skin accumulates close to elastic fibers [31]. It has been suggested that the amyloid component normally present on elastic fibers may serve as a ligand for the amyloid–elastic fiber association [32]. Meratoja and Tarkkanen [30] showed amyloid positive material in sites atypical for PEX disease, such as the ciliary body stroma, sclera, and cornea, in eyes with PEX. Besides its presence in the eye the PEX material is found in many other parts of the body such as the eyes, skin, heart, lungs, liver, kidney, gall bladder, blood vessels, optic nerves, and meninges [26,33,34].

PEX is a heterogeneous group of disorders with both Mendelian and multifactorial traits. Even within individual families, there can be large variations in the phenotypic presentation of gene mutations. Therefore, multifactorial etiologies must be involved in PEX development. This can include polygenic and environmental factors [35]. Some genes may act as susceptibility factors that allow other genes or environmental influences to produce PEX. Further, familial aggre-gation and the increased frequency of PEX in relatives of affected subjects compared with relatives of unaffected subjects [36,37] suggest an underlying genetic component [38]. The main problems with studies on the genetic background of PEX have been the asymptomatic nature of PEX and late age of onset which make it difficult to collect multi-generation families with several affected individuals for linkage and association studies. A wide variety of inheritance models have been suggested depending on the study material [39] and, of these, the autosomal dominant mode of inheritance with incomplete penetrance has received the most support [40,41]. However, most of these studies investigating PEX inheritance have been based on small pedigrees making hypotheses about the inheritance model uncertain. Thorleifsson et al. [42] explained the genetic aetiology of PEX in virtually all instances. In Iceland and Sweden, the high-risk haplotype is very common with a frequency that averages about 50% in the general population; approximately 25% are homozygous (two copies) for the haplotype with the highest risk.

Apolipoprotein E (APOE) is the major apolipoprotein in the central nervous system, which plays important role in the uptake and redistribution of cholesterol within neuronal network [43]. Immunologically, APOE is present in many cerebral and systemic amyloidoses; such as late-onset Alzheimer's disease, Down's syndrome, and prion disorders. It is thought that APOE can promote the aggregation of amyloidogenic proteins into the β-pleated sheet conformation that is typical of all amyloid deposits, and is directly involved in the amyloid deposition and fibril formation [44,45]. This widespread association of APOE with biochemi-cally diverse amyloids has led scientists to postulate a more general role for it in the process of amyloid formation.

APOE is synthesized by Muller cells (the predominant glial cells of the retina) and released into the vitreous and then transported into the optic nerve through anterograde rapid transport where it has an important role in axonal nutrition [46]. It has been suggested that APOE plays a role in neuronal survival following ischemia and other chemical insults and particular APOE isoform may be related to neuronal degeneration in glaucoma [47]. APOE, is a 34-kDa glycosylated protein, composed of 299 amino acids encoded by a four exon polymorphic gene on chromosome 19q13.2. The gene encoding APOE has three polymorphic variants in human designated as $\epsilon2$, $\epsilon3$, and $\epsilon4$. These variants differ from one another by the presence of either C or T nucleotide at codons 112 and 158. These three alleles encode different APOE isoforms which vary significantly in structure and function including receptor binding capacity and lipid metabolism [48]. As each individual human being carries two allelic copies in a gene, six possible genotypes ($\epsilon2/\epsilon2$, $\epsilon3/\epsilon3$, $\epsilon2/\epsilon3$, $\epsilon3/\epsilon4$, $\epsilon2/\epsilon4$, and $\epsilon4/\epsilon4$) are formed by different combinations of these three alleles. The frequency of these genotypes differ significantly among different ethnic groups, however, APOE ε3/ε3 is the most predominant genotype and ε3 the most common allele in majority of populations [49-51]. The ε3 allele is considered to be the ancestral allele; and ε2 and ε4 are considered as variants, on the basis of single point mutations. Global studies on the APOE locus have shown highly significant variations in the allele frequencies of ε2, ε3, and ε4 [52-58].

The complex genetic contributions to glaucoma and PEX have been attributed to the effects of individual causative mutations as well as interactions of multiple genes with a variety of environmental factors. However, most of the identified genes do not appear to have a major role in the complex phenotype. Recent whole genome–association studies have successfully identified a number of single nucleotide polymorphisms as genetic factors conferring susceptibility to complex diseases, such as age-related macular degeneration, and it is expected that this will be a useful approach for glaucoma and PEX as well.

Earlier studies clearly point towards a possible association between APOE alleles and glaucoma. However, the results of these studies are contradictory. Some investigators suggested positive association [47,59,60] while others have shown no link at all [61-63]. Moreover, earlier studies were mainly restricted to white populations from Australia [47], United Kingdom [62,63] and Sweden [61] with only few reports from other ethnic groups restricted to Chinese and Japanese [59,60,64,65]. Similarly APOE polymorphism and the presence of ε 2 alleles have been reported to be significantly associated with the development of PEX in Turkish patients [66]. However, APOE genotypes and PEX seems to differ among study populations and no significant differences in allele and genotype frequencies between PEX and control were observed in European patients from Norway [67] and Germany [68]. Moreover, the information about the association of APOE alleles with glaucoma and PEX in Arabs is very limited. Therefore, this study on underlying genetics in these complex disorders will help analyze the genetic aspect of PEX and glaucoma in Saudi patients. In this study, we evaluated the possible association of alleles/genotypes of APOE with primary glaucoma (POAG and PACG) and PEX in Saudi population.

2. Methods

2.1. Subjects

The present study was undertaken to evaluate the association of APOE allele and genotype in Saudi primary glaucoma and pseudoexfoliation syndrome patients. A total of 200 unrelated Saudi patients with primary glaucoma [primary open angle glaucoma (POAG) and primary angle closure glaucoma (PACG)] and 51 pseudoexfoliation syndrome (PEX) were recruited from ophthalmology clinic of the Riyadh Military Hospital, Saudi Arabia. The glaucoma patient group consisted of 100 males and 100 females, with age at diagnosis ranging from 30 to 78 years (mean ± SD: 58±14.4). The control group consisted of 200 unrelated subjects, with 160 males and 40 females, ages ranging from 20 to 58 years (mean ± SD: 45±11.6). The diagnosis of PG was based on clinical observations:

A comprehensive eye examination was done that included best-corrected visual acuity (BCVA) measurements using logarithm of the minimum angle of resolution (logMAR) 4-m charts (Light House Low Vision Products, New York, NY), applanation tonometry, gonioscopy, dilated fundus examination, optic disc photography, and visual field (VF) examination. On gonioscopy, an angle was considered occludable if the pigmented trabecular meshwork was not visible in >180° of angle in dim illumination. Laser iridotomy was performed in subjects with occludable angles after consent was obtained, and they had the rest of the examination on some other day.

2.2. Visual fields

Automated VFs were performed for all the subjects with BCVA of 4/16 (logMAR 0.6) or better, using frequency-doubling perimetry (Carl Zeiss Meditec, Inc., Dublin, CA). All eligible subjects underwent C-20-1 screening (if the results were unreliable or abnormal, the test was repeated) and the N-30 threshold test. The reliability criteria were no fixation or false-positive errors for the C-20-1 screening test and < 20% fixation errors and <33% false-positive and false-negative errors for the threshold N-30 test. Visual fields with no depressed points to any level of sensitivity were considered to be normal. A provisional diagnosis of suspected glaucoma was made when the subject had one or more of the following conditions: intraocular pressure (IOP) ≥ 21 mmHg in either eye; vertical cup-to-disc ratio (VCDR) ≥ 0.7 in either eye or CDR asymmetry ≥ 0.2; and focal thinning, notching, or a splinter hemorrhage. All these subjects were asked to perform a threshold VF test using the Swedish interactive threshold algorithm Standard 30-2 program (model 750, Carl Zeiss Meditec). A glaucomatous field defect was diagnosed using a single reliable threshold VF examination of the central 30° (Swedish interactive threshold algorithm Standard 30-2). The field was considered to be abnormal if the glaucoma Hemi-field test results were outside normal limits and ≥3 abnormal contiguous non-edge points (except the nasal horizontal meridian) were depressed to $P<5\%$ [69]. Reliability criteria were as recommended by the instrument's algorithm (fixation losses <20%; false-positive and false-negative < 33%).

2.3. Diagnostic definitions

The distribution of VCDR and IOP was obtained from those subjects with reliable and normal supra-threshold VF testing using frequency-doubling perimetry. Cases of glaucoma were defined using the International Society of Geographical and Epidemiologic Ophthalmology classification [70]. Glaucoma was classified according to 3 levels of evidence. In category 1, diagnosis was based on structural and functional evidence. It required CDR or CDR asymmetry ≥ 97.5th percentile for the normal population or a neuroretinal rim width reduced to ≥ 0.1 CDR (between 11- and 1-o'clock or 5- and 7-o'clock) with a definite VF defect consistent with glaucoma using the Swedish interactive threshold algorithm 30-2. Category 2 was based on advanced structural damage with unproved field loss. This included those subjects in whom VFs could not be determined or were unreliable, with CDR or CDR asymmetry ≥ 99.5th percentile for the normal population. Lastly, category 3 consisted of persons with an IOP ≥ 99.5th percentile for the normal population, whose optic discs could not be examined because of media opacities.

Blindness was defined as a best-corrected logMAR visual acuity of < 2/40 (log MAR 1.3) and/or constriction of the VF to <10° from fixation in the better eye [71]. Hyperopia was defined as spherical equivalent > 0.50 diopter (D) in a phakic eye [72]. Diabetes mellitus was detected based on current use of antidiabetic medication and/or random blood sugar level > 200 mg/dl [73]. Thus the primary Glaucoma patients were separated in two groups (POAG and PACG) as follows:

POAG: Anterior chamber angles open and appearing normal by gonioscopy, typical features of glaucomatous optic disc as defined earlier, and visual field defects corresponding to the optic disc changes.

PACG: At least two of the criteria mentioned: glaucomatous optic disc damage or glaucomatous visual field defects in combination with anterior chamber angle partly or totally closed, appositional angle closure or synechiae in angle, absence of signs of secondary angle closure (e.g., uveitis, lens related glaucoma; microspherophakia; evidence of neovascularization in the angle and associated retinal ischemia or congenital angle anomalies). Patients with signs of intracranial disease that would cause optic nerve atrophy in x-ray computerized tomography or magnetic resonance imaging were excluded.

Diagnosis of PEX among Saudi patients visiting Primary Care Clinics of Riyadh Military Hospital was undertaken by a team of ophthalmologists. Patients visiting primary care clinic were offered free eye examination to exclude the presence of PEX. Consent was obtained from the patients after describing them the features of PEX syndrome. Patients who suffered ocular trauma or with active eye condition, and/or has undergone ocular surgery were excluded from this study.

All patients were subjected to interviews and initial evaluation was performed by the ophthalmic assistant (OA). Demographic data were collected, complaints of the eye and family history of eye problems were recorded. Visual acuity was recorded. After the preliminary examination and interview all patients were examined by an ophthalmologist for identifying the factors for PEX syndrome by the external eye examination: PEX flakes on pupil margin (undilated examination), Iris transillumination defects, evaluation of anterior chamber depth by Van Herick's technique, measurement of intraocular pressure, poor pupil dilation, and examination of the crystalline lens surface after papillary dilation for the presence of PEX material. After identification of PEX, the patients were short listed and further rechecking and confirmation of PEX syndrome was performed by (1) slit lamp examination of the anterior segment which included flakes on the pupillary margin, iris transillumination defects, flare in the A/C and corneal edema, (2) measurement of intraocular pressure (IOP) with Goldman tanometer (3) gonioscopy to record angle depth PEX flakes and/or hyperpigmentation on the trabecular meshwork which was followed by examination after dilation which included Poor pupillary dilation, flakes on the anterior lens capsule, posterior synechiae, lens opacity, phacodenesis and lens subluxation, bilaterality and symmetry and optic nerve head cupping. Out of 51 confirmed cases of PEX 25 were males and 26 females. The average age of PEX positive males and females patients was 70.43±9.62 years and 65.56±7.45 years respectively.

Venous blood was collected from the confirmed PEX and PG patients as well as healthy controls, stored at -20ºC before extraction of DNA. The study protocol was approved by the

Ethics Committee of the Hospital, and written informed consent was obtained from all study participants.

2.4. Genotyping

The genotypes of the APOE polymorphisms were determined using APOE StripAssay™ kit based on polymerase chain reaction (PCR) and reverse-hybridization technique (ViennaLab Labordiagnostika GmbH, Vienna, Austria). The procedure included three steps: (1) DNA isolation, (2) PCR amplification using biotinylated primers, (3) hybridization of amplification product to a test strip containing allele-specific oligonucleotide probes immobilizd as an array of parallel lines. Bound biotinylated sequences were detected using streptavidin- alkaline phosphatase and color substrates. To cross-check the results the genotypes of the APOE polymorphisms were also determined by PCR and restriction fragment length polymorphism (RFLP) technique. Primers were designed on the basis of the sequence data for APOE available in the GenBank to amplify the coding sequence of APOE. PCR was performed using PuRe Taq Ready-To-Go PCR Beads (Amersham, USA) with following primers:

Forward primer:	5- GAC GCG GGC ACG GCT GTC CAA GGA GCT GCA GGC
	GAC GCA GGC CCG GCT GGA CGC GGA CAT GGA GGA-3
Backward primer:	5 - AGG CCA CGC TCG ACG CCC TCG CGG GCC CCG GCC
	TGG TAC ACT-3

Genomic DNA was extracted from whole blood using a commercial kit (Qiamp; Qiagen, Hiden, Germany). The 200–300 ng of genomic DNA was used as a template in 25 μl reaction. Genomic DNA was amplified for 40 cycles. Each cycle consisted of: 94 °C for 30 sec, 68 °C for 10 sec, 72 °C for 1 min; PCR products obtained were separated by electrophoresis on 1.5% agarose gel in TAE buffer, visualized by ethidium bromide fluorescence. Fragments with the expected size were cut from the gel, purified using GFX PCR DNA Gel band purification kit (Amersham, USA). Purified DNA was digested with *Cfo* I (Hha I) enzyme, separated by agarose gel electrophoresis to identify the genotype. On the basis of size and number of various fragments generated, APOE genotypes were determined as $\varepsilon2/\varepsilon2$ with 144 bp and 96 bp, $\varepsilon3/\varepsilon3$ with 144 bp and 48 bp, $\varepsilon4/\varepsilon4$ with 72 bp and 48 bp, $\varepsilon2/\varepsilon3$ with 144 bp, 96 bp and 48 bp, $\varepsilon3/\varepsilon4$ with 144 bp, 72 bp and 48 bp, and $\varepsilon2/\varepsilon4$ with 144 bp, 96 bp, 72 bp and 48 bp fragments. The prevalence of various genotypes in patients and controls was determined. Complete matching of results was obtained following both of the above mentioned procedures.

2.5. Statistical analysis

Frequencies of various alleles and genotypes for each polymorphism were compared between patients and controls and analyzed by Fisher's exact test and the P-values < 0.05 were considered as significant. The strength of the association of disease with respect to a particular allele/ genotype is expressed by odd ratio interpreted as *relative risk* (RR) according to the method of Woolf as outlined by Schallreuter *et al* [74]. The RR was calculated only for those alleles and genotype which were increased or decreased in patients as compared to normal Saudis. The RR was calculated for all the subjects using the formula given below:

$RR = (a) \times (d)/(b) \times (c)$

a = number of patients with expression of allele or genotype

b = number of patients without expression of allele or genotype

c = number of controls with expression of allele or genotype

d = number of controls without expression of allele or genotype.

Etiologic Fraction (EF): The EF indicates the hypothetical genetic component of the disease. Values 0.0-0.99 are of significance. It was calculated for positive association (RR>1) using the following formula [75].

$EF = (RR-1)f/RR$, where $f = a/a+c$

Preventive Fraction (PF): The PF indicates the hypothetical protective effect of one specific antigen for the disease. It was calculated for negative association only where RR<1 using following formula [75].

$PF = (1-RR)f/RR (1-f) + f$, where $f = a/a+c$

Values <1.0 indicated the protective effect of the genotype/ allele against the manifestation of disease.

3. Results

Out of 200 PG patients 134 were diagnosed as having POAG and 66 as having PACG. Diagnosis of POAG was based on category 1 in 20 subjects (14.93 %) and category 2 in 114 subjects (85.07 %). Between category 1 and category 2 there was no significant different in age, IOP and gender distribution. One subject was blind in both eyes and 1 subject had unilateral blindness due to POAG. There were 66 subjects with PACG. Diagnosis was based on category 1 in 16 subjects (24.24%), category 2 in 46 subjects (69.70%), and category 3 in 4 subjects (6.06%). Three subjects (4.55 %) bilaterally, 4 (6.06 %) were unilaterally blind due to PACG.

The results of frequency of APOE alleles and genotypes in the PG patients and the control subjects are summarized in Tables 1, 2,3,4,5 and 6. The frequency of the ε3 alleles was significantly lower in the glaucoma patients (86.5 %) compared to the control subjects (95.75 %, P=0.0001, RR=0.284, PF=0.544). On the other hand the frequencies of the ε4 allele was significantly higher in the glaucoma patients as compared to controls (12.25% vs 4.25%, P=0.0001, RR=3.145, EF=0.506). The allele ε2 was present only in 5 patients while totally absent in control groups (Table 1).

Allele	Glaucoma (N=400)		Control (N=400)		P-value	RR	EF*/PF
	Number	Frequency (%)	Number	Frequency(%)			
ε4	49	12.25	17	4.25	0.0001‡	3.145	0.506*
ε3	346	86.50	383	95.75	0.0001‡	0.284	0.544
ε2	5	1.25	0	0.0	0.030‡	-	-

N, number of alleles; RR, relative risk; EF, etiological fraction; PF, preventive fraction; ‡, statistically significant

Table 1. Distribution of APOE allele frequencies in glaucoma patients and matched control subjects.

Our study on various genotypes of APOE also showed variations in patient and control groups (Table 2). The prevalence of ε3/ε3, ε3/ε4, ε4/ε4, ε2/ε3, and ε2/ε4 was 75.5, 20.5, 1.5,1.5 and 1.0% in patients and 91.5, 8.5, 0,0 and 0 % in control group respectively.

Genotype	Glaucoma (N=200)		Control (N=200)		P-value	RR	EF*/PF
	Number	Frequency (%)	Number	Frequency (%)			
ε3/ε3	151	75.50	183	91.50	0.0001‡	0.286	0.530
ε3/ε4	41	20.50	17	8.50	0.0006‡	2.775	0.491*
ε4/ε4	3	1.50	0	0.0	0.1240	-	-
ε2/ε3	3	1.50	0	0.0	0.1240	-	-
ε2/ε4	2	1.00	0	0.0	0.2493	-	-
ε2/ε2	0	0.0	0	0.0	-	-	-

N, number of subjects; RR, relative risk; EF, etiological fraction; PF, preventive fraction; ‡, statistically significant

Table 2. Distribution of APOE genotypes in glaucoma patients and matched controls

Though the frequency of ε3/ε3 genotype was higher in both the test and control Saudi population, the statistical analysis of data showed strongly significant difference in ε3/ ε3 genotype frequencies between patients and controls (P=0.0001, RR=0.286, PF=0.53). The difference in the frequencies of the second common genotype (ε3/ ε4) was also statistically significant between the two groups (P=0.0006) being more in glaucoma patients. Genotypes ε4/ε4, ε2/ε3 were found only in 1.5% and ε2/ε4 in 1% of patients while being completely absent in the controls (P=0.124). The genotypes ε2/ε2 was absent in both patient and control groups. These results indicated that allele ε4 and genotype ε3/ ε4 are associated with glaucoma and can be a risk factor while allele ε3 and genotype ε3/ ε3 may be protective in Saudis. The frequencies of various genotypes and alleles were not significantly different in male and female patients clearly indicating that gender plays no role in genotype/ allele distributions among populations (Table 3).

Genotype/Allele	Male (N=100)		Female (N=100)		P-value
	Number	Frequency (%)	Number	Frequency (%)	
ε3/ε3	71	71.00	80	80.00	0.143
ε3/ε4	26	26.00	15	15.00	0.079
ε4/ε4	0	0.0	3	3.00	0.123
ε2/ε3	2	2.00	1	1.00	0.623
ε2/ε4	1	1.00	1	1.00	0.999
ε3	170	85.00	176	88.00	0.385
ε4	27	13.50	22	11.00	0.451
ε2	3	1.50	2	1.00	0.685

N, number of subjects

Table 3. Distribution of APOE genotypes and alleles in male and female glaucoma patients

Though the distribution of APOE genotypes and alleles was not significantly different in two types of glaucoma (Table 4) however when compared with controls separately, significant difference was found in the frequencies of genotypes ε3/ε4, ε3/ε3 and alleles ε4 and ε3 in POAG and controls.

Genotype/Allele	Open angle glaucoma (134) N (%)	Angle closure glaucoma (66) N (%)	P-value
ε3/ε4	30 (22.39)	11 (16.66)	0.456
ε4/ε4	3 (2.24)	00	0.552
ε3/ε3	98 (73.13)	53 (80.30)	0.298
ε2/ε3	2 (1.49)	1 (1.52)	1.000
ε2/ε4	1 (0.75)	1 (1.52)	0.552
ε4	37 (13.81)	12 (9.09)	0.197
ε2	3 (1.12)	2 (1.52)	0.666
ε3	228 (85.07)	118(89.39)	0.277

N, number of subjects

Table 4. Comparison of APOE genotype/ allele frequencies in patients with POAG and PACG

The frequency of genotype ε3/ ε4 and ε 4 allele was significantly more ($P= 0.0006$ and 0.0001 respectively) in POAG patients as compared to controls (Table 5).

Genotype/Allele	Open angle glaucoma (134) N (%)	Controls (200) N (%)	p-value	RR	EF*/PF
ε3/ε4	30 (22.39)	17 (8.50)	0.0006⁺	3.105	0.432*
ε4/ε4	3 (2.24)	00	0.063	-	-
ε3/ε3	98 (73.13)	183 (91.50)	0.0001⁺	0.252	0.507
ε2/ε3	2 (1.49)	00	0.160	-	-
ε2/ε4	1 (0.75)	00	0.401	-	-
ε4	37 (13.81)	17(4.25)	0.0001⁺	3.608	0.495*
ε2	3 (1.12)	00	0.064	-	
ε3	228 (85.07)	383 (95.75)	0.0001⁺	0.253	0.524

N, number of subjects; RR, relative risk; EF, etiological fraction; PF, preventive fraction; ⁺, statistically significant

Table 5. Distribution of APOE genotype/ allele frequencies in patients with POAG and matched controls

The frequency of allele ε3 and ε3/ε3 genotype was significantly higher in controls (P=0.0001). Similarly, the frequency of various genotypes of APOE differ between PACG and controls but the differences were not statistically significant except for ε3/ε3(P=0.022) (Table 6). However, the frequency of allele ε4 was higher in PACG whereas ε3 in controls indicating that the allele ε4 is also significantly associated with PACG in Saudis while genotype ε3/ε3 and allele ε3 may be protective.

Genotype/Allele	Angle closure glaucoma (66) N (%)	Controls (200) N (%)	P-value	RR	EF*/PF
ε3/ε4	11 (16.66)	17 (8.50)	0.067	2.152	0.210*
ε4/ε4	0	00	-	-	-
ε2/ε3	1 (1.52)	00	0.248	-	-
ε2/ε4	1 (1.52)	00	0.248	-	-
ε3/ε3	53 (80.30)	183 (91.50)	0.022⁺	0.378	0.269
ε4	12 (9.09)	17(4.25)	0.045⁺	2.252	0.229*
ε2	2 (1.52)	00	0.061	-	-
ε3	118(89.39)	383 (95.75)	0.010⁺	0.374	0.282

N, number of subjects; RR, relative risk; EF, etiological fraction; PF, preventive fraction;

Table 6. Distribution of APOE genotype/ allele frequencies in patients with PACG and matched controls

Over all prevalence of PEX in our study was 3.03%. Unilateral PEX was noted in 38% while bilateral PEX in 62% of the PEX patients (Figures.1 & 2). However, there was no significant difference in the prevalence of PEX in male and female. Prevalence distribution of PEX with the age in Saudi population is summarized in (Table 7). The prevalence of PEX varied from 0.50% to 25% in various age groups. The majority of the patients screened was in the age group of 50-60 years followed by those from <50 years, 61-70 years, 71-80 years and 81-100 years groups. The prevalence of PEX increased with progressing of age.

Age group (years)	Patients screened (N)	PEX positive patients (N)	Frequency of PEX (%)
<50	600	3	0.50
51-60	850	27	3.17
61-70	200	16	8.00
71-80	30	4	13.33
81-100	4	1	25
Total	1684	51	3.03

N, number of patients

Table 7. Age specific prevalence of PEX in Saudi patients

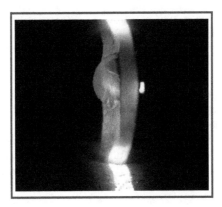

Figure 1. Showing massive PEX material in the papillary area forming a membrane like deposit

The results of frequency of APOE alleles and genotypes in the PEX patients and the control subjects are summarized in Tables 8 and 9. The frequency of the ε3 alleles was significantly lower in the PEX patients (82.35 %) compared to the control subjects (95.75 %, P=0.0001, RR=0.207, PF=0.373). On the other hand the frequencies of the ε2 and ε4 allele were significantly higher in the PEX patients as compared to controls (2.94% vs 0.00%, P=0.0081 and 14.70% vs 4.25%, P=0.0004, RR=3.884, EF=0.347 respectively). The allele ε2 was absent in control group (Table 8).

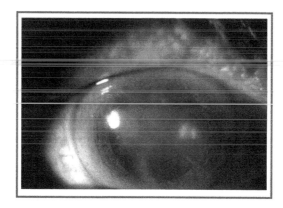

Figure 2. Shows deposition of PEX material more peripherally indicating wide pupillary excursion

Allele	Pseudoexfoliation (N=102)		Control (N=400)		P-value	RR	EF*/PF
	Number	Frequency (%)	Number	Frequency(%)			
ε4	15	14.70	17	4.25	0.0004⁺	3.884	0.347
ε3	84	82.35	383	95.75	0.0001⁺	0.207	0.373
ε2	3	2.94	0	0.0	0.0081⁺	-	-

N, number of subjects; RR, relative risk; EF, etiological fraction; PF, preventive fraction; ⁺, statistically significant

Table 8. Distribution of APOE allele frequencies in PEX patients and matched controls

Our study on various genotypes of APOE also showed variations in PEX patient and control groups (Table 9). The prevalence of ε3/ε3, ε3/ε4, ε4/ε4, ε2/ε3 and ε2/ε4 was 70.58, 21.56, 1.96, 1.96 and 3.92% in patients and 91.5, 8.5, 0, 0, and 0 % in control group respectively. Though the frequency of ε3/ε3 genotype was high in both the test and control Saudi population, the statistical analysis of data showed significant difference in ε3/ ε3 genotype frequencies between patients and controls, being more in controls than patients ($P=0.0002$, RR=0.222, PF=0. 363). The difference in the frequencies of the second common genotype ε3/ ε4 was also statistically significant between the two groups and was found to be increased in PEX patient group ($P=0.012$, RR=2.96, EF=0.259). Genotypes ε4/ε4, ε2/ε3 and ε2/ε4 were found only in patients while being completely absent in the controls. The genotype ε2/ε2, was absent in both the groups (Table 9).

These results indicated that alleles ε4 and ε2 and genotype ε3/ ε4 and ε2/ε4 were associated with PEX and can be a risk factor while allele ε3 and genotype ε3/ ε3 may be protective in Saudis. The frequencies of various genotypes and alleles were almost similar in male and female patients clearly indicating that gender plays no role in genotype/ allele distributions among populations.

Genotype	Pseudoexfoliation (N=51)		Control (N=200)		P-value	RR	EF*/PF
	Number	Frequency (%)	Number	Frequency (%)			
ε3/ε3	36	70.58	183	91.50	0.0002+	0.222	0.363
ε3/ε4	11	21.56	17	8.50	0.012+	2.960	*0.259
ε4/ε4	1	1.96	0	0.0	0.203	-	-
ε2/ε2	0	0	0	0.0	-	-	-
ε2/ε3	1	1.96	0	0.0	0.203	-	-
ε2/ε4	2	3.92	0	0.0	0.040+	-	-

N, number of subjects; RR, relative risk; EF, etiological fraction; PF, preventive fraction; +, statistically significant

Table 9. Distribution of APOE genotype frequencies in PEX patients and matched controls

4. Discussion

The result of this study showed a very high frequency (95.75%) of allele ε3, very low frequency (4.25%) of ε4 and absence of allele ε2 in control population. Global studies on APOE locus have shown highly significant variations in allele frequencies among various populations. Studies from various geographical locations and ethnicities have reported a wide range of frequencies of ε2 (0-12%), ε3 (75-90 %) and ε4 (6-20%) [52-58]. The differences in the APOE genotype/allele frequencies in different populations may be attributed to environmental factors as well as genetic differences. The ε3 allele is the most frequent in all the human groups, especially in populations with a long established agricultural economy, whereas APOE ε4 allele remains higher in populations where the economy of foraging still exists or food supply is/was scarce and sporadically available [76]. Data on APOE allele frequencies collected from literature showed that the APOE allele distributions were different between North and South Europe. Additionally, compared to northern European countries, Mediterranean countries such as Italy, Turkey and Greece had lower frequencies of APOE- ε2 and ε4 alleles [77-79].

Results of present study revealed significant differences in the frequencies of ε3 and ε4 alleles in glaucoma patient as compared to control groups (Table 1). Allele ε3 being more common in controls while ε4 was predominant in glaucoma patients suggesting that the inheritance of the ε4 allele might be a risk factor whereas ε3 might exert a protective effect for glaucoma in Saudi population. Neuroprotective effect of ε3 is also evident from several earlier studies. APOE has an isoform specific effect on neuronal growth with ε3 stimulating neuronal elongation and neurite outgrowth on dorsal root ganglion [80]. In individuals with acute cerebral ischemia, such as an intracerebral hemorrhage, the ε3 allele confers a much higher survival and functional recovery whereas ε4 leads higher rate of disability and mortality [81]. Our results clearly suggest that presence of ε4 is associated with high risk of both POAG and PACG. Vickers et al [47] also reported an association between the ε4 allele and NTG in the Tasmanian population. Recently, Yaun et al [65] reported that the ε4 may be a latent risk factor in developing primary glaucoma in Chinese population. On the other hand Liew et al [82] found a weak association between APOE ε4 and retinal microvascular degeneration. Contrary to these findings a decrease risk of NTG in Chinese [59,60] and POAG in Japanese with ε4 allele [64] has been reported, whereas some investigators reported no link between APOE polymorphism and glaucoma [61,62].

Besides glaucoma, APOE ε4 allele has been identified as a genetic susceptibility factor for a variety of neurodegenerative disorders in diverse ethnic populations [83-86]. APOE ε4 allele has also been associated with early age-at-onset of AD in a dose dependent manner [87,88]. Interestingly, a high incidence of glaucoma in AD patients clearly suggests a close association between ophthalmic and neurodegenerative disorders [89,90]. It has been hypothesized that the cellular mechanisms involved in the degeneration of optic nerve cells in glaucoma are quite similar to the neurodegenerative changes in AD [47,91,92]. APOE allele ε4 is also strongly linked with increased risk of Parkinson's disease, schizophrenia and coronary artery disease [93-99]. Possession of the ε4 allele is also associated with a retarded recovery after traumatic head injury [100,101]. The exact mechanism by which APOE ε4 exerts its deleterious effect is far from clear. However, APOE alleles has been reported to modulate the biological functions of APOE in part by altering the binding of the different lipoprotein lipid classes [93]. Individuals carrying the ε4 allele have higher plasma and neuronal levels of cholesterol as compared to individuals with ε2 or ε3. APOE immunoreactivity has been localized to basal laminar deposits and soft drusen in age related macular degeneration [102]. APOE has also been localized to the Müller cells (specialized retinal glia) [46,102] and this protein may be increased in Müller cells in glaucomatous eyes [103], indicating that this glial cell may have a role in the retinal response to glaucomatous injury.

On the other hand, earlier genetic studies support the concept that APOE would directly be involved in the amyloid deposition and fibril formation; and they suggest a close association between one of the main isoforms of APOE encoded by the ε4 allele and both familial and sporadic late-onset Alzheimer's disease (AD) [44,45]. In addition, deposits in various amyloidoses and prion diseases such as Down's syndrome, cystatin C-related Icelandic-type hereditary amyloid angiopathy, Creutzfeldt-Jakob disease, Lewy body dementia, dementia in Parkinson's disease include both biochemically and immunohistochemically detectable amounts of APOE [104-107].

The higher frequency of ε3/ ε3 in controls as compared to the patients indicated a protective effect of ε3/ ε3 on development of glaucoma in Saudis. Though the genotypes ε4/ε4, ε2/ ε3 and ε2/ε4 were only found in glaucoma patients and completely absent in normal Saudi population however, the differences were statistically insignificant. The genotypes ε2/ε2, was absent in both patients and control group. Earlier studies on APOE polymorphism in general healthy population also showed absence of genotypes containing ε2 allele among Saudis [51,108] as well as Native Americans [109].

This study showed that prevalence of PEX in Saudi Population was 3.03%. No significant difference was found in prevalence of PEX between male and female whereas the rate of prevalence varied in different age group. the prevalence of PEX increased with progressing of age. Earlier investigators from Saudi Arabia using a very small hospital based study reported overall prevalence of PEX as 9.3% [110]. PEX occurs worldwide, although reported prevalence rates vary extensively with geographical location, as well as with ethnicity [21,111]. The prevalence of PEX varies significantly among Asians. The prevalence of PEX has been reported to be 3.01% and 6.28% in two different age groups in Southern Indian population [112], 6.45 % in Pakistani population [113], 3.4% in Japanese [114], 0.4% in Chinese [115] and 0.2 to 0.7% in Chinese Singaporeans [116]. In Scandinavia, the prevalence among persons over age 60 varies from over 20% in Finland to about 25% in Iceland. Aasved [117] found prevalence of 6.3%, 4.0%, and 4.7% in persons over age 60 in Norway, England, and Germany, respectively. Forsius [118] studied prevalence in patients over age 60 years in varied groups and found prevalence ranging from 0% in Greenland Eskimos to 21% in Icelanders. Lantukh and Piatin [119] found a low prevalence in native Siberian Tchutchee, but a much higher rate among immigrants to the area indicating ethnic variations. Similarly in New Mexico, Spanish-American men are nearly six times as likely to develop PEX than are non-Spanish-Americans [120].

The prevalence of PEX may also vary within the same country in similar environments and over short distances as found in present study. Similarly, in France the prevalence in over age 70 years varies from 3.6% in Toulon to 20.6% in Brest [121]. Ringvold et al [122] also found rates of 10.2%, 19.6%, and 21.0% in three closely situated municipalities in central Norway. The reasons underlying true variations, both from one population to another and within more or less homogeneous populations, remain to be explained. Geographic distribution patterns may perhaps be explained either by regional gene pools or by environmental influences. Persons living at lower latitudes (Greece, Saudi Arabia, and Iran) appear to develop PEX at younger ages [123]. Exposure to sunlight (ultraviolet radiation) may or may not be implicated. Forsius and Lukka [124] found no PEX in Eskimos versus 20% among Lapps living at the same latitude.

Similar to our observations, the prevalence of PEX increases with age in most of the studies [112,114,117]. Forsius [125] found PEX incidence to double every decade after age 50. These variations in prevalence rates may consequently be caused, to varying degrees, by genuine differences in genetic, ethnic and environmental factors and by methodological differences in age and sex distribution, diagnostic criteria, experience of the examiners in diagnosing the syndrome and the thoroughness of their examination [126].

This study also indicated that allele ε4 was associated with PEX and can be a risk factor while allele ε3 may be protective for PEX similar to PG in Saudi patients. Allele ε2 was found in only 2.94% of the PEX while totally absent in controls. Contrary to our results, Yilmaz et al [66] reported a close association of ε2 allele with PEX in Turkish population. According to them PEX have significantly higher frequency of ε2 allele (50%). In their study the frequency of genotypes carrying ε2 allele was also significantly higher in PEX. They have suggested that especially when ε2 allele is heterozygous, the possibility of developing PEX increases which could be an indicator for pathogenicity when this allele frequency is over 30% in the PEX group. In our study ε2/ ε3 and ε2/ ε4 genotypes are found only in 1 and 2 cases respectively. As the genotype frequencies are low in these groups, it is difficult to make general conclusion on statistically insignificant data.

On the other hand our results for APOE polymorphism in PEX indicated that genotype ε3/ ε4 was also associated with PEX ($P=0.012$) and can be a risk factor while genotype ε3/ ε3 may be protective for PEX (P=0.0002) similar to PG in Saudi patients. In addition, the control group had a significantly higher frequency of the ε3 allele (95.75%) than the PEX group (82.35%), showing that this allele had a protective effect for developing the disease (P=0.0001). This is in agreement with Yilmaz et al [66] who reported a protective role of APOE ε3 allele in patients with exfoliation syndrome in Turkish population. However there are reports indicating no association of APOE genotypes and PEX in Germans or Italians [68] and Norwegians [67].

In the literature, ε 4 allele has been shown to be risky for developing amyloidoses in AD [44,45,104,106,107]. Yilmaz et al [66] suggested PEX to belong to the amyloidosis group depending on the deposition of amyloid or amyloid-like material throughout the body. As stated earlier inheritance of the ε4 allele has also been associated with elevated risk to Alzheimer's disease. In this regard, it is interesting that visual deficits have been reported in Alzheimer's disease cases. However, there are conflicting reports as to whether visual field loss observed in a relatively high proportion of Alzheimer's disease cases is associated with retinal or central damage [127-129]. It has also been noted that both Alzheimer's disease and Parkinson's disease cases have increased glaucomatous retinal changes [90]. In the light of the these findings, there may be similar cellular processes involving APOE related to neuronal damage. It has been argued that both Alzheimer's disease and glaucoma/PEX are ultimately axon damaging conditions and it is how nerve cells respond to this injury that leads to overall neuronal degeneration and the clinical picture of progressive loss of function [130]. Müller cells that express particular APOE isoforms may thus have an important role in regulating the response of retinal ganglion cells to injury. However, it cannot be ruled out that APOE may be acting centrally to promote β-amyloid fibril formation in structures such as the lateral geniculate nucleus [131] and that these plaques are causing damage to retinal axons and visual pathways. In this regard, it would be intriguing to determine whether glaucoma and PEX cases may have a higher incidence of Alzheimer-type dementia.

The result of this study suggests that APOE alleles may influence the risk of glaucoma and PEX. The inheritance of the ε4 allele is associated with elevated risk of POAG, PACG and PEX and ε3 may exert protection for both type of glaucoma as well as PEX. Genotypes containing allele ε2 (ε2/ε3, ε2/ε4) were found only in small number of patients (3POAG, 2 PACG and 1PEX) whereas altogether absent in Saudi normal population so it is difficult to derive any conclusion. Further studies involving larger number of patients from different race/tribes of Saudi Arabia are warranted to reach any definite conclusion as the APOE allele frequencies from same population (Turkish) reported by different authors are not uniform [66,132,133]. These differences in the distribution of APOE allele and genotype in single population in different studies have been attributed to geographical/ racial differences and/ or variations in genotyping methodology.

Though the inheritance of the ε4 allele seems to be associated with elevated risk of primary glaucoma and PEX in our Saudi population. However, it will be important to replicate these results in populations from other geographical locations of Saudi Arabia. The significance of inheritance of these APOE allelic isoforms has yet to be established, as is the case for the potential role of this protein in many other neurodegenerative conditions, but it may be linked with associated hypertension, formation of central β-amyloid deposits or a more general role in the regulation of lipids following axonal injury. However, our results together with similar data elucidated a potential overlap between the degenerative pathways underlying glaucoma/ PEX and Alzheimer-type dementia and brain injury.

5. Conclusion

This study clearly showed that the APOE polymorphism represents a major risk factor for ophthalmic/neurodegenerative diseases and this study together with previous studies pointed to a possible association between APOE alleles and PG/PEX in defined populations. However, the association between APOE genotype and PG/PEX seems to differ among studied populations, indicating a modifying rather than a direct genetic effect. Although our results indicated ε4 allele to be significantly associated with the development of primary glaucoma (POAG and PACG) and PEX in a Saudi population. Further studies are warranted to understand the role of APOE allelic isoforms in various ethnic populations and to predict the predisposition to degenerative eye diseases like PEX and glaucoma.

Acknowledgements

The authors would like to thank S. Sadaf Rizvi and Mohammad Al-Asmari for their help in laboratory work.

Author details

Najwa Mohammed Al-Dabbagh[1], Sulaiman Al-Saleh[1], Nourah Al-Dohayan[1], Misbahul Arfin[2], Mohammad Tariq[2] and Abdulrahman Al-Asmari[2*]

*Address all correspondence to: abdulrahman.alasmari@gmail.com

1 Department of Ophthalmology, Riyadh Military Hospital Riyadh, Saudi Arabia

2 Research Center, Riyadh Military Hospital Riyadh, Saudi Arabia

References

[1] Quigley HA, Broman AT. The number of people with glaucoma worldwide in 2010 and 2020. British Journal of Ophthalmology 2006;90: 262-267.

[2] He M, Foster PJ, Huang W, Zheng Y, Freidman DS, et al. Prevalence and Clinical characteristics of Glaucoma in Adult Chinese: A population based study in Liwan

District, Guangzhou. Investigative Ophthalmology & Visual Science 2006;47: 2782-2788.

[3] Wong TY, Loon SC, Saw SM. The epidemiology of age related eye diseases in Asia. British Journal of Ophthalmology 2006;90: 506-511.

[4] Sakata K, Sakata LM, Sakata VM, Santini, Hopker LM. Prevalence of Glaucoma in a South Brazilian Population: Projeto Glaucoma. Investigative ophthalmology & visual Science 2007;48: 4974-4979.

[5] Cedrone C, Mancino R, Cerulli A, Cesareo M, Nucci C. Epidemiology of primary glaucoma : prevalence, incidence, and blinding effects. Progress in Brain Research 2008;173: 3-14.

[6] Vijaya L, George R, Arvind H, Baskaran M, Ramesh V. Prevalence of primary angle-closure disease in an urban South Indian population and comparison with a rural population. The Chennai glaucoma study. Ophthalmology 2008;115(4): 655-660.

[7] Vijaya L, George R, Baskaran M , Arvind H, Raju P. Prevalence of primary open angle glaucoma in an Urban South Indian population and comparison with a rural population. The Chennai glaucoma study. Ophthalmology 2008;115(4): 648-654.

[8] Pekmezci M, Vo B, Lim AK, Hirabayashi D, Tanaka GH. The characteristics of glaucoma in Japanese Americans. Archives of Ophthalmology 2009;127: 167-171.

[9] Kwon YH, Fingert JH, Kuehn MH, Alward WL. Primary open angle glaucoma. New England Journal of Medicine 2009;360: 1113-1124.

[10] Eid TM, El-Harwary I, El-Menawy W. Prevalence of glaucoma types and legal blindness from glaucoma in the Western region of Saudi Arabia: a hospital based study. International Ophthalmology 2009;29: 477-483.

[11] McKinnon SJ, Goldberg LD, Peeples P, Walt JG, Bramley TJ. Current management of glaucoma and the need for complete therapy. The American Journal of Managed Care 2008;14(1 Suppl): S20-7.

[12] Savini G, Zanini M, Carelli V, Sadun AA, Ross-Cisneros FN, et al. Correlation between retinal nerve fibre layer thickness and optic nerve head size: an optical coherence tomography study. British journal of Ophthalmology 2005;89(4): 489-492.

[13] Gordon W C, Bazan NG. Cellular organization and biochemistry of the retina. London: Chapman and Hall;1997.

[14] Yu DY, Cringle SJ. Oxygen distribution and consumption within the retina in vascularised and avascular retinas and in animal models of retinal disease. Progress in Retinal and Eye Research 2001;20: 175-208.

[15] Fliesler SJ, Anderson RE. Chemistry and metabolism of lipids in the vertebrate retina. Progress in Lipid Research 1983;22: 79-131.

[16] Gordiyenko N, Campos M, Lee JW, Fariss R N, Sztein J, et al. RPE cells internalize low-density lipoprotein (LDL) and oxidized LDL (oxLDL) in large quantities in vitro and in vivo. Investigative Ophthalmology & Visual Science 2004;45: 2822-2829.

[17] Tserentsoodol N, Sztein J, Campos M, Gordiyenko NV, Fariss RN, et al. Uptake of cholesterol by the retina occurs primarily via a low density lipoprotein receptor-mediated process. Molecular Vision 2006;12: 1306-1318.

[18] Fliesler SJ, Florman R, Rapp LM, Pittler SJ, Keller RK. In vivo biosynthesis of choles-terol in the rat retina. Febs Letters 1993;335: 234-238.

[19] Fourgeux C, Bron A, Acar N, Creuzot-Garcher C, Bretillon L. 24S-hydroxycholesterol and cholesterol-24S-hydroxylase (CYP46A1) in the retina: from cholesterol homeosta-sis to pathophysiology of glaucoma. Chemistry and Physics of Lipids 2011;164(6): 496-499.

[20] Tielsch JM, Sommer A, Katz J, Royall RM, Quigley HA, et al. Racial variations in the prevalence of primary open-angle glaucoma. The Baltimore Eye Survey. Journal of the American Medical Association 1991;266: 369-374.

[21] Ritch R, Schlötzer-Schrehardt U. Exfoliation syndrome. Survey of Ophthalmology 2001;45: 265-315.

[22] Li ZY, Streeten BW, Wallace RN. Association of elastin with pseudoexfoliative mate-rial: an immunoelectron microscopic study. Current Eye Research 1988;7: 1163-1172.

[23] Netland PA, Ye H, Streeten BW, Hernandez M R. Elastosis of the lamina cribrosa in pseudoexfoliation syndrome with glaucoma. Ophthalmology 1995;102: 878-886.

[24] Dark AJ, Streeten BW, Cornwall CC. Pseudoexfoliative disease of the lens: a study in electron microscopy and histochemistry. British Journal of Ophthalmology 1977;61: 462-472.

[25] Morrison JC, Green WR. Light microscopy of the exfoliation syndrome. Acta Oph-thalmologica (Copenh.) 1988;184: 5-27.

[26] Streeten BW, Li ZY, Wallace RN, Eagle RC Jr, Keshgegian AA. Pseudoexfoliative fi-brillopathy in visceral organs of a patient with pseudoexfoliation syndrome. Ar-chives of Ophthalmology 1992;110: 1757-1762.

[27] Bertelsen TI, Ehlers N. Morphological and histochemical studes on fibrillopathia epi-thelocapsularis. Acta Ophthalmologica (Copenh) 1969;47: 476-488.

[28] Ringvold A. Light and electron microscopy of the anterior iris surface in eyes with and without pseudo-exfoliation syndrome. Graefe's Archive For Clinical and Experi-mental Ophthalmology 1973;188:131-137.

[29] Davanger M, Pedersen OO. Pseudo-exfoliation on the anterior lens surface. Demon-stration and examination of an interfibrillar ground substance. Acta Ophthalmologi-ca 1975;53: 3-18.

[30] Meretoja J, Tarkkanen A. Occurrence of amyloid in eyes with pseudoexfoliation. Ophthalmic Research 1977;9: 80-91.

[31] Yanagihara M, Kato F, Shikano Y, Fukushima N, Mori S. Intimate structural association of amyloid and elastic fibers in systemic and cutaneous amyloidoses. Journal of Cutaneous Pathology 1985;12(2): 110-116.

[32] Winkelmann RK, Peters MS, Venencie PY. Amyloid elastosis. A new cutaneous and systemic pattern of amyloidosis. Archives of Dermatology 1985;121(4): 498-502.

[33] Streeten BW, Dark AJ, Wallace RN, Li ZY, Hoepner JA. Pseudoexfoliative fibrillopathy in the skin of patients with ocular pseudoexfoliation. American Journal of Ophthalmology 1990;110: 490-499.

[34] Schlötzer-Schrehardt U, Dörfler S, Naumann GO. Immunohistochemical localization of basement membrane components in pseudoexfoliation material of the lens capsule. Current Eye Research 1992;11: 343-355.

[35] Wani FR, Romana M, Singh T, Wani IR, Wani IR, et al. Prevalence of Exfoliative Glaucoma among Kashmiri Population: A Hospital Based Study. International Journal of Health Sciences (Qassim) 2009;3(1): 51–57.

[36] Pohjanpelta P, Hurskainen L. Studies on relatives of patients with glaucoma simplex and patients with pseudoexfoliation of the lens capsule. Acta Ophthalmologica (Copenh) 1972;50(2): 255-261.

[37] Tarkkanen A. Pseudoexfoliation of the lens capsule. Acta Ophthalmologica. 1962;71: 1-98.

[38] Allingham RR, Loftsdottir M, Gottfredsdottir MS, Thorgeirsson E, Jonasson F, et al. Pseudoexfoliation syndrome in Icelandic families. British Journal of Ophthalmology 2001;85: 702-707.

[39] Damji KF, Bains HS, Stefansson E, Loftsdottir M, Sverrisson T, et al. Is pseudoexfoliation syndrome inherited? A review of genetic and nongenetic factors and a new observation. Ophthalmic Genetics 1998;19: 175-185.

[40] Forsius HR, Fellman JO, Eriksson AW. Genetics of exfoliation syndrome (pseudoexfoliation of the lens). New Trends in Ophthalmology 1993;3: 135-139.

[41] Lemmelä S, Forsman E, Sistonen P, Eriksson A, Forsius H, et al. Genome-wide scan of exfoliation syndrome. Investigative Ophthalmology & Visual Science 2007;48(9): 4136-4142.

[42] Thorleifsson G, Magnusson KP, Sulem P, Walters GB, Gudbjartsson DF, et al. Common sequence variants in the LOXL1 gene confer susceptibility to exfoliation glaucoma. Science 2007;317: 1397-1400.

[43] Laws SM, Hone E, Gandy S, Martins RN. Expanding the association between the APOE gene and the risk of Alzheimer's disease: possible roles for APOE promoter

polymorphisms and alterations in APOE transcription. Journal of Neurochemistry 2003;84: 1215-1236.

[44] Strittmatter WJ, Weisgraber KH, Huang DY, Dong LM, Salvesen GS, et al. Binding of human apolipoprotein E to synthetic amyloid beta peptide: isoform-specific effects and implications for late-onset Alzheimer disease. Proceedings of the National Academy of Sciences of the United States of America 1993;90(17): 8098-8102.

[45] Castano EM, Prelli F, Wisniewski T, Golabek A, Kumar RA, et al. Fibrillogenesis in Alzheimer's disease of amyloid beta peptides and apolipoprotein E. Biochemical Journal 1995;306: 599-604.

[46] Amaratunga A, Abraham CR, Edwards RB, Sandell JH, Schreiber BM, et al. Apolipoprotein E is synthesized in the retina by Muller glial cells, secreted into the vitreous, and rapidly transported into the optic nerve by retinal ganglion cells. Journal of Biological Chemistry 1996;271: 5628-5632.

[47] Vickers JC, Craig JE, Stankovich J, McCormak GH, West AK, et al. The apolipoprotein epsilon4 gene is associated with elevated risk of normal tension glaucoma. Molecular Vision 2002;8: 389-393.

[48] Artiga MJ, Bullido MJ, Sastre I, Recuero M, García MA. Allelic polymorphisms in the transcriptional regulatory region of apolipoprotein E gene. Febs Letters 1998;421: 105-108.

[49] Yin R, Pan S, Wu J, Lin W, Yang D. Apolipoprotein E gene polymorphism and serum lipid levels in the Guangxi Hei Yi Zhuang and Han populations. Experimental Biology and Medicine (Maywood) 2008;233: 409-418.

[50] Raygani VA, Kharrazi H, Rahimi Z, Pourmotabbed T. Frequencies of apolipoprotein E polymorphism in a healthy Kurdish population from Kermanshah, Iran. Human Biology 2007;79: 579-587.

[51] Al-Dabbagh NM, Al-Dohayan N, Arfin M, Tariq M. Apolipoprotein E polymorphisms and primary glaucoma in Saudis. Molecular Vision 2009;15: 912-919.

[52] Gerdes LU, Klausen LC, Sihm I, Faergeman O. Apolipoprotein E polymorphism in a Danish population compared to findings in 45 other study populations around the world. Genetic Epidemiology 1992;9: 155-167.

[53] Mastana SS, Calderon R, Pena J, Reddy PH, Papiha SS. Antrhopology of the apolipoprotein E (Apo E) gene: low frequency of Apo E4 allele in Basques and in tribal (Baiga) populations of India. Annals of Human Biology 1998;25: 137-143.

[54] Corbo RM, Scacchi R, Mureddu L, Mulas G, Castrechini S, et al. Apolipoprotein B, apolipoprotein E, and angiotensin-converting enzyme polymorphisms in 2 Italian populations at different risk for coronary artery disease and comparison of allele frequencies among European population. Human Biology 1999;71: 933-945.

[55] Singh P, Singh M, Gerdes U, Mastana SS. Apolipoprotein E polymorphism in India: high APOE*E3 allele frequency in Ramgarhia of Punjab. Anthropologischer Anzeiger 2001;59: 27-34.

[56] Singh PP, Singh M, Mastana SS. APOE distribution in world populations with new data from India and the UK. Annals of Human Biology 2006;33: 279-308.

[57] Raygani AV, Zahrai M, Raygani AV, Doosti M, Javadi E, et al. Association between apolipoprotein E polymorphism an Alzheimer disease in Tehran, Iran. Neuroscience Letters 2005;375: 1-6.

[58] Svobodova h, Kucera F, Stule T, Vrablik M, Amartuvshin B, et al. Apolipoprotein E gene polymorphism in the Mongolian population. Folia Biologica (Praha) 2007;53: 138-142.

[59] Fan BJ, Wang DY, Fan DS, Tam PO, Lam DS, et al. SNPs and interaction analyses of myocilin, optineurin, and apolipoprotein E in primary open angle glaucoma patients. Molecular Vision 2005;11: 625-631.

[60] Lam CY, Fan BJ, Wang DY, Tam PO, Yung Tham CC, et al. Association of apolipoprotein E polymorphisms with normal tension glaucoma in a Chinese population. Journal of Glaucoma 2006;15: 218-222.

[61] Zetterberg M, Tasa G, Palmer MS, Juronen E, Teesalu P, et al. Apolipoprotein E polymnorphisms in patients with primary open-angle glaucoma. American Journal of Ophthalmology 2007;143: 1059-1060.

[62] Lake S, Liverani D, Desai M, Casson R, James B, et al. Normal tension glaucoma is not associated with the common apolipoprotein E gene polymorphisms. British Journal of Ophthalmology 2004;88: 491-493.

[63] Ressiniotis T, Griffiths PG, Birch M, Keers S, Chimnery PF. The role of apolipoprotein E gene polymorphisms in primary open-angle glaucoma. Archives of Ophthalmology 2004;122: 258-261.

[64] Mabuchi F, Tang S, Ando D, Yamakita M, Wang J, et al. The apolipoprotein E gene polymorphism is associated with open angle glaucoma in the Japanese population. Molecular Vision 2005;11: 609-612.

[65] Yuan HP, Xiao Z, Yang BB. A study on the association of apolipoprotein E genotypes with primary open-angle glaucoma and primary angle-closure glaucoma in northeast of China. Zhonghua Yan Ke Za Zhi 2007;43: 416-420.

[66] Yilmaz A, Tamer L, Aras Ates N, Camdeviren H, Degirmenci U. Effects of apolipoprotein E genotypes on the development of exfoliation syndrome. Experimental Eye Research 2005;80: 871-875.

[67] Ritland JS, Utheim TP, Utheim OA, Espeseth T, Lydersen S, et al. Effects of APOE and CHRNA4 genotypes on retinal nerve fibre layer thickness at the optic disc and

on risk for developing exfoliation syndrome. Acta Ophthalmologica Scandinavica 2007;85(3): 257-261.

[68] Krumbiegel M, Pasutto F, Mardin CY, Weisschuh N, Paoli D, et al. Apolipoprotein E genotypes in pseudoexfoliation syndrome and pseudoexfoliation glaucoma. Journal of Glaucoma 2010;19: 561-565.

[69] Anderson DR, Patella VM. Automated static perimetry. St. louis, MO: Mosby; 1999. p10-35.

[70] Foster PJ, Buhrmann R, Quigley HA, Johnson GJ. The definition and classification of glaucoma in prevalence surveys. British Journal of Ophthalmology 2002;86(2): 238-242.

[71] Vijay L, George R, Arvind H, Baskaran M, Raju P, et al. Prevalence and causes of blindness in the rural population of the Chennai Glaucoma study. British Journal of Ophthalmology 2006;90: 407-410.

[72] Attebo K, Ivers RQ, Mitchell P. Refractive errors in an older population: the Blue Mountains Eye Study. Ophthalmology 1999;106(6): 1066-1072.

[73] Lamb EJ, Day AP. New diagnostic criteria for diabetes mellitus: are we any further forward? Annals of Clinical Biochemistry 2000;37(5): 588-592.

[74] Schallreuter KU, Levenig C, Kuhnl P, Loliger C, Hohl-Tehari M, et al. Histocompatability antigens in vitiligo: Hamburg study on 102 patients from Northern Germany. Dermatology 1993;187: 186-192.

[75] Savejgaard A, Platz P, Ryder LP. HLA and disease A survey. Immunological Reviews 1982;70: 193-218.

[76] Corbo RM, Schachi R. Apolipoprotein distribution around the world. Is APOE 4 a thrifty allele? Annals of Human Genetics 1999;63: 301-310.

[77] Lehtinen S, Luoma P, Lehtimaki T, Nayha S, Hassi J, et al. Differences in genetic variations of apolipoprotein E in Lapps and Finns. Atherosclerosis 1994;109: 263-268.

[78] Corbo RM, Scacchi R, Mureddu L, Mulas G, Alfano G. Apolipoprotein E polymorphism in Italy investigated in native plasma by a simple polyacrylamide gel isoelectric focusing technique. Comparison with frequency data of other European populations. Annals of Human Genetics 1995;59: 197-209.

[79] Sklavounou E, Economou-Peterse, Karadima G, Panas M, Avramopoulos D, et al. Apolipoprotein E polymorphism in the Greek population. Clinical Genetics 1997;52: 216-218.

[80] Nathan BP, Bellosta S, Sanan DA, Weisgraber KH, Mahley RW, et al. Differential effects of apolipoprotein E3 and E4 on neuronal growth in vitro. Science 1994;264: 850-852.

[81] Roses AD, Saunders AM. ApoE, Alzheimer's disease, and recovery from brain stress. Annals of the New York Academy of Sciences 1997;826: 200-212.

[82] Liew G, Shankar A, Wang JJ, Klein R, Bray MS, et al. Apolipoprotein E gene polymorphisms and retinal vascular signs: the atherosclerosis risk in communities (ARIC) study. Archives of Ophthalmology 2007;125: 813-818.

[83] Hong CJ, Liu TY, Liu HC, Wang SJ, Fuh JL, et al. Epsilon 4 allele of apolipoprotein E increases risk of Alzheimer's disease in a Chinese population. Neurology 1996;46: 1749-1751.

[84] Katzman R, Zhang MY, Chen PJ, Gu N, Jiang S, et al. Effects of apolipoprotein E on dementia and aging in the Shanghai Survey of Dementia. Neurology 1997;49: 779-785.

[85] Lehmann DJ, Smith AD, Combrinck M, Barnetson L, Joachim C. Apoliporpotein E epsilon 2 may be a risk factor for sporadic frontotemporal dementia. Journal of Neurology, Neurosurgery and Psychiatry 2000;69: 404-405.

[86] Mak YT, Chiu H, Woo J. Apolipoprotein E genotype and Alzheimer's disease in Hong Kong elderly Chinese. Neurology 1996;46: 146-149.

[87] Farrer LA, Cupples LA, Haines JL, Hyman B, Kukull WA, et al. Effects of age, sex, and ethnicity on the association between apolipoprotein E genotype and Alzheimer disease. A Meta-Analysis. APOE and Alzheimer Disease Meta Analysis Consortium. Journal of the American Medical Association 1997;278: 1349-1356.

[88] Tilley L, Morgan K, Grainger J, Marsters P, Morgan L, et al. Evaluation of polymorphisms in the presenilin-1 gene and the butyrylcholinesterase gene as risk factors in sporadic Alzheimer's disease. European Journal of Human Genetics 1999;7: 659-663.

[89] Bayer AU, Ferrari F. Severe progression of glaucomatous optic neuropathy in patients with Alzheimer's disease. Eye 2002;16: 201-212.

[90] [90]Bayer AU, Keller ON, Ferrari F, Maag KP. Association of glaucoma with neurodegenerative diseases with apoptotic cell death: Alzheimer's disease and Parkinson's disease. American Journal of Ophthalmology 2002;133: 135-137.

[91] McKinnon SJ. Glaucoma: ocular Alzheimer's disease? Frontiers in Bioscience 2003;8: 1140-1156.

[92] Tatton W, Chen D, Chalmers-Redman R, Wheeler L, Nixon R, et al. Hypothesis for a common basis for neuroprotection in glaucoma and Alzheimer's disease: anti-apoptosis by alpha-2-adrenergic receptor activation. Survey of Ophthalmology 2003;48: 25-37.

[93] Strittmatter WJ, Roses AD. Apolipoprotein E and Alzheimer's disease. Annual Review of Neuroscience 1996;19: 53-77

[94]   Saunders AM, Schmader K, Breitner JC, Benson MD, Brown WT. Apolipoprotein E e4 allele distributions in late-onset Alzheimer's disease and in other amyloid-forming diseases. Lancet 1993;342: 710-711.

[95]   [95]Saunders AM, Strittmatter WJ, Schmechel D, George-Hyslop PH, Pericak-Vance MA, et al. Association of apolipoprotein E allele epsilon 4 with late-onset familial and sporadic Alzheimer's disease. Neurology 1993;43: 1467-1472.

[96]   Corder EH, Saunders AM, Strittmatter WJ, Schmechel DE, Gaskell PC, et al. Gene dose of apolipoprotein E type-4 allele and the risk of Alzheimer's disease in late onset families. Science 1993;261: 921-923.

[97]   Harrington CR, Roth M, Xuereb JH, McKema PJ, Wischik CM. Apolipoprotein E type epsilon 4 allele frequency is increased in patients with schizophrenia. Neuroscience Letters 1995;202(1-2): 101-104.

[98]   Liu W, Breen G, Zhang J, Li S, Gu N, et al. Association of APOE gene with schizophrenia in Chinese: a possible risk factor in times of malnutrition. Schizophrenia Research 2003;62: 225-230.

[99]   Papapetropoulos S, Farrer MJ, Stone JT, Milkovic NM, Ross OA, et al. Phenotypic associations of tau and ApoE in Parkinson's disease. Neuroscience Letters 2007; 414(2): 141-144.

[100] Teasdale GM, Nicoll JA, Murray G, Fiddes M. Association of apolipoprotein E polymorphism with outcome after head injury. Lancet 1997;350: 1069-1071.

[101] Friedman JS, Walter MA. Glaucoma genetics, present and future. Clinical Genetics 1999;55: 71-79.

[102] Klaver CC, Kliffen M, van Duijn CM, Hofman A, Cruts M, et al. Genetic association of apolipoprotein E with age-related macular degeneration. American Journal of Human Genetics 1998; 63: 200-206

[103] Kuhrt H, Härtig W, Grimm D, Faude F, Kasper M, Reichenbach A. Changes in CD44 and ApoE immunoreactivities due to retinal pathology of man and rat. Journal für Hirnforschung 1997;38(2): 223-229.

[104] Wisniewski T, Frangione B. Apolipoprotein E: a pathological chaperone protein in patients with cerebral and systemic amyloid. Neuroscience Letters 1992;135: 235-238.

[105] Arai H, Muramatsu T, Higuchi S, Sasaki H, Trojanowski JQ. Apolipoprotein E gene in Parkinson's disease with or without dementia. Lancet 1994;344(8926): 889

[106] Benjamin R, Leake A, Ince PG, Perry RH, McKeith IG, et al. Effects of apolipoprotein E genotype on cortical neuropathology in senile dementia of the Lewy body and Alzheimer's disease. Neurodegeneration 1995;4: 443-448.

[107] Schupf N, Kapell D, Lee JH, Zigman W, Canto B. Onset of dementia is associated with apolipoprotein E epsilon4 in Down's syndrome. Annals of Neurology 1996; 40: 799-801.

[108] Al-Khedhairy AA. Apolipoprotein E polymorphism in Saudis. Molecular Biology Reports 2004;31: 257-260.

[109] Gamboa R, Hernandez-Pacheco G, Hesiquio R, Zuniga J, Masso F, et al. Apolipoprotein E polymorphism in the Indian and Mestizo population of Mexico. Human Biology 2000;72: 975-981.

[110] Summanen P, Tonjum AM. Exfoliation syndrome among Saudis. Acta Ophthalmologica 1988;184(Suppl): 107-111.

[111] Desai MA, Lee RK. The medical and surgical management of pseudoexfoliation glaucoma. International Ophthalmology Clinics 2008;48(4): 95-113.

[112] Thomas R, Kumar RS, Chandrasekhar G, Parikh R. Applying the recent clinical trials on primary open angle glaucoma: the developing world perspective. Journal of Glaucoma 2005;14(4): 324-7.

[113] Rao RQ, Arain TM, Ahad MA. The prevalence of pseudoexfoliation syndrome in Pakistan. Hospital based study. BMC Ophthalmology 2006;6: 27.

[114] Miyazaki M, Kubota T, Kubo M, Kiyohara Y, Iida M, Nose Y, Ishibashi T.The prevalence of pseudoexfoliation syndrome in a Japanese population: the Hisayama study. J Glaucoma. 2005;14(6): 482-484.

[115] Young AL, Tang WW, Lam DS.The prevalence of pseudoexfoliation syndrome in Chinese people. British Journal of Ophthalmology 2004;88(2): 193-195.

[116] Foster PJ, Sheah SKL. The prevalence of pseudoexfoliation syndrome in Chinese people: the Tanjong Pagar Survey. Briitish Journal of Ophthalmology 2005;89: 239-240.

[117] Aasved H. Prevalence of bibrilopathia epitheliocapsularies (pseudoexfoliation) and capsular glaucoma. Transaction of Ophthalmological Society UK 1975; 99: 293-295.

[118] Forsius H. Prevalence of pseudoexfoliation of the lens in Finns, Lapps, Icelanders, Eskimos and Russinas. Transaction of Ophthalmological Society UK1979;99: 296-298.

[119] Lantukh VV, Piatin MM. Features of ocular pathology among the indigenous inhabitants of Chukotka. Vestnik Oftalmologii 1982; 18-20.

[120] Ringvold A, Blika S, Elsas T. The middle-Norway eye-screening study. III. The prevalence of capsular glaucoma is influenced by blood-group antigens. Acta Ophthalmologica (Copenh)1993; 71: 207-213.

[121] Colin J, Le Gall G, Le Jeune B, Cambria MD. The prevalence of exfoliation syndrome in different areas of France. Acta Ophthalmologica1988;184(Suppl): 86-89.

[122] Ringvold A, Blika S, Elsas TL The prevalence of pseudoexfolation in three separate municipalities of Middle-Norway. A preliminary report. Acta Ophthalmologica 1987;182(Suppl): 17-20.

[123] Ringvold A: Epidemiology of the pseudo-exfoliation syndrome. Acta Ophthalmologica Scandinavica 1999;77:371-375.

[124] Forsius H, Lukka H. Pseudoexfoliation of the anterior capsule of the lens in Lapps and Eskimos. Canadian Journal of Ophthalmology 1973; 8:274-277.

[125] Forsius H. Exfoliation syndrome in various ethnic populations. Acta Ophthalmologica 1988;184(Suppl): 71-85.

[126] Ritch R. Exfoliation syndrome and occludable angles. Transactions of American Ophthalmology Society1994;92: 845-944

[127] Hinton DR, Sadun AA, Blanks JC, Miller CA. Optic-nerve degeneration in Alzheimer's disease. New England Journal of Medicine 1986;315: 485-487.

[128] Sadun AA, Bassi CJ. Optic nerve damage in Alzheimer's disease. Ophthalmology 1990; 97: 9-17.

[129] Davies DC, McCoubrie P, McDonald B, Jobst KA. Myelinated axon number in the optic nerve is unaffected by Alzheimer's disease. British Journal of Ophthalmology 1995;79: 596-600.

[130] Vickers JC, Lazzarini RA, Riederer BM, Morrison JH. Intraperikaryal neurofilamentous accumulations in a subset of retinal ganglion cells in aged mice that express a human neurofilament gene. Experimental Neurology 1995;136(2): 266-269.

[131] Leuba G, Saini K. Pathology of subcortical visual centres in relation to cortical degeneration in Alzheimer's disease. Neuropathology and Applied Neurobiology 1995;21: 410-422.

[132] Brega A, Scacchi R, Cuccia M, Kirdar B, Peloso G. Study of 15 protein polymorphisms in a sample of the Turkish population. Human Biology 1998;70: 715-728

[133] Attila G, Acartürk E, Eskandari G, Akpinar O, Tuli A, et al. Effects of apolipoprotein E genotypes and other risk factors on the development of coronary artery disease in Southern Turkey. Clinica Chimica Acta 2001;312: 191-196.

Chapter 8

Neuroprotection in Glaucoma

Sotiria Palioura and Demetrios G. Vavvas

Additional information is available at the end of the chapter

1. Introduction

Glaucoma is a distinctive group of optic neuropathies characterized by progressive degeneration of neuronal tissue due to death of retinal ganglion cells, with accompanying gradual visual field loss. [1, 2] It is the leading cause of irreversible blindness worldwide [3] and complex genetic and environmental risk factors have been implicated in its progression. [4-7] Neuroprotection for glaucoma refers to any intervention that aims either to prevent optic nerve damage and retinal ganglion cell death or to preserve already diseased neuronal tissue and its function, with the ultimate goal of maintaining vision. Thus, neuroprotective agents can be thought of as pharmacological antagonists of intracellular injury and death pathways.

Agents that lower the intra-ocular pressure (IOP) have been shown to slow glaucoma progression in several controlled clinical trials and even arrest the progression in some cases [8-10], yet their effectiveness is limited in preventing retinal ganglion cell loss. Retinal ganglion cell damage in glaucoma is not confined to the neurons that are insulted primarily, but neighboring neurons are injured secondarily as well. [11] Therefore, efforts that focus on discovering alternative therapeutic approaches independent of IOP reduction have placed neuroprotective treatment modalities at the frontiers of glaucoma research.

2. Apoptosis and necrosis in glaucoma

Apoptosis and necrosis constitute the two major pathways to cell death. [12] In 1972, Kerr, Wyllie and Currie used the Greek term 'apoptosis' (from the Greek: dropping off of petals from plants) to describe a specific morphological aspect of cell death. [13] Apoptosis is accompanied by rounding-up of the cell, reduction of cellular volume, chromatin condensation, and engulfment by resident phagocytes. Apoptosis is the best-characterized type of programmed cell death, and these morphological changes are largely mediated by the activation of the caspase family of cysteine proteases. [14] In contrast, 'necrosis' (from the Greek: death) is associated with a gain in cell volume, swelling of organelles, plasma membrane rupture and subsequent release of intracellular contents with ensuing inflammation. Until recently necrosis had been considered a passive, unregulated form of cell death. New evidence indicates that some forms of necrosis can be induced by regulated signal transduction pathways such as those mediated by receptor interacting protein kinases (RIP Kinases). RIP kinases cross talk with caspases and lie downstream of cell death signals such as the Fas Ligand or the Tumor Necrosis Factor-α (TNF-α). [15] This programmed form of necrosis is termed programmed necrosis or necroptosis. [12, 16, 17]

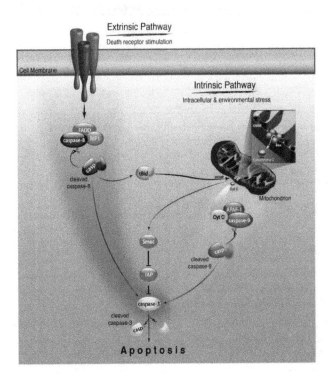

Figure 1. The extrinsic pathway is initiated by binding of death ligands such as TNF-α and Fas ligand to their cell-surface death receptors such as TNF receptor and Fas. The death domains of these receptors recruit adaptor molecules like FADD and caspase-8, which leads to the activation of caspase-8. Activated caspase-8 cleaves the effector caspases such as caspase-3, thereby activating them and inducing apoptosis. The extrinsic pathway interacts with the intrinsic pathway via caspase-8-mediated cleavage of Bid. The intrinsic pathway is initiated by release of mitochondrial intermembrane proteins such as cytochrome c and Smac/Diablo into the cytosol. Released cytochrome c forms an apoptosome with Apaf-1 and caspase-9, which leads to caspase-9 activation. Smac/Diablo enhances caspase activation through the neutralization of IAP proteins.

Cysteine aspartate-specific proteases or caspases are central to the execution of apoptosis. Their activation occurs mainly through two distinct pathways: extrinsic and intrinsic (Fig. 1). [18] The extrinsic pathway is initiated by binding of extracellular death ligands such as TNF-α and Fas ligand to their cell-surface death receptors, TNF receptor and Fas. [19] The death domains of these receptors recruit adaptor molecules like Fas-associated death domain (FADD) and caspase-8, forming the death inducing signaling complex (DISC). [20] The formation of DISC leads to activation of caspase-8, which in turn mediates cleavage of effector caspases. The extrinsic pathway can cross-talk with the intrinsic pathway through caspase-8-mediated cleavage of Bid, aBH3-only member of the Bcl-2 family of proteins. [21, 22] Bid cleavage releases a truncated fragment that triggers the release of mitochondrial proteins, thereby initiating the intrinsic caspase cascade as described below.

The intrinsic pathway is mediated by mitochondria. [23] In response to intracellular and environmental stress, mitochondria release inter-membrane proteins such as cytochrome c and second mitochondria-derived activator of caspases (Smac)/direct inhibitor of apoptosis-binding protein with low pI (Diablo) into the cytosol. Released cytochrome c triggers the formation of an apoptosome along with apoptotic protease activating factor-1 (Apaf-1) and caspase-9 in the presence of ATP, which leads to caspase-9 activation. [24] Smac/Diablo enhances caspase activation through the neutralization of inhibitor of apoptosis (IAP) (Fig. 1). [25, 26]

Necrosis is mainly regulated by a set of protein Kinases called RIP Kinases. RIP1 switches its function to a regulator of cell death when it is deubiquitinated by A20 or cylindromatosis (CYLD). [27, 28] Deubiquitination of RIP1 abolishes its ability to activate NF-κB after TNF-α stimulation, and leads to the formation of cytosolic DISC with FADD and caspase-8, the so-called complex II. [29] As described above in caspase signaling, DISC formation leads to caspase-8 activation and subsequent apoptosis. In contrast to TNF signaling, Fas directly recruits RIP1, FADD and caspase-8 to the plasma membrane and forms DISC (Fig. 2). [30] During apoptosis, RIP1 is cleaved and inactivated by caspases. [31] Although many cell lines are protected against death receptor-induced apoptosis by use of pan-caspase inhibitors, Vercammen and others found that, in mouse L929 fibrosarcoma cells, caspase inhibition does not prevent TNF- or Fas-induced cell death and the cells acquire a necrotic morphology. [32, 33] In 2000, Holler and others discovered that RIP1 kinase is a key molecule that induces necrotic cell death mediated by death receptors. [34]

In 2005, Degterev, Yuan, and others using chemical library screening, identified small compounds named necrostatins that specifically inhibit death receptor- mediated necrosis. [16] Necrostatins have been shown to specifically inhibit RIP1 kinase phosphorylation during necrosis without affecting death receptor-induced NF-κB activation. [35] RIP1 kinase activity appears to be important for necrosome formation, as necrostatin-1 abolishes the formation of the RIP1-RIP3 complex and RIP3 kinase phosphorylation during necrosis. [36, 37] Cho and others propose that another unknown kinase activated by RIP1 may mediate RIP3 phosphorylation, based on the findings that ectopically expressed RIP1 does not phosphorylate RIP3. [36] The activities of RIP1 and RIP3 may be mutually regulated in a necrosome signaling complex. RIPK activation leads likely to increased reactive oxygen species (ROS) production. Activated RIP3 interacts with metabolic enzymes such as glycogen phosphorylase (PYGL), glutamate-ammonia ligase (GLUL) and glutamate dehydrogenase 1 (GLUD1). [38] Activation of these enzymes eventually stimulates the Krebs cycle and oxidative phosphorylation, thereby increasing mitochondrial ROS production. Secondly, after TNF-α stimulation, RIP1 forms a complex with TNFR, Riboflavin kinase, and NADPH oxidase 1. [39, 40] NADPH oxidase is the best characterized non-mitochondrial source of ROS and forms a membrane bound enzyme complex with p22phox and Rac. [41] Thirdly, RIP1 kinase activates autophagic degradation of catalase, which converts hydrogen peroxide to water and oxygen, thereby increasing ROS accumulation. [42] More recently, activation of the necrosome has shown to interact with the mixed lineage kinase domain-like (MLKL) and phosphoglycerate mutase 5 (PGAM5) resulting in the fusion of mitochondria and necrotic cell death. [43, 44]

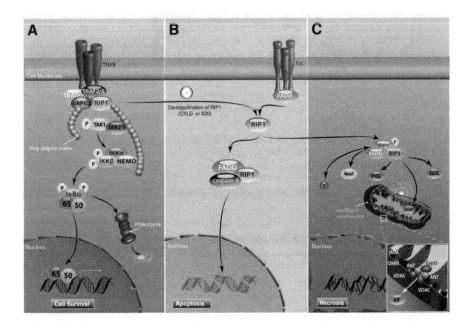

Figure 2. Schematic of the RIPK signaling pathway.
A, In response to TNF-α stimulation, RIP1 is recruited to TNFR and forms a membrane associated complex I with TRADD, TRAF2/5 and cIAP1/2, which in turn leads to polyubiquitination of RIP1 and pro-survival NF-κB activation.
B, RIP1 switches function to a regulator of cell death when RIP1 is unubiquitinated by A20 or CYLD. Deubiquitination of RIP1 leads to the formation of cytosolic DISC with FADD and caspase-8, the so-called complex II. In contrast to TNF signaling, Fas stimulation directly forms DISC. Activation of caspase-8 in DISC leads to apoptosis induction. During apoptosis, RIP1 is cleaved and inactivated by caspase-8. C, In conditions where caspases are blocked or cannot be activated efficiently, RIP1 binds to RIP3, and both RIP1 and RIP3 kinases are phosphorylated at the RIP1-RIP3 complex. RIP1 kinase phosphorylation is critical for necrosis induction. In response to TNF-α, RIP1 binds to NADPH oxidase 1 and produces superoxide. Activated RIP3 binds to PYGL, GLUL and GLUD1 and increases the production of mitochondrial ROS. ROS overproduction leads to mitochondrial dysfunction, resulting in the release of mitochondrial pro-death proteins. Activation of the necrosome has been shown to interact with mixed lineage kinase domain-like (MLKL) and phosphoglycerate mutase 5 (PGAM5) resulting in the fusion of mitochondria and necrotic cell death

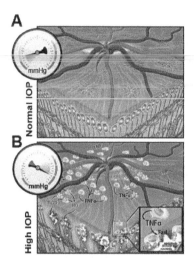

Figure 3. Schematic of changes in animal models of high IOP mediated optic nerve damage. A, In normal IOP micro-glia are quiescent and cells are in normal state. B, Elevated IOP leads to increased numbers of activated microglia with amoeboid morphology around the optic nerve head. These microglia appear to secrete TNF-α leading to RGC death. Other molecules, including FasL on microglia, nitric oxide (NO), and reactive oxygen species (ROS) may also play a role in RGC death. Changes in blood supply and ischemia also contribute to the death of RGCs.

In chronic glaucoma, apoptosis of retinal ganglion cells has been shown as the main path-way to cell death. [2, 45, 46] The exact mechanism though is not clear. Since a significant proportion of patients who suffer from glaucoma have high IOP, it has been hypothesized that high IOP induces stress to retinal ganglion cells either directly [47, 48] or indirectly to their axons at the lamina cribrosa [49] thus leading to apoptosis. However, although high IOP has been thought to be the main causative factor, the fact that glaucoma can occur in the presence of IOP within the normal range, while can be absent in a subset of subjects with high IOP indicates that the underlying etiology of this disease remains unknown and in es-sence fail to fully fulfill Koch's postulates [50, 51].

Mechanisms believed to cause stress to retinal ganglion cells and to initiate the apoptotic cascade include: biomechanical stress [52, 53], excitotoxicity [54-57], tissue hypoxia [58, 59], altered nutritional blood supply [60, 61], mitochondrial dysfunction [62-65], Müller glial cell activation [66], protein misfolding [67-69], oxidative stress [70, 71], dysfunctional autoim-munity [72], neurotrophin deprivation [73, 74], and inflammation. [75, 76]

3. Animal models

Animal experimental models in glaucoma research are produced by inducing either an ele-vation in intraocular pressure or damage to the axons of retinal ganglion cells. [77] Several methods have been employed to raise intraocular pressure in animal models. They range from obliteration of episcleral vessels [78] to iatrogenic sclerosis of the trabecular mesh-work (laser-induced [79] or through retroinjection of hypertonic saline into the limbal plexus [80]) or to mechanical obstruction of the trabecular meshwork with polystyrene beads. [81] Direct damage to retinal ganglion cell axons can be achieved via axotomy or crushing of axons. Retinal ganglion cell death occurs in 1-2 weeks from the time of optic nerve transection or crushing of axons in a fairly predictable fashion. [82] Interestingly, there is a specific mouse strain (DBA/J2) which inherently produces a much slower degeneration of retinal ganglion cells; a process thought to more closely mimic human disease than other induced mouse models of glaucoma. [83] Mutations in the transmembrane glycoprotein Gpnmb (premature stop codon at position 150 -GpnmbR150X) and the presence of the Tyrp1b gene allele (the b mutation is in a heme-associated domain and renders the protein susceptible to rapid proteolytic degradation) in the DBA/2J mouse model are thought to cause pigment dispersion and iris atrophy respectively. Both proteins are highly expressed in melanocytes and are involved in melanin and cell growth regulation. The decreased levels of Gpnmb and Tyrp1 lead to cell death and abnormal melanin content release that deposits onto the trabecular meshwork resulting in elevated IOP. [84] Of note, these mutations have not been shown to cause glaucoma in patients.

The ideal animal model should manifest slow focal injury to retinal ganglion cell axons at the optic nerve head that leads to sectoral death of retinal ganglion cells without loss of other retinal neurons. [77] The currently used animal models for glaucoma research are far from ideal and their limitations are partly responsible for the failure to translate results from the bench to the bedside. For the elevated IOP models, it is clear that there are different susceptibilities of retinal ganglion cell damage among different species (mice, rats, monkeys) and among different strains or age of the same species. [51, 85, 86] For the axotomy models, acute damage to retinal ganglion cell axons is different from the slow progression seen clinically in glaucoma, and thus it remains unclear whether studies with these models can safely reproduce glaucomatous damage as it occurs in humans. [82] For the DBA/2J mouse, there is significant variability in glaucoma progression among animals and between eyes of the same animal, which renders any comparison study particularly difficult. [77]

An inherent limitation of using animal models for the study of any human disease process is that animal models often lack the heterogeneity, compounded comorbidities, and polypharmacy that are present in human pathologic conditions. Moreover, it is difficult to extrapolate from animal studies what the appropriate dose of a putative neuroprotective agent would be in human subjects since pre-clinical studies rarely assess for a dose-response curve, therapeutic index, and central nervous system penetration. [87, 88]

4. Success in the lab

Efforts in pre-clinical studies have targeted the various mechanisms that produce axonal degeneration and retinal ganglion cell death and have led to the discovery of an array of neu roprotective agents. [89] First, apoptosis of retinal ganglion cells has been inhibited in the lab through the use of anti-excitotoxic agents that primarily inhibit or interfere with the glutamate excitotoxic cascade. [90] Glutamate is a natural neurotransmitter that is required by the organism for proper cell signaling including retinal ganglion cells. Glutamate acts through many types of glutamate receptors/ion channels. One of these receptors/ion channels is the N-methyl-D-aspartate (NMDA) type, which leads to calcium flux upon activation. Persistent activation of this channel by glutamate or NDMA leads to excitotoxicity. Glutamate induced excitotoxicity has been shown in some but not all animal models and elevated glutamate levels have been detected in some but not all studies (reviewed in [91]). Memantine is an uncompetitive antagonist of the N-methyl-D-aspartate (NMDA) type of glutamate receptor/channel. It can only bind to this ion channel in its "open" state, that is after glutamate has already bound to its receptor and has caused the channel to open. [92] Studies on several animal models of glaucoma have supported the neuroprotective role of memantine on retinal ganglion cells. [93]. Activated glutamate receptor leads to increased calcium flux. Calcium levels are important in many neuronal signaling events and aberrant calcium levels are thought to be important mediators of neuronal cell death. Increased levels of intracellular calcium can be very detrimental to the health of the cell. Most recently, inhibitors of the L-type voltage-gated calcium channel, clinidipine [94] and lomerizine [95] as well as the alpha-2 adrenergic agonist brimonidine [96] have also been shown to limit glutamate-induced excitotoxicity. Although the exact mechanism of action of brimonidine remains unknown, intraperitoneal pre-treatment with brimonidine has been shown by several groups to increase survival of retinal ganglion cells after optic nerve or retinal injury in animal models of NDMA excitotoxicity, optic nerve crush and ischemia. [97-100]

Antiapoptotic strategies utilize neurotrophins [101] or aim at the activation of Bcl-2 antiapoptotic pathways. [102] Neurotrophins are factors that signal the survival and growth of neurons. The first neurotrophin to be discovered was Nerve Growth Factor (NGF) in the 1960s. In 1986 Levi-Montalcini and Cohen shared the Nobel prize "for their discovery of growth factors for neurons." Neurotrophins are peptides that bind to cell surface receptors and activate survival signals, thus suppressing the apoptotic process (Fig. 4). [80, 103, 104] Exogenous administration of brain-derived neurotrophic factor (BDNF) or nerve growth factor (NGF) has delayed but not prevented retinal ganglion cell death. [105-108] Injection of BDNF, ciliary neurotrophic factor (CNTF), neurotrophin-4 (NT-4), fibroblast growth factor-2 (FGF-2), and neurturin (a ligand for a glial cell line-derived neurotrophic factor family related receptor A2 - GFRA2) into the vitreous has also increased survival of retinal ganglion cells. [105, 109, 110] Neurotrophin delivery and overexpression via viral vector delivery seems to promote survival of retinal ganglion cells even further. [106] Finally, agents that interact with the two major neurotrophin cell surface receptor systems, tropomyosin-related kinase (Trk) receptor and p75 neurotrophin receptor (p75NTR), can also prolong survival of retinal neuronal tissue (Fig. 4). [111-113] Neurotrophins are difficult to be used in clinics because of their polypeptidic nature: they are destroyed in the acidic milieu of the stomach, while their size hinders their ability of crossing the blood-brain barrier. Thus, special techniques have to be invented, such as intravitreal implants of cells producing these molecules locally, such as the CNTF producing cells by Neurotech (Cumberland, RI, USA)

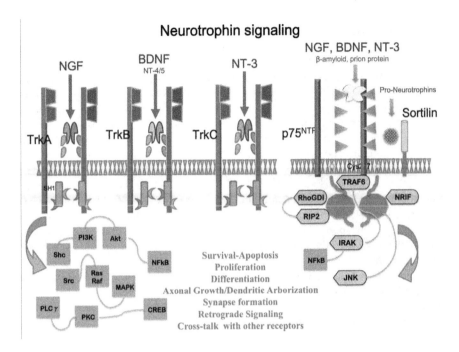

Neurotrophin signaling

Figure 4. Neurotrophin Signaling Summary. (courtesy of Dr A. Gravanis). Neurotrophins include the first to be discovered: Nerve Growth Factor (NGF) as well as Brain Derived Neurotrophic Factor (BDNF) and Neurotrophin 3 and 4 (NT-3 and NT-4). There are two classes of receptors for neurotrophins: p75 and the "Trk" family of Tyrosine kinase receptors. P75 can bind all factors, whereas Trk receptors are specific for their ligands. Binding of neurotrophins to their receptors leads to activation of many pro-survival signals including PI3K, Akt, and MAPK among others.

Tumor necrosis factor-alpha (TNF-α) can lead to death of retinal ganglion cells by inducing mitochondrial damage and activation of caspases. [114] Inhibition of TNF-α via the use of etanercept [115] or an anti-TNF-α neutralizing antibody [116] can protect retinal ganglion cells in mouse models of glaucoma.

Providing free radical scavengers, such as coenzyme Q10 [117, 118] or thioredoxin [119], or inhibiting the formation of free radicals by blocking the action of nitric oxide synthase [120] has shown promise as an alternative neuroprotective strategy. Inflammatory and immune mechanisms also play a role in glaucomatous damage of retinal ganglion cells. [121] Immunomodulation [122], inhibition of calcineurin by tacrolimus [123], and subcutaneous injection of granulocyte-colony stimulating factor [124] also have neuroprotective potential in glaucoma.

Other mechanisms that have been investigated in the lab with encouraging results include the use of mesenchymal stem cells, which are thought to exert their effect through production of neurotrophins or stimulation of inflammation [125, 126]. A recent study has shown that amyloid β (Aβ) is found to be elevated in an animal model of ocular hypertension induced glaucoma and that inhibition of the generation of amyloid β led to preservation of

RGCs. [67] Other studies have shown that treatment with minocycline reduces RGC death in experimental glaucoma. [127] The antiapoptotic effects of minocycline are not very clear and seem to be pleiotropic. They are exerted, at least in part, by modulating inflammation and metalloproteinases and by reducing mitochondrial calcium overloading. Minocycline stabilizes the mitochondrial membrane and inhibits release of cytochrome c and other apoptotic factors into the cytoplasm, thus resulting in decreased caspase activation and nuclear damage. Minocycline also exerts caspase-independent neuroprotective effects including upregulation of anti-apoptotic factor Bcl-2. Another promising agent is Rasagiline, a monoamine oxidase inhibitor that has been found have neuroprotective and anti-apoptotic effects partially through increase in the mitochondrial family of Bcl-2 proteins, prevention in the fall in mitochondrial membrane potential, prevention of the activation of caspase 3, and of translocation of glyceraldehyde-3-phosphate dehydrogenase from the cytoplasm to the nucleus. It can also affect the secretion of amyloid precursor protein (APP) and it has been shown to delay RGC cell death in experimental glaucoma [128]. However, it has to be noted that it has not taken approval by the United States Food and Drug Administration in a Parkinson's disease trial. Erythropoietin (EPO) activates the NF-κB pathway and results in prosurvival and anti-oxidant enzyme upregulation and has been shown to be protective of RGC in the DBA/2J mouse of pigmentary glaucoma [129]. Citicholine (cytidine 5'-diphosphocholine) which exhibits neuroprotective effects by preserving cardiolipin and sphingomyelin among other actions, has been tested in patients with anterior ischemic optic neuropathy and showed preliminary benefits. [130]

5. Difficulties in designing a clinical trial

Over the last 30 years, numerous pharmacologic agents and gene therapeutic approaches have been shown to be neuroprotective in animal models of retinal and optic nerve injury. To date, none of the trials on neuroprotection of the visual system have shown efficacy and none of the agents developed in the laboratory have translated into a definitive clinical treatment. [131] There are several reasons for the universal failure of clinical trials to confirm preclinical results; they stem from the nature of glaucoma itself and from the poor design of previous neuroprotective trials. [51, 131] First, the long, slow course of glaucomatous optic neuropathy hinders our efforts to measure whether an improvement in progressive worsening has been achieved and asks for a design of therapeutic trials that last several years. Second, the rate of worsening varies among patients and thus a larger sample size is required to account for this inherent variability in disease progression. Third, the current standard of outcome measurement remains visual field testing and this carries a significant test-retest variance even among patients who are adept in taking the test. Fourth, any neuroprotection clinical trial would have to include patients that are already on topical medications that lower IOP. IOP-lowering agents have proven effective in slowing glaucoma progression in several controlled clinical trials [8-10] and it would be unethical to preclude neuroprotection study patients from using IOP-lowering medications.

6. Failed and ongoing trials

Success in the lab has not paralleled success in neuroprotection clinical trials. A Cochrane review in 2010 failed to identify any neuroprotection studies with significant results. [132] The largest neuroprotection study to date consisted of two industry-supported, parallel, randomized, phase III clinical trials on oral memantine in patients with chronic progressive open angle glaucoma. A total of 2,200 patients were enrolled into the trials at 89 sites and they were followed for at least 4 years. Despite the success of memantine in animal models of glaucoma, both clinical trials failed to show efficacy with respect to their primary outcome measures. The results of these two trials are as of yet unpublished and only two press releases hinted on their results. [133] The first release stated, "Two measures of visual function were selected in the statistical analysis plan to assess the efficacy of memantine in glaucoma. The functional measure chosen as the endpoint (glaucomatous field progression) did not show a benefit of memantine in preserving visual function. In a number of analyses using the secondary functional measure, memantine demonstrated a statistically significant benefit of the high-dose compared to placebo." The second release stated, "Allergan unmasked the second Phase III clinical trial examining the safety and efficacy of oral memantine as a treatment for glaucoma. Although the study showed that the progression of disease was significantly lower in patients receiving the higher dose of memantine compared to patients receiving the low dose of memantine, there was no significant benefit compared to patients receiving placebo. Therefore, the study failed to meet its primary endpoint and to sufficiently replicate the results of the first Phase III trial." In going forward, knowing the specifics of these trials and the reasons for failure would facilitate a more well-thought design of future trials; yet, the results remain unpublished.

The second most studied agent in neuroprotection trials is the highly selective alpha-2 adrenergic agonist, brimonidine, which had also shown great promise in animal studies. The first trial included 9 patients with Leber's hereditary optic neuropathy in whom use of brimonidine after loss of vision in one eye failed to prevent loss of vision in the second eye, which naturally occurs within weeks to months after first eye involvement. [134] The second trial also failed to show efficacy of brimonidine in aiding recovery of vision loss in patients with anterior ischemic optic neuropathy, though the trial itself may have been underpowered. [135]

The last trial assessing the neuroprotective effects of brimonidine was the Low-Pressure Glaucoma Treatment Study, which recruited patients with normal-tension glaucoma and randomized them to either treatment with brimonidine or with timolol. [136] Timolol has no neuroprotective properties and it thus served as a control for the pressure-lowering effects of brimonidine. However, the IOP was only minimally lowered in both groups, which raises concerns about patient adherence to the treatment regimen. [51] Results of the trial were published in 2011 and showed that low-pressure glaucoma patients treated with brimonidine were less likely to have visual field progression than patients treated with timolol. [137]

A review of ongoing trials at clinicaltrials.gov revealed one phase I trial that is still recruiting patients and aims to investigate the safety and efficacy of the NT-501 clinical neurotrophic factor (CNTF) implant in patients with chronic progressive open angle glaucoma (trial identifier: NCT01408472).

7. Hope for success

Designing neuroprotection trials in glaucoma is challenging. Modifications in study design, patient selection, and outcome measures can aid in the clinical testing of neuroprotective agents with positive pre-clinical results. [51] Instead of the standard randomized controlled clinical trial prototype, neuroprotection trials in glaucoma may be served better by using a so-called futility design strategy. Detection of beneficial agents with robust treatment effects in a short period of time in a single treatment group (i.e. there is no need for a control group) are advantages of futility design. Clearly, a major disadvantage of this approach is the inability to adequately assess for side effects and time-dependent treatment effects in a trial that has fewer patients and a shorter testing time frame. [138, 139] In addition, selection of patients whose disease is rapidly can maximize the opportunity to detect differences after the use of neuroprotective agents. Older age, higher baseline intraocular pressure, bilateral disease, low perfusion pressure, presence of exfoliation, disc hemorrhages, and thinner central corneal thickness are all risk factors for rapid progression and should be used in the selection of the study population in neuroprotection trials. [51, 140] The agent in question also should reach its target tissue(s), the retina and optic nerve head. Steps should be taken to ensure patient adherence with medication administration or the results of any neuroprotective trial that is performed on a background of co-administered IOP-lowering therapy are deemed to be confounded. [141]. If the IOP is reduced to an identical degree, while one agent (like brimonidine or other neuroporotectant) shows fewer injuries to the visual fields, this would indirectly support the additional neuroprotective effect of the agent on top of its IOP lowering effects.

In terms of endpoints for such trials, visual field testing is likely more suitable than structural measures since it has been employed extensively to measure progression of disease. Its disadvantages of high variability in some test point areas, the patient effort it requires, and the insensitivity to show the earliest stages of damage are well known. Nevertheless, it has been well established as a method to assess glaucoma progression. Given the lack of reliable software to measure progression using structural tests, such as the Heidelberg Retinal Tomograph or Optical Coherence Tomography, visual field testing remains the most reliable endpoint to use. If structural measures are to be used in the future, one should keep in mind that the more optic nerve damage present at the outset, the less sensitive structural change will be. [51]

8. Conclusion

Novel neuroprotective agents and mechanisms show promise in pre-clinical studies and animal models. However, translating these findings into effective treatments still remains a challenge. This challenge can be met by a careful study design, appropriate selection of the study population, and use of better outcome measures and clinical end points. In addition, the various laboratory investigations suggest that there are multiple pathways that play a role in the loss of retinal ganglion cells. It is thus necessary to espouse combinatorial treatment approaches, if we want to successfully provide neuroprotection in the clinical setting.

Acknowledgements

We would like to thank Aristomenis Thanos for his assistance with the figures included in this chapter.

Author details

Sotiria Palioura[1] and Demetrios G. Vavvas[2]*

*Address all correspondence to: Demetrios_Vavvas@meei.harvard.edu

1 Department of Ophthalmology, Massachusetts Eye and Ear Infirmary, Harvard Medical School, Boston, MA, USA

2 Angiogenesis Laboratory Retina Service, Department of Ophthalmology, Massachusetts Eye and Ear Infirmary, Harvard Medical School, Boston, MA, USA

References

[1] Gupta N, Ang LC, Noel de Tilly L, Bidaisee L, Yucel YH. Human glaucoma and neural degeneration in intracranial optic nerve, lateral geniculate nucleus, and visual cortex. British J Ophthalmol. 2006;90(6):674-8.

[2] Quigley HA, Nickells RW, Kerrigan LA, Pease ME, Thibault DJ, Zack DJ. Retinal ganglion cell death in experimental glaucoma and after axotomy occurs by apoptosis. Invest Ophthalmol Vis Sci 1995;36(5):774-86.

[3] Quigley HA, Broman AT. The number of people with glaucoma worldwide in 2010 and 2020. British J Ophthalmol. 2006;90(3):262-7.

[4] Fingert JH, Heon E, Liebmann JM, Yamamoto T, Craig JE, Rait J, et al. Analysis of myocilin mutations in 1703 glaucoma patients from five different populations. Human Molecul Genetics. 1999;8(5):899-905.

[5]   Libby RT, Gould DB, Anderson MG, John SW. Complex genetics of glaucoma sus-
      ceptibility. Ann Rev Genomics Human Genetics. 2005;6:15-44.

[6]   Mabuchi F, Tang S, Kashiwagi K, Yamagata Z, Iijima H, Tsukahara S. The OPA1
      gene polymorphism is associated with normal tension and high tension glaucoma.
      Am J Ophthalmol. 2007;143(1):125-30.

[7]   Ray K, Mukhopadhyay A, Acharya M. Recent advances in molecular genetics of
      glaucoma. Mol Cel Biochem. 2003;253(1-2):223-31.

[8]   Group CN-TGS. Comparison of glaucomatous progression between untreated pa-
      tients with normal-tension glaucoma and patients with therapeutically reduced in-
      traocular pressures. Collaborative Normal-Tension Glaucoma Study Group. Am J
      Ophthalmol. 1998;126(4):487-97.

[9]   Heijl A, Leske MC, Bengtsson B, Hyman L, Bengtsson B, Hussein M. Reduction of in-
      traocular pressure and glaucoma progression: results from the Early Manifest Glau-
      coma Trial. Arch Ophthalmol. 2002;120(10):1268-79.

[10] Kass MA, Heuer DK, Higginbotham EJ, Johnson CA, Keltner JL, Miller JP, et al. The
      Ocular Hypertension Treatment Study: a randomized trial determines that topical
      ocular hypotensive medication delays or prevents the onset of primary open-angle
      glaucoma. Arch Ophthalmol. 2002;120(6):701-13.

[11] Baltmr A, Duggan J, Nizari S, Salt TE, Cordeiro MF. Neuroprotection in glaucoma -
      Is there a future role? Exp Eye Res. 2010;91(5):554-66.

[12] Kroemer G, Galluzzi L, Vandenabeele P, Abrams J, Alnemri ES, Baehrecke EH, et al.
      Classification of cell death: recommendations of the Nomenclature Committee on
      Cell Death 2009. Cell Death Differ. 2009;16(1):3-11.

[13] Kerr JF, Wyllie AH, Currie AR. Apoptosis: a basic biological phenomenon with wide-
      ranging implications in tissue kinetics. British J Cancer. 1972;26(4):239-57.

[14] Riedl SJ, Shi Y. Molecular mechanisms of caspase regulation during apoptosis. Na-
      ture Rev Mol Cell Biol. 2004;5(11):897-907.

[15] Vandenabeele P, Galluzzi L, Vanden Berghe T, Kroemer G. Molecular mechanisms of
      necroptosis: an ordered cellular explosion. Nature Rev Mol Cell Biol. 2010;11(10):
      700-14.

[16] Degterev A, Huang Z, Boyce M, Li Y, Jagtap P, Mizushima N, et al. Chemical inhibi-
      tor of nonapoptotic cell death with therapeutic potential for ischemic brain injury.
      Nat Chem Biol. 2005;1(2):112-9.

[17] Chan FK, Shisler J, Bixby JG, Felices M, Zheng L, Appel M, et al. A role for tumor
      necrosis factor receptor-2 and receptor-interacting protein in programmed necrosis
      and antiviral responses. J Biol Chem. 2003;278(51):51613-21.

[18] Bredesen DE, Rao RV, Mehlen P. Cell death in the nervous system. Nature. 2006;443(7113):796-802.

[19] Nagata S. Apoptosis by death factor. Cell. 1997;88(3):355-65.

[20] Peter ME, Krammer PH. The CD95(APO-1/Fas) DISC and beyond. Cell Death Different. 2003;10(1):26-35.

[21] Luo X, Budihardjo I, Zou H, Slaughter C, Wang X. Bid, a Bcl2 interacting protein, mediates cytochrome c release from mitochondria in response to activation of cell surface death receptors. Cell. 1998;94(4):481-90.

[22] Li H, Zhu H, Xu CJ, Yuan J. Cleavage of BID by caspase 8 mediates the mitochondrial damage in the Fas pathway of apoptosis. Cell. 1998;94(4):491-501.

[23] Wang X. The expanding role of mitochondria in apoptosis. Gen Develop. 2001;15(22): 2922-33.

[24] Li P, Nijhawan D, Budihardjo I, Srinivasula SM, Ahmad M, Alnemri ES, et al. Cytochrome c and dATP-dependent formation of Apaf-1/caspase-9 complex initiates an apoptotic protease cascade. Cell. 1997;91(4):479-89.

[25] Du C, Fang M, Li Y, Li L, Wang X. Smac, a mitochondrial protein that promotes cytochrome c-dependent caspase activation by eliminating IAP inhibition. Cell. 2000;102(1):33-42.

[26] Verhagen AM, Ekert PG, Pakusch M, Silke J, Connolly LM, Reid GE, et al. Identification of DIABLO, a mammalian protein that promotes apoptosis by binding to and antagonizing IAP proteins. Cell. 2000;102(1):43-53.

[27] Shembade N, Ma A, Harhaj EW. Inhibition of NF-kappaB signaling by A20 through disruption of ubiquitin enzyme complexes. Science. 2010;327(5969):1135-9.

[28] Wright A, Reiley WW, Chang M, Jin W, Lee AJ, Zhang M, et al. Regulation of early wave of germ cell apoptosis and spermatogenesis by deubiquitinating enzyme CYLD. Develop Cell. 2007;13(5):705-16.

[29] Micheau O, Tschopp J. Induction of TNF receptor I-mediated apoptosis via two sequential signaling complexes. Cell. 2003;114(2):181-90.

[30] Stanger BZ, Leder P, Lee TH, Kim E, Seed B. RIP: a novel protein containing a death domain that interacts with Fas/APO-1 (CD95) in yeast and causes cell death. Cell. 1995;81(4):513-23.

[31] Lin Y, Devin A, Rodriguez Y, Liu ZG. Cleavage of the death domain kinase RIP by caspase-8 prompts TNF-induced apoptosis. Gen Develop. 1999;13(19):2514-26.

[32] Vercammen D, Beyaert R, Denecker G, Goossens V, Van Loo G, Declercq W, et al. Inhibition of caspases increases the sensitivity of L929 cells to necrosis mediated by tumor necrosis factor. J Exp Med. 1998;187(9):1477-85.

[33] Vercammen D, Brouckaert G, Denecker G, Van de Craen M, Declercq W, Fiers W, et al. Dual signaling of the Fas receptor: initiation of both apoptotic and necrotic cell death pathways. J Expe Med. 1998;188(5):919-30.

[34] Holler N, Zaru R, Micheau O, Thome M, Attinger A, Valitutti S, et al. Fas triggers an alternative, caspase-8-independent cell death pathway using the kinase RIP as effector molecule. Nature Immunol. 2000;1(6):489-95.

[35] Degterev A, Hitomi J, Germscheid M, Ch'en IL, Korkina O, Teng X, et al. Identification of RIP1 kinase as a specific cellular target of necrostatins. Nat Chemical Biol. 2008;4(5):313-21.

[36] Cho YS, Challa S, Moquin D, Genga R, Ray TD, Guildford M, et al. Phosphorylation-driven assembly of the RIP1-RIP3 complex regulates programmed necrosis and virus-induced inflammation. Cell. 2009;137(6):1112-23.

[37] He S, Wang L, Miao L, Wang T, Du F, Zhao L, et al. Receptor interacting protein kinase-3 determines cellular necrotic response to TNF-alpha. Cell. 2009;137(6):1100-11.

[38] Zhang DW, Shao J, Lin J, Zhang N, Lu BJ, Lin SC, et al. RIP3, an energy metabolism regulator that switches TNF-induced cell death from apoptosis to necrosis. Science. 2009;325(5938):332-6.

[39] Kim YS, Morgan MJ, Choksi S, Liu ZG. TNF-induced activation of the Nox1 NADPH oxidase and its role in the induction of necrotic cell death. Mol Cell. 2007;26(5): 675-87.

[40] Yazdanpanah B, Wiegmann K, Tchikov V, Krut O, Pongratz C, Schramm M, et al. Riboflavin kinase couples TNF receptor 1 to NADPH oxidase. Nature. 2009;460(7259): 1159-63.

[41] Sumimoto H. Structure, regulation and evolution of Nox-family NADPH oxidases that produce reactive oxygen species. FEBS J. 2008;275(13):3249-77.

[42] Yu L, Wan F, Dutta S, Welsh S, Liu Z, Freundt E, et al. Autophagic programmed cell death by selective catalase degradation. Proc Nat Acad Sci USA. 2006;103(13):4952-7.

[43] Sun L, Wang H, Wang Z, He S, Chen S, Liao D, et al. Mixed lineage kinase domain-like protein mediates necrosis signaling downstream of RIP3 kinase. Cell. 2012;148(1-2):213-27.

[44] Wang Z, Jiang H, Chen S, Du F, Wang X. The mitochondrial phosphatase PGAM5 functions at the convergence point of multiple necrotic death pathways. Cell. 2012;148(1-2):228-43.

[45] Kerrigan LA, Zack DJ, Quigley HA, Smith SD, Pease ME. TUNEL-positive ganglion cells in human primary open-angle glaucoma. Arch Ophthalmol. 1997;115(8):1031-5.

[46] Quigley HA. Glaucoma: macrocosm to microcosm the Friedenwald lecture. Invest Ophthalmol Vis Sci. 2005;46(8):2662-70.

[47] Guo L, Moss SE, Alexander RA, Ali RR, Fitzke FW, Cordeiro MF. Retinal ganglion cell apoptosis in glaucoma is related to intraocular pressure and IOP-induced effects on extracellular matrix. Invest Ophthalmol Vis Sci. 2005;46(1):175-82.

[48] Kwon YH, Fingert JH, Kuehn MH, Alward WL. Primary open-angle glaucoma. N Engl J Med. 2009;360(11):1113-24.

[49] Howell GR, Libby RT, Jakobs TC, Smith RS, Phalan FC, Barter JW, et al. Axons of retinal ganglion cells are insulted in the optic nerve early in DBA/2J glaucoma. J Cell Biol. 2007;179(7):1523-37.

[50] Sommer A. Intraocular pressure and glaucoma. Am J Ophthalmol. 1989;107(2):186-8.

[51] Quigley HA. Clinical trials for glaucoma neuroprotection are not impossible. Curr Opin Ophthalmol. 2012;23(2):144-54.

[52] Burgoyne CF, Downs JC. Premise and prediction-how optic nerve head biomechanics underlies the susceptibility and clinical behavior of the aged optic nerve head. J Glaucoma. 2008;17(4):318-28.

[53] Sigal IA, Ethier CR. Biomechanics of the optic nerve head. Exp Eye Res. 2009;88(4): 799-807.

[54] Dreyer EB, Zurakowski D, Schumer RA, Podos SM, Lipton SA. Elevated glutamate levels in the vitreous body of humans and monkeys with glaucoma. Arch Ophthalmol. 1996;114(3):299-305.

[55] Guo L, Salt TE, Maass A, Luong V, Moss SE, Fitzke FW, et al. Assessment of neuroprotective effects of glutamate modulation on glaucoma-related retinal ganglion cell apoptosis in vivo. Invest Ophthalmol Vis Sci. 2006;47(2):626-33.

[56] Osborne NN, Ugarte M, Chao M, Chidlow G, Bae JH, Wood JP, et al. Neuroprotection in relation to retinal ischemia and relevance to glaucoma. Surv Ophthalmol. 1999;43 Suppl 1:S102-28.

[57] Salt TE, Cordeiro MF. Glutamate excitotoxicity in glaucoma: throwing the baby out with the bathwater? Eye (Lond). 2006;20(6):730-1.

[58] Kaur C, Foulds WS, Ling EA. Hypoxia-ischemia and retinal ganglion cell damage. Clin Ophthalmol. 2008;2(4):879-89.

[59] Tezel G, Yang X, Luo C, Cai J, Kain AD, Powell DW, et al. Hemoglobin expression and regulation in glaucoma: insights into retinal ganglion cell oxygenation. Invest Ophthalmol Vis Sci. 2010;51(2):907-19.

[60] Costa VP, Arcieri ES, Harris A. Blood pressure and glaucoma. British J Ophthalmol. 2009;93(10):1276-82.

[61] Leske MC. Ocular perfusion pressure and glaucoma: clinical trial and epidemiologic findings. Curr Opin Ophthalmol. 2009;20(2):73-8..

[62] Mittag TW, Danias J, Pohorenec G, Yuan HM, Burakgazi E, Chalmers-Redman R, et al. Retinal damage after 3 to 4 months of elevated intraocular pressure in a rat glaucoma model. Invest Ophthalmol Vis Sci. 2000;41(11):3451-9.

[63] Tatton WG, Chalmers-Redman RM, Sud A, Podos SM, Mittag TW. Maintaining mitochondrial membrane impermeability. an opportunity for new therapy in glaucoma? Surv Ophthalmol. 2001;45 Suppl 3:S277-83.

[64] Tezel G, Yang X. Caspase-independent component of retinal ganglion cell death, in vitro. Invest Ophthalmol Vis Sci. 2004;45(11):4049-59.

[65] Hisatomi T, Nakazawa T, Noda K, Almulki L, Miyahara S, Nakao S, et al. HIV protease inhibitors provide neuroprotection through inhibition of mitochondrial apoptosis in mice. J Clin Invest. 2008;118(6):2025-38.

[66] Lebrun-Julien F, Duplan L, Pernet V, Osswald I, Sapieha P, Bourgeois P, et al. Excitotoxic death of retinal neurons in vivo occurs via a non-cell-autonomous mechanism. J Neurosc. 2009;29(17):5536-45.

[67] Guo L, Salt TE, Luong V, Wood N, Cheung W, Maass A, et al. Targeting amyloid-beta in glaucoma treatment. Proc Nat Acad Sci USA. 2007;104(33):13444-9.

[68] McKinnon SJ, Lehman DM, Kerrigan-Baumrind LA, Merges CA, Pease ME, Kerrigan DF, et al. Caspase activation and amyloid precursor protein cleavage in rat ocular hypertension. Invest Ophthalmol Vis Sci. 2002;43(4):1077-87.

[69] Yoneda S, Hara H, Hirata A, Fukushima M, Inomata Y, Tanihara H. Vitreous fluid levels of beta-amyloid((1-42)) and tau in patients with retinal diseases. Japan J Ophthalmol. 2005;49(2):106-8.

[70] Ko ML, Peng PH, Ma MC, Ritch R, Chen CF. Dynamic changes in reactive oxygen species and antioxidant levels in retinas in experimental glaucoma. Free Rad Biol Med. 2005;39(3):365-73.

[71] Tezel G. Oxidative stress in glaucomatous neurodegeneration: mechanisms and consequences. Progr Ret Eye Res. 2006;25(5):490-513.

[72] Wax MB. The case for autoimmunity in glaucoma. Exp Eye Res. 2011;93(2):187-90.

[73] Cui Q, Harvey AR. At least two mechanisms are involved in the death of retinal ganglion cells following target ablation in neonatal rats. J Neurosci. 1995;15(12):8143-55.

[74] Rudzinski M, Wong TP, Saragovi HU. Changes in retinal expression of neurotrophins and neurotrophin receptors induced by ocular hypertension. J Neurobiol. 2004;58(3):341-54.

[75] Tezel G, Li LY, Patil RV, Wax MB. TNF-alpha and TNF-alpha receptor-1 in the retina of normal and glaucomatous eyes. Invest Ophthalmol Vis Sci. 2001;42(8):1787-94.

[76] Tezel G, Yang X, Luo C, Peng Y, Sun SL, Sun D. Mechanisms of immune system activation in glaucoma: oxidative stress-stimulated antigen presentation by the retina and optic nerve head glia. Invest Ophthalmol Vis Sci. 2007;48(2):705-14.

[77] Danesh-Meyer HV. Neuroprotection in glaucoma: recent and future directions. Curr Opin Ophthalmol. 2011;22(2):78-86.

[78] Danias J, Shen F, Kavalarakis M, Chen B, Goldblum D, Lee K, et al. Characterization of retinal damage in the episcleral vein cauterization rat glaucoma model. Exp Eye Res. 2006;82(2):219-28.

[79] Levkovitch-Verbin H, Quigley HA, Martin KR, Valenta D, Baumrind LA, Pease ME. Translimbal laser photocoagulation to the trabecular meshwork as a model of glaucoma in rats. Invest Ophthalmol Vis Sci. 2002;43(2):402-10.

[80] Johnson EC, Guo Y, Cepurna WO, Morrison JC. Neurotrophin roles in retinal ganglion cell survival: lessons from rat glaucoma models. Exp Eye Res. 2009;88(4):808-15.

[81] Sappington RM, Carlson BJ, Crish SD, Calkins DJ. The microbead occlusion model: a paradigm for induced ocular hypertension in rats and mice. Invest Ophthalmol Vis Sci. 2010;51(1):207-16.

[82] Levkovitch-Verbin H, Quigley HA, Kerrigan-Baumrind LA, D'Anna SA, Kerrigan D, Pease ME. Optic nerve transection in monkeys may result in secondary degeneration of retinal ganglion cells. Invest Ophthalmol Vis Sci. 2001;42(5):975-82.

[83] John SW, Smith RS, Savinova OV, Hawes NL, Chang B, Turnbull D, et al. Essential iris atrophy, pigment dispersion, and glaucoma in DBA/2J mice. Invest Ophthalmol Vis Sci. 1998;39(6):951-62.

[84] Anderson MG, Smith RS, Hawes NL, Zabaleta A, Chang B, Wiggs JL, et al. Mutations in genes encoding melanosomal proteins cause pigmentary glaucoma in DBA/2J mice. Nature Gen. 2002;30(1):81-5.

[85] Cone FE, Gelman SE, Son JL, Pease ME, Quigley HA. Differential susceptibility to experimental glaucoma among 3 mouse strains using bead and viscoelastic injection. Exp Eye Res. 2010;91(3):415-24.

[86] Chrysostomou V, Trounce IA, Crowston JG. Mechanisms of retinal ganglion cell injury in aging and glaucoma. Ophthalm Res. 2010;44(3):173-8.

[87] Faden AI. Neuroprotection and traumatic brain injury: theoretical option or realistic proposition. Curr Opin Neurol. 2002;15(6):707-12.

[88] Tolias CM, Bullock MR. Critical appraisal of neuroprotection trials in head injury: what have we learned? NeuroRx. 2004;1(1):71-9.

[89] Lebrun-Julien F, Di Polo A. Molecular and cell-based approaches for neuroprotection in glaucoma. Optom Vis Sci. 2008;85(6):417-24.

[90] Levin LA. Retinal ganglion cells and neuroprotection for glaucoma. Surv Ophthalmol. 2003;48 Suppl 1:S21-4.

[91] Lipton SA. Possible role for memantine in protecting retinal ganglion cells from glaucomatous damage. Surv Ophthalmol. 2003;48 Suppl 1:S38-46.

[92] Hare WA, WoldeMussie E, Weinreb RN, Ton H, Ruiz G, Wijono M, et al. Efficacy and safety of memantine treatment for reduction of changes associated with experimental glaucoma in monkey, II: Structural measures. Invest Ophthalmol Vis Sci. 2004;45(8):2640-51.

[93] Lagreze WA, Knorle R, Bach M, Feuerstein TJ. Memantine is neuroprotective in a rat model of pressure-induced retinal ischemia. Invest Ophthalmol Vis Sci. 1998;39(6): 1063-6.

[94] Sakamoto K, Kawakami T, Shimada M, Yamaguchi A, Kuwagata M, Saito M, et al. Histological protection by cilnidipine, a dual L/N-type Ca(2+) channel blocker, against neurotoxicity induced by ischemia-reperfusion in rat retina. Exp Eye Res. 2009;88(5):974-82.

[95] Fitzgerald M, Payne SC, Bartlett CA, Evill L, Harvey AR, Dunlop SA. Secondary retinal ganglion cell death and the neuroprotective effects of the calcium channel blocker lomerizine. Invest Ophthalmol Vis Sci. 2009;50(11):5456-62.

[96] Saylor M, McLoon LK, Harrison AR, Lee MS. Experimental and clinical evidence for brimonidine as an optic nerve and retinal neuroprotective agent: an evidence-based review. Arch Ophthalmol. 2009;127(4):402-6.

[97] Dong CJ, Guo Y, Agey P, Wheeler L, Hare WA. Alpha2 adrenergic modulation of NMDA receptor function as a major mechanism of RGC protection in experimental glaucoma and retinal excitotoxicity. Invest Ophthalmol Vis Sci. 2008;49(10):4515-22.

[98] Ma K, Xu L, Zhang H, Zhang S, Pu M, Jonas JB. Effect of brimonidine on retinal ganglion cell survival in an optic nerve crush model. Am J Ophthalmol. 2009;147(2): 326-31.

[99] Goldenberg-Cohen N, Dadon-Bar-El S, Hasanreisoglu M, Avraham-Lubin BC, Dratviman-Storobinsky O, Cohen Y, et al. Possible neuroprotective effect of brimonidine in a mouse model of ischaemic optic neuropathy. Clin Exp Ophthalmol. 2009;37(7): 718-29.

[100] Hernandez M, Urcola JH, Vecino E. Retinal ganglion cell neuroprotection in a rat model of glaucoma following brimonidine, latanoprost or combined treatments. Exp Eye Res. 2008;86(5):798-806.

[101] Saragovi HU, Hamel E, Di Polo A. A neurotrophic rationale for the therapy of neurodegenerative disorders. Curr Alzh Res. 2009;6(5):419-23.

[102] Koriyama Y, Tanii H, Ohno M, Kimura T, Kato S. A novel neuroprotective role of a small peptide from flesh fly, 5-S-GAD in the rat retina in vivo. Brain Res. 2008;1240:196-203.

[103] Cooper NG, Laabich A, Fan W, Wang X. The relationship between neurotrophic factors and CaMKII in the death and survival of retinal ganglion cells. Progr Brain Res. 2008;173:521-40.

[104] Weber AJ, Harman CD, Viswanathan S. Effects of optic nerve injury, glaucoma, and neuroprotection on the survival, structure, and function of ganglion cells in the mammalian retina. J Physiol. 2008;586:4393-400.

[105] Parrilla-Reverter G, Agudo M, Sobrado-Calvo P, Salinas-Navarro M, Villegas-Perez MP, Vidal-Sanz M. Effects of different neurotrophic factors on the survival of retinal ganglion cells after a complete intraorbital nerve crush injury: a quantitative in vivo study. Exp Eye Res. 2009;89(1):32-41.

[106] Pease ME, Zack DJ, Berlinicke C, Bloom K, Cone F, Wang Y, et al. Effect of CNTF on retinal ganglion cell survival in experimental glaucoma. Invest Ophthalmol Vis Sci. 2009;50(5):2194-200.

[107] Fu QL, Hu B, Wu W, Pepinsky RB, Mi S, So KF. Blocking LINGO-1 function promotes retinal ganglion cell survival following ocular hypertension and optic nerve transection. Invest Ophthalmol Vis Sci. 2008;49(3):975-85.

[108] Quigley HA, McKinnon SJ, Zack DJ, Pease ME, Kerrigan-Baumrind LA, Kerrigan DF, et al. Retrograde axonal transport of BDNF in retinal ganglion cells is blocked by acute IOP elevation in rats. Invest Ophthalmol Vis Sci. 2000;41(11):3460-6.

[109] Grozdanic SD, Lazic T, Kuehn MH, Harper MM, Kardon RH, Kwon YH, et al. Exogenous modulation of intrinsic optic nerve neuroprotective activity. Graefe's Arch Clin Exp Ophthalmol. 2010;248(8):1105-16.

[110] Weber AJ, Viswanathan S, Ramanathan C, Harman CD. Combined application of BDNF to the eye and brain enhances ganglion cell survival and function in the cat after optic nerve injury. Invest Ophthalmol Vis Sci. 2010;51(1):327-34.

[111] Park KJ, Grosso CA, Aubert I, Kaplan DR, Miller FD. p75NTR-dependent, myelin-mediated axonal degeneration regulates neural connectivity in the adult brain. Nature Neurosci. 2010;13(5):559-66.

[112] Lebrun-Julien F, Morquette B, Douillette A, Saragovi HU, Di Polo A. Inhibition of p75(NTR) in glia potentiates TrkA-mediated survival of injured retinal ganglion cells. Mol Cel Neurosci. 2009;40(4):410-20.

[113] Bai Y, Xu J, Brahimi F, Zhuo Y, Sarunic MV, Saragovi HU. An agonistic TrkB mAb causes sustained TrkB activation, delays RGC death, and protects the retinal structure in optic nerve axotomy and in glaucoma. Invest Ophthalmol Vis Sci. 2010;51(9): 4722-31.

[114] Tezel G. TNF-alpha signaling in glaucomatous neurodegeneration. Progr Brain Res. 2008;173:409-21.

[115] Roh M, Zhang Y, Murakami Y, Thanos A, Lee SC, Vavvas DG, et al. Etanercept, a Widely Used Inhibitor of Tumor Necrosis Factor-alpha (TNF- alpha), Prevents Retinal Ganglion Cell Loss in a Rat Model of Glaucoma. PloS One. 2012;7(7):e40065.

[116] Nakazawa T, Nakazawa C, Matsubara A, Noda K, Hisatomi T, She H, et al. Tumor necrosis factor-alpha mediates oligodendrocyte death and delayed retinal ganglion cell loss in a mouse model of glaucoma. J Neurosci. 2006;26(49):12633-41.

[117] Nucci C, Tartaglione R, Cerulli A, Mancino R, Spano A, Cavaliere F, et al. Retinal damage caused by high intraocular pressure-induced transient ischemia is prevented by coenzyme Q10 in rat. Internat Rev Neurobiol. 2007;82:397-406.

[118] Russo R, Cavaliere F, Rombola L, Gliozzi M, Cerulli A, Nucci C, et al. Rational basis for the development of coenzyme Q10 as a neurotherapeutic agent for retinal protection. Progr Brain Res. 2008;173:575-82.

[119] Munemasa Y, Ahn JH, Kwong JM, Caprioli J, Piri N. Redox proteins thioredoxin 1 and thioredoxin 2 support retinal ganglion cell survival in experimental glaucoma. Gene Ther. 2009;16(1):17-25.

[120] Neufeld AH. Pharmacologic neuroprotection with an inhibitor of nitric oxide synthase for the treatment of glaucoma. Brain Res Bul. 2004;62(6):455-9.

[121] Wax MB, Tezel G. Immunoregulation of retinal ganglion cell fate in glaucoma. Exp Eye Res. 2009;88(4):825-30.

[122] Bakalash S, Kessler A, Mizrahi T, Nussenblatt R, Schwartz M. Antigenic specificity of immunoprotective therapeutic vaccination for glaucoma. Invest Ophthalmol Vis Sci. 2003;44(8):3374-81.

[123] Huang W, Fileta JB, Dobberfuhl A, Filippopolous T, Guo Y, Kwon G, et al. Calcineurin cleavage is triggered by elevated intraocular pressure, and calcineurin inhibition blocks retinal ganglion cell death in experimental glaucoma. Proc Nat Acad Sci USA. 2005;102(34):12242-7.

[124] Frank T, Schlachetzki JC, Goricke B, Meuer K, Rohde G, Dietz GP, et al. Both systemic and local application of granulocyte-colony stimulating factor (G-CSF) is neuroprotective after retinal ganglion cell axotomy. BMC Neurosci. 2009;10:49.

[125] Bull ND, Irvine KA, Franklin RJ, Martin KR. Transplanted oligodendrocyte precursor cells reduce neurodegeneration in a model of glaucoma. Invest Ophthalmol Vis Sci. 2009;50(9):4244-53.

[126] Johnson TV, Bull ND, Hunt DP, Marina N, Tomarev SI, Martin KR. Neuroprotective effects of intravitreal mesenchymal stem cell transplantation in experimental glaucoma. Invest Ophthalmol Vis Sci. 2010;51(4):2051-9.

[127] Levkovitch-Verbin H, Kalev-Landoy M, Habot-Wilner Z, Melamed S. Minocycline delays death of retinal ganglion cells in experimental glaucoma and after optic nerve transection. Arch Ophthalmol. 2006;124(4):520-6.

[128] Levkovitch-Verbin H, Vander S, Melamed S. Rasagiline-induced delay of retinal ganglion cell death in experimental glaucoma in rats. J Glaucoma. 2011;20(5):273-7.

[129] Zhong L, Bradley J, Schubert W, Ahmed E, Adamis AP, Shima DT, et al. Erythropoietin promotes survival of retinal ganglion cells in DBA/2J glaucoma mice. Invest Ophthalmol Vis Sci. 2007;48(3):1212-8.

[130] Parisi V, Coppola G, Ziccardi L, Gallinaro G, Falsini B. Cytidine-5'-diphosphocholine (Citicoline): a pilot study in patients with non-arteritic ischaemic optic neuropathy. Eur J Neurol. 2008;15(5):465-74.

[131] Danesh-Meyer HV, Levin LA. Neuroprotection: extrapolating from neurologic diseases to the eye. Am J Ophthalmol. 2009;148(2):186-91 e2.

[132] Sena DF, Ramchand K, Lindsley K. Neuroprotection for treatment of glaucoma in adults. Cochrane Database Syst Rev. 2010(2):CD006539.

[133] Inc. A. Press releases on Memantine Trials. http://wwwallergancom/newsroom/indexhtm.

[134] Newman NJ, Biousse V, David R, Bhatti MT, Hamilton SR, Farris BK, et al. Prophylaxis for second eye involvement in leber hereditary optic neuropathy: an open-labeled, nonrandomized multicenter trial of topical brimonidine purite. Am J Ophthalmol. 2005;140(3):407-15.

[135] Wilhelm B, Ludtke H, Wilhelm H. Efficacy and tolerability of 0.2% brimonidine tartrate for the treatment of acute non-arteritic anterior ischemic optic neuropathy (NAION): a 3-month, double-masked, randomised, placebo-controlled trial. Graefe's Archive Clin Exp Ophthalmol. 2006;244(5):551-8.

[136] Krupin T, Liebmann JM, Greenfield DS, Rosenberg LF, Ritch R, Yang JW. The Low-pressure Glaucoma Treatment Study (LoGTS) study design and baseline characteristics of enrolled patients. Ophthalmology. 2005;112(3):376-85.

[137] Krupin T, Liebmann JM, Greenfield DS, Ritch R, Gardiner S. A randomized trial of brimonidine versus timolol in preserving visual function: results from the Low-Pressure Glaucoma Treatment Study. Am J Ophthalmol. 2011;151(4):671-81.

[138] Schwid SR, Cutter GR. Futility studies: spending a little to save a lot. Neurology. 2006;66(5):626-7.

[139] Tilley BC, Palesch YY, Kieburtz K, Ravina B, Huang P, Elm JJ, et al. Optimizing the ongoing search for new treatments for Parkinson disease: using futility designs. Neurology. 2006;66(5):628-33.

[140] Leske MC, Heijl A, Hyman L, Bengtsson B, Dong L, Yang Z. Predictors of long-term progression in the early manifest glaucoma trial. Ophthalmology. 2007;114(11): 1965-72.

[141] Nordstrom BL, Friedman DS, Mozaffari E, Quigley HA, Walker AM. Persistence and adherence with topical glaucoma therapy. Am J Ophthalmol. 2005;140(4):598-606.

Chapter 9

Strategies for Neuroprotection in Glaucoma

Lizette Mowatt and Maynard Mc Intosh

Additional information is available at the end of the chapter

1. Introduction

Glaucoma has long been considered an irreversible progressive optic neuropathy with associated visual loss. Elevated intraocular pressure (IOP) was once considered the main modifiable risk for progression of glaucoma and has been the target for treatment. The pathogenesis of glaucoma was originally based on the mechanical and vascular dysregulation theory, however, this has evolved over the past decade. With the classification of low tension glaucoma, it is now recognized that the damage that occurs in the optic disc is not directly due to the elevated IOP and may be independent of this risk factor. Even though clinicians may aim for a target pressure, progression of optic disc cupping and visual field loss can still continue despite normal IOPs.

In contemplating a systematic approach to neuroprotection, the main areas to target include 1) neurotoxic agents such as nitric oxide and glutamate, 2) deprivation of internal neurotrophic factors 3) balancing self-repair with self-destruction in ocular nerve tissue and, 4) ocular blood flow and combating ischemia [1,2,3]. Focus in this chapter is dedicated to reviewing the mechanisms involved in the pathophysiology of neurodegeneration, target processes that offer neuroprotection, and the chemical and genetic interventions bearing potential for increasing retinal ganglion cell (RGC) survival. Glaucoma has cellular and molecular neurodegenerative pathways akin to those of other neurodegenerative disorders such as alzheimer's and parkinsons, which increases the accessibility to possible treatment options.

Gene therapy targets increased conventional and uveoscleral outflow, reduced aqueous production and prevention of wound healing in addition to neuroprotection. Interfering with the apoptosis cycle by gene therapy has also being considered by increasing neurotrophic factors [4]. Intravitreal injections of brain-derived neurotrophic factor (BDNF), a neurotrophin that improves neurogenesis and survival are being studied. Interestingly it has recently been noted in animal models that short periods of hyperglycemia may be protective to the retinal ganglion cells during periods of elevated intra ocular pressure [5].

Neuroprotection is the strategy to prevent retinal ganglion cell death. There have been several methods, many still experimental, aimed at reducing glutamate excitotoxicity, nitric oxide, free radical production and tumour necrosis factor (TNF) inhibition [1-4,6]. With the latest research, glaucoma, which was once thought to be an optic neuropathy, then a retinal disease, is now being considered a neurodegenerative disease, like alzheimer and parkinson [7].

This chapter will review the present pathophysiology theories of neurodegeneration in glaucoma and highlight the latest updates in neuroprotection strategies, mechanisms that block apoptosis and improving the survival and functionality of the retinal ganglion cell.

2. Retinal ganglion cell death

The neurodegeneration seen in glaucoma is as an end result of apoptosis (programmed cell death) of the retinal ganglion cell (RGC). When the retinal ganglion cell dies, there is a degenerative change along the axon with the resulting clinical findings including thinning of the retinal nerve fiber layer (objectively measured by Optical Coherence Tomography, Heidelberg Retinal Tomography or GDx) and increased optic disc cupping. Retinal ganglion cell apoptosis results in visual field loss and ultimately loss of vision in glaucoma. There are several etiologies for retinal ganglion cell (RGC) death which occurs with and without elevated intraocular pressures.

Retinal ganglion cell apoptosis is thought to be a result of several factors:

- increased intraocular pressure (IOP)
- glutamate excitotoxicity
- oxidative stress: free radical induced apoptosis (nitric oxide)
- neurotrophic factors deprivation
- glial cell activation
- abnormal immune response
- hypo perfusion

The glutamate and nitric oxide (NO) theories were the early proposed mechanisms for neurodegeneration. There is a proposed oxidative component which results in oxidative stress on the RGC due to increased IOP and hypoxia leading to apoptosis.

3. Increased intraocular pressure

Although neurodegeneration theories were considered because of progression despite normal IOPs, increased IOP does have a role in RGC death. Increased IOP can block axonal transport of the excitotoxic transmitter, glutamate, at the level of the lamina cribrosa, leading to deprivation of neurotrophic factors. It is also theorized that a secondary release or decreased uptake of glutamate via the müller cells is another cause for retinal ganglion cell apoptosis. It has been noted that retinal ganglion cell death has been associated with elevated IOP with positive correlation with an increase in matrix metallopetidase- 9 (MMP-9) activity (P<0.001), tissue inhibitor of matrix metalloproteinase (TIMP-1) (P<0.05) and collagen 1 (P<0.01) [8].

With increased IOP, structural changes occur in the optic nerve head. There are several proposed theories for this effect. The mechanical bowing of the lamina cribrosa and loss of the axons may occur because of the hypo perfusion secondary to increased IOP. Optic nerve damage may be more prominent in hypotensive patients which may in part be due reduced perfusion and resulting oxidative stress from the induced hypoxia associated with reduced blood flow. In addition to this elevated IOP results in remodelling of the lamina cribrosa which may be a result of an increased synthesis of extracellular matrix ; matrix metalloproteases (MMP), collagen I and IV and elastin [9-11].

The upregulation of MMP may be due to either the vascular insufficiency with resulting ischemia or secondary to increased endothelin and TNF α production [12]. There is a significant correlation between MMP-9 activity and both RGC apoptosis (P <0.001) and loss of laminin (P <0.01) [8,9]. This change in the structure of the lamina cribosa may result in damage to the retinal ganglion cell axons as they traverse it [13]. Astrocyte activation can result from ischemia, increased hydrostatic pressure or damaged axons and this can propagate the process of structurally changing the lamina cribrosa, resulting in further damage to the transversing ganglion cell axons [14,15].

4. Glutamate

Glutamate is an excitatory neurotransmitter that is continuously released by photoreceptors and OFF bipolar cells in the dark which results in the dark current. Light stimuli starts the process of phototransduction which leads to reduced glutamate concentration in the synaptic cleft. Glutamate transporters allow for the uptake of glutamate by müller cells which is converted by glutamine synthetase into glutamine which is then released by the glial cells. This glutamine is taken up by the neurons and hydrolysed by glutaminase to glutamate again. Glutamate allows the influx of calcium, resulting in high intracellular calcium levels which promote apoptosis. Glutamate in excess is neurotoxic, due to its induced excitotoxicity. The glutamate-glutamine cycle allows for natural homeostasis between the neurons and the glial cells (Figure 1).

Glutamate is released from degenerating cells or reduced uptake from müller's cells can increase the presence of glutamate. RGC may undergo apoptosis directly because of increased glutamate excitotoxicity. Müller cells can be injured by the excess glutamate which results in a secondary RGC death [16].

Glutamate ionotropic receptors are found on the post synaptic bipolar, horizontal, amacrine and ganglion cells. They are gating cation channels that are classified into 3 groups; N-methyl-D-aspartate (NMDA) receptors, α-amino-3-hydroxy-5-methyl-4-isoxazolepropionic acid

(AMPA) receptors and kainite receptors. In view of this glutamate receptor antagonists have been found to reduce the neurotoxic effect of increased glutamate levels.

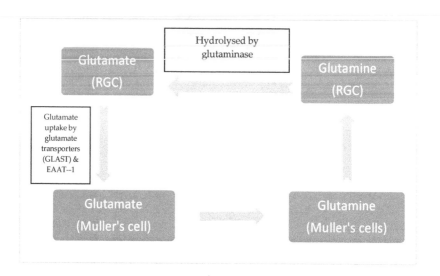

Figure 1. The glutamate-glutamine cycle (RGC= Retinal Ganglion cell, GLAST = Glutamate Aspartate transporter, EAAT-1 =Excitatory Amino Acid Transporter))

Increased glutamate has been noted in the vitreous of glaucoma patients [17]. However the glutamate transporters; glutamate aspartate transporter (GLAST) and excitatory amino acid transporter-1 (EAAT-1) are localized exclusively to müller's cells and glutamate transporter -1 (GLT-1) and excitatory amino acid transporter- 2 (EAAT-2) in the brain, decreased with increasing IOPs [18,19,20] (Figure 1). Therefore, the increase IOP effect on the glutamate transporters can further aggravate glutamine neurotoxicity.

Mice deficient in excitatory amino acid carrier-1 (EAAC1) or GLAST had RGC apoptosis in the absence of elevated IOP. Neuronal EAAC1 does not play a direct role in glutamate transport but transports cysteine much more than GLAST. This is important for the glutathione synthesis. Lack of glutathione made the RGCs more susceptible to oxidative stress [21].

5. Glutamate receptor antagonists

The NMDA ionotropic glutamate receptor has been shown to have an important role in the mechanisms of certain CNS disorders, eg alzheimer's and parkinson's disease as seen in rat and human models [22,23,24]. Glutamate opens calcium and sodium channels after binding to the NMDA receptor, which results in a high intracellular influx of calcium which starts the cascade of apoptosis. Therefore, NMDA receptor blockers have been investigated for counteracting possible glutamate excitotoxicity.

5.1. Memantine

Memantine, is a NMDA receptor blocker which is approved in the USA for dementia associated with alzheimer's disease. Although oral memantine clinically showed a protective effect on visual function and structural damage on macaque monkeys, it did not persist in long term treatment (>5 months) on ERG findings [25,26]. It has been used at doses of 4mg/kg po daily reaching concentrations of 0.3-1.8uM in the monkey vitreous [25,26]. The second phase III clinical trial showed that although the progression of disease was significantly lower in patients receiving the higher dose of memantine compared to patients receiving the low dose of memantine, there was no significant benefit compared to patients receiving placebo [27].

Latest animal studies have shown that using memantine in monkeys will result in an overall higher mean multifocal visual evoked potential (VEP) amplitudes than the non treated memantine monkeys when experimental glaucoma has been induced [28]. However it was not significant from baseline in the former. The use of the GDx in future studies will also allow more sensitive changes in retinal nerve fiber layer to be detected however, this may not directly be translated into functional damage, which in humans can be assesed with visual fields.

5.2. Eliprodil

This NMDA antagonist acts at the polyamine binding site of the NMDA receptor (NR2B subunit), blocking voltage dependent calcium channels. It has been shown to be neuroprotective in cultured neurons of brain and retina from excitotoxic and ischemia damage at doses of 1-10mg/kg [29]. Eliprodil has shown reduction in the NMDA currents by 78% in a glutamate induced cytotoxicity model [30]. Although there has been promise of this drug in animal studies, clinical trials have not been undertaken for glaucoma in humans.

5.3. Nitric oxide

Nitric oxide (NO) is a neurotransmitter, vasodilator and neuromodulator and can be neurotoxic. Nitric oxide is found at the post junctional area of glutaminergic junctions (rods, bipolar, amacrine and ganglion cells) and acts as an intracellular mediator for glutamate. Excessive production of nitric oxide by astrocytes has been shown to play a role in cell death in both the optic nerve head and the RGC [2,3,6,31,32]. Reactive oxidative species (ROS) may play a role in neurodegeneration as a result of apoptosis (Figure 2).

5.3.1. Oxidative stress

Nitric oxide is produced by nitric oxide synthase (NOS-2). NOS has 3 isoforms inducible NO (iNO), endothelial NO (eNO) and neuronal NO (nNO). These oxidize L-arginine to L-citrulline, producing NO. Nitric oxide freely diffuses to adjacent neurons and combines with O2 – to form peroxynitrite anions (ONOO-) which is a potential toxin, setting into motion neuronal apoptosis. It can be induced by injury or cytokines, such as interleukin 1 beta, tumour necrosis factor alpha, resulting in high concentrations of nitric oxide [32,33]. Increased levels of NOS are seen in the optic nerve head of glaucoma patients [32]. Tumour necrosis factor (TNF) α is upregulated in the glaucomatous optic nerve head and induces NOS in the astrocytes [34].

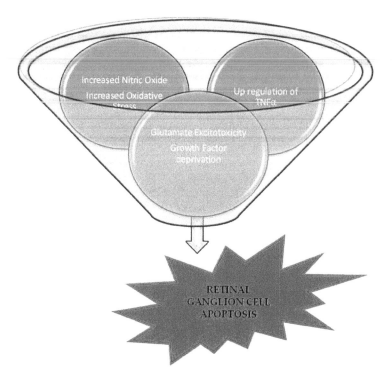

Figure 2. Multiple mechanisms for neurodegeneration which may be aggravated by vascular dysregulation, hypoxia and elevated IOP

nNO and iNO are expressed in reactive astrocytes. Increased NO reacts with a superoxide anion which can be toxic to the axons of the retinal ganglion cell. Motallebipour et al, showed a genetic association between iNO and primary open angle glaucoma (POAG) using genetic analysis and nuclear factor [35]. iNO is located in the astrocytes and microglial in the optic nerve head and expresses more activity with exposure to increased intraocular pressure and cytokines. This results in increased in NO production and the induction of the apoptotic cascade [36]. The NO oxide has its effect in both the astrocytes of the optic nerve head and the pericytes of the vasculature [32].

5.3.2. Vascular modulation

The endothelial NO synthase (eNOS) is expressed in the trabecular membrane and schlem's canal cells. eNOS produces nitric oxide which regulates the vascular tone causing smooth muscle relaxation and relaxation of the trabecular meshwork which improves aqueous humour outflow [37]. Elevation of the IOP increases the shear stress which activates eNOS which results in increase in the pressure dependent outflow.

5.3.3. The future

Krauss 2011 and Impagnatiello 2011 have had success in lowering IOP in preclinical trials with a nitric oxide donating prostaglandin F2 agonist (BOL-303259-X) more than with latanoprost (prostaglandin F2 agonist) alone [38,39]. Fabrizi 2012, also had some success with combining a carbonic anhydrase inhibitor with a nitric oxide moiety, NCX250 in lowering IOP compared with the a carbonic anhydrase inhibitor alone [40].

6. Alpha adrenergic receptor agonist

α2 adrenergic agonists are a known group of anti glaucoma drugs that inhibit adenylate cyclase, reducing cAMP, thereby decreasing aqueous production. They also act by increasing uveoscleral outflow. α_{2A} receptors can be found in non pigmented ciliary epithelium, α_{2B} receptors on neuronal dendrites and α_{2C} receptors on photoreceptors cell bodies and inner segments [41]. α_2 agonists have been shown to have secondary neuroprotective effects [42,43,44].

6.1. Brimonidine

α2 adrenergic receptors can modulate the release of neurotransmitters such as glutamate [45]. NMDA receptors when stimulated results in an increase in intracellular Ca2+ and an inward current in the RGC. Brimonidine, an α2 agonist, can block the NMDA receptors which results in controlling the intracellular calcium, hereby allowing neuroprotection [23,46]. Brimonidine is also thought to up regulate brain derived neurotrophic factor (BDNF), activating anti apoptotic genes and the cell survival signaling pathway. It is also thought to modulate the N methyl-D-aspartate receptors [43,46-48].

Brimonidine is also known to upregulate not only BDNF, but prosurvival factors, such as anti apoptotic factors B-cell lymphoma -2 (Bcl-2) and B-cell lymphoma extra large (bcl-xl), basic fibroblastic growth factor (bFGF) and extracellular signal regulated kinases (ERKs). These actions assist in the prevention of neuronal death and promotes cell survival [49].

7. Selective beta receptor blockade

Beta blockers have a long history of use in reducing the IOP in glaucoma by reducing the production of aqueous humour. Levobetaxolol, timolol and metipranolol have been shown to have secondary neuroprotective effect by reducing sodium and calcium influx, which reduces the release of glutamate with levobetaxolol being more effective than timolol [50,51,52].

7.1. Betaxolol

Betaxolol has been shown to reduce the spontaneous firing rate by suppressing glutamate-gated current and in effect Na currents in the ganglion cells [52]. By doing this it also reversibly blocks the voltage gated calcium current. High intracellular calcium can be neurotoxic. Due to the Ca2+ channel blockage activity by the selective beta 1 beta blocker, betaxolol exerts a neuroprotective effect on the retinal ganglion cells. This effect can be seen at 2-50uM concentration [53]. Timolol is not effective even in higher concentrations (100uM) and clinically betaxolol is more efficacious in preserving visual fields in glaucoma patients compared to timolol [54]. It has been demonstrated in human cryopreserved retinal arterioles that intraluminal bextaolol caused a significant greater dilatation than timolol, this may be due to the selective nature of the beta blocker [55]

Betaxolol 0.5% also upregulates the neurotrophic factor BDNF in retinal glia cells [56]. By its action on vascular smooth muscle relaxation this improves blood flow and reduces ischemia induced RGC apoptosis [52, 57]. Retinal ganglion cells protection has been shown using rat experimental model and the preservation of the a and b waves in the electroretinogram in both ischemic-reperfusion and glutamate toxicity models [56,57,58]. This has also been seen in light response experiments on tiger salamander flat mounted retinas [53].

8. Calcium channel blockade

As high intracellular calcium can be neurotoxic reducing this effect can be neuroprotective to the cells. This effect can be seen in both beta blockers and alpha agonists [2] (Table 1).

9. Prostaglandin analogs

Prostaglandin analogs are known as a first line treatment for reducing the IOP. However, latanoprost and bimatoprost acid have shown a neuroprotective on hypoxic induced or glutamate exocitoxity on RGCs [58,59]. This was IOP independent and is not thought to be associated with normal mechanism to lower IOP [59]. Acting via prostaglandin F2 receptors, it has been suggested that latanoprost may have a COX 2 feedback inhibition resulting in neuroprotection [58]. It has also been shown that it inhibits inducible NOS [56]. Latanoprost may also be combined with the NO moiety as previously mentioned [38,39]. Further, it has been theorized that it may have an anti apoptotic effect through the inhibition of caspase-3 [58,60].

10. Carbonic anhydrase inhibitors

The hypotensive effect of carbonic anhydrase inhibitors is a result of reduction of aqueous humour production at the ciliary epithelium level. However in cultured retinal cells, RGC death is prevented by dorzolamide because of its anti-apoptotic pathway [60].

NEUROPROTECTION STRATEGIES	Substances studied	General Method of Action
Glutamate Receptor Antagonists • NMDA receptors	Memantine Eliprodil	Reduces glutamate excitotoxicity and neurotoxicity
Nitric Oxide Synthase Inhibitors	Combinations of nitric oxide donating prostaglandin F2 agonist and with a carbonic anhydrase inhibitor (experimental)	Reduce oxidative stress
Beta blockade	Selective Beta Blockade (Betaxolol)	Reduces IOP Reduce glutamate production Upregulates BDNF Calcium channel blockade
Alpha adrenergic agonists	Alpha 2 agonist (Brimonidine)	Reduces IOP Reduce glutamate production Upregulates BDNF Calcium channel blockade Increases anti apoptotic genes
Prostaglandin analogue	Latanoprost acid Bimatoprost acid Tafluprost acid	Reduces IOP Inhibition of COX-2 activity Possible caspase 3 inhibition
Carbonic Anhydrase Inhibitor	Dorzolamide	Reduces IOP Reduces apoptosis
Neurotrophic factors (BDNF and CNTF)	Brain Derived Neurotrophic Factor Ciliary Derived Neurotrophic Factor	suppress the intrinsic apoptosis whilst activating the survival signals
Antioxidants: Reactive Oxygen species scavengers	Melatonin Vitamin E Co Q10 cofactor Manganese Tetrakis (in vitro)	activates anti oxidative enzymes Neutralizes free radicals. Oxidative stress can damage the trabecular meshwork, optic nerve head and retina.
Immunmodulators Anti Inflammatory agents TNF- α Inhibitors	Cop-1(glatiramer acetate) Ethanrecept Agmatine, an aminoguanidine Aspaminergic agent GLC756	Immunization can modulate immune function
Gene Therapy (Mitochondrial Augmentation)	Cycloheximide (CHX)	inducing neuroprotective genes including bcl-2
Apoptosis Inhibitors Inhibition of cytochrome c release Caspase inhibitors	Deprenyl BIRC4	Increase mitochondrial expression of bcl-2 and bcl-x, suppresses bax. Improved neuronal survival
Hypo perfusion	Gingko Bilboa IOP lowering medications	Improved blood flow

Table 1. Pharmacological neuroprotection strategies

11. Antioxidants

Numerous studies have shown that mitochondrial metabolism results in the release of reactive oxidative species that cause damage to lipids, protein, resulting in cell death and neurode-generation [61]. Hypoxia and ischemia are found to play an important role in the cascade of events leading to oxidative stress, and stimulating delta-opioid receptors (DOR) [62]. DOR has been proven to reduce the build-up of harmful free radicals, glutamate, and pro-inflammatory cytokines [62]. It has been shown that naloxone, an opioid blocker given intraperitoneally 6mg/kg in rabbits can reduce the retinal thickness thinning caused by ischemia [63]. Morphine has been used to pharmacological pre condition rabbit retina and has been shown to reduce acute IOP induced damage [64]

11.1. Coenzyme Q10 (Co Q10)

Coenzyme Q10, either on its own or in combination with vitamin E (alpha -tocopherol) have been shown to reduce intravitreal NMDA mediated damage in mice when adminsitered orally in 10mg/kg dosage [65]. In addition to its effect against oxidative stress its positive effect on the mitochondria may assist in the energy levels within the neuron, protecting it from apoptosis [66]. The RGC requires energy produced from mitochondria to ensure the conduction of currents and normal function of the RGC. Agents that promote the ganglion cell mitochondrial energy production may be neuroprotective in glaucoma. Oral alpha-lipoic acid and nicotinamide have been suggested for further assessment for their neuroprotective effect on light induced neuronal apoptosis [67].

Ginkgo biloba may be useful for treating dementia associated with alzheimer and for vascular insufficiency. Although the mechanism of action remains unknown for its use in glaucoma, it is thought that it causes intracellular signaling and neutralizes reactive oxygen species [13, 68, 69]. It has been shown to reduce the RGC axonal loss in mice compared to controls in a dose dependent manner after intragastral administration [68]. In one prospective randomized placebo controlled cross over trial, Ginkgo biloba extract was used 40mg tds orally for 4 weeks, which resulted in a statistically significant decrease in the corrected pattern standard deviation in visual fields of those patients [70].

Visual field defects have been noted to improve in patients with normal tension glaucoma after 4 weeks on gingko biloba and no ocular nor systemic adverse events occurred. Ginkgo biloba may exert multifactorial mechanisms which include increase ocular blood flow, anti oxidant activity, nitric oxide inhibition and improved cognitive function due to improved cerebral blood flow [70]. *Manganese Tetrakis* (4-benzoyl acid) porphyrin, a cell superoxide scavenger can prevent NO mediated motor neuron death in vitro [3]. *Cyclohex-imide (CHX)*, a protein synthesis inhibitor has been used in doses of 50-500nM, to prevent neuronal death and protects against oxidative insults by inducing neuroprotective genes including bcl-2 [3].

12. Neurotrophic factors

12.1. Brain derived neurotrophic factor

Brain derived neurotropic factor is a neurotrophin derived from the brain (produced in the lateral geniculate body of primates) which moves in a retrograde fashion to bind TrkB receptors on RGC cell body and axon. Its retrograde transport is obstructed in acute and chronic glaucoma models, hence apoptosis occurs, as its neurotrophic support is important in RGC survival [13].

Eyes with chronic glaucoma exhibit loss of physiological neurotrophin levels particularly BDNF. Intravitreal injections of neurotrophins, eg BDNF has shown a reduction in apoptotic RGC death in adult rat models [71]. A recent study considered the cost effective use of serum BDNF as a biomarker for early POAG as its levels were significantly decreased in glaucoma patients compared with controls [72].

12.1.1. Role in neuroprotection

BDNF acts through Trk B receptors; phosphorylating kinase enzyme, activating phosphoino-sitol 3-kinase thereby inhibiting the activation of capsase 3, an important link in the apoptosis pathway (Figure 3). Experimentally BDNF has shown little effect on RGC survival in a single dose, but repeated intravitreal injections as well as virally mediated over expression has been shown to slow RGC loss [4]. It has been used at doses of 25-100ug/kg in clinical trials [73]

12.2. Ciliary derived neurotrophic factor

Ciliary derived neurotrophic factor (CNTF) is a secretor- protein expressed in cells of all retinal layers and the optic nerve head. The protein shows increased expression in retinal and optic nerve injuries, and is reduced in the presence of increased IOP [4]. The protein demonstrates neuroprotection in virally-mediated overexpression after intravitreal injection. In one study by Pease et al, CNTF showed a 15% less axonal death in experimental induced glaucoma, which was statistically significant over combined CNTF- BDNF and BDNF alone [74]. Intraocular delivery of neurotrophins, BDNF and CNTF, intravitreal or by viral transfer may be a potential future development for neuroprotection [4].

13. Immune modulation

13.1. Anti-inflammatory agents

There is an inflammatory component to the neuronal retinal degeneration in glaucoma [75-78]. Studies have proved an age related susceptibility of glaucoma victims to progressive nerve damage and RGC loss even with single digit IOP [4]. Researchers have also established elements of the complement pathway such as C1q, as markers for astrocyte destruction that may result in RGC apoptosis [78]. Thus, the future of glaucoma therapy lies in employing additional modalities based on proven mechanisms of RGC loss.

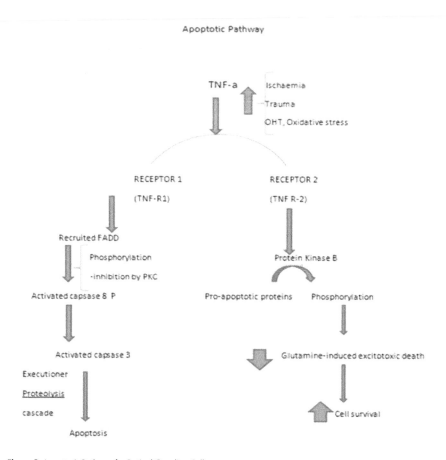

Figure 3. Apoptosis Pathway for Retinal Ganglion Cells

13.2. Tumour Necrosis Factor α (TNF α)

Progression of optic nerve axonal degeneration and retinal ganglion cell (RGC) apoptosis, have been shown to be responsible for progressive visual field loss in glaucoma, with or without ocular hypertension. One mechanism has been linked to tumor necrosis factor (TNF-α) in tissue around the optic nerve head demonstrated during immunostaining of mouse specimen [77]. This protein is a pro-inflammatory cytokine produced in response to trauma and inflammation and can start the apoptotic cascade [77] (Figure 3). TNF-α, secreted by damaged glials cells and through the binding of TNF receptor-1 (TNF-R1) starts the apoptotic process stimulating caspase ultimately leading to RGC death [79] (Figure 1). However the binding of the TNF-R1 receptor also triggers via heat shock proteins and activation of transcription factor NF-KB, a cell survival pathway. TNF- α levels if at best optimized (kept low) create a homeostasis that facilitates a balance between neuroprotection and neurodegeneration [75,79].

TNF- α is one of a 19-member family of ligands that exert their inflammatory activities through 29 receptors, triggering a cascade of inflammatory responses. TNF- α has been found to be upregulated in neurodegenerative diseases such as parkinson's and alzheimer's disease. In studies on the brain tissue of Alzheimer's patients, TNF- α, a mediator of chronic inflammation, has been detected in increased levels [76].

TNF- α in some studies was found in high concentration after laser-induced OHT, along with increased macrophage/microglia near the optic nerve head [77]. The levels of TNF α surpassed those in other inflammatory processes not involving ocular hypertension, validating the protein as a likely mediator of the RGC death, and hence a target for gene therapy. The increase in microglia population in the vitreous surface around the optic nerve head also alludes to an inflammation theory of glaucomatous optic nerve and RGC damage [77]. Research in alzheimer's has established TNF-α as a mediator of chronic inflammation with detection of increased levels in the brain of victims of this neurodegenerative disorder [76]. Serum amyloid A, is another acute-phase inflammatory marker discovered in the retina and trabecular meshwork of glaucoma eyes [78]. An understanding of the molecular processes in parallel disorders will influence the outlook on the future of glaucoma management.

Agarwal et al 2012, reported on extensive research evidence in support of the role of TNF-α in glaucomatous optic nerve degeneration and RGC apoptosis [75]. Research involved eyes with POAG, NTG and exfoliative glaucoma, with cataract eyes as controls [75]. Results showed marked elevation in TNF- α in aqueous samples of all glaucoma groups compared with controls. In addition, optic nerve degeneration and RGC loss were demonstrated in eyes subject to intravitreal injection of TNF- α.

13.2.1. How does TNF- α work?

Under normal conditions there is greater expression of TNF-R1 over TNF- α. Stress factors such as trauma, ischaemia, and elevated hydrostatic pressure result in an increase in expression of TNF-R1 and TNF- α. These have been shown to have several roles including pro-apoptotic and neuroprotective properties depending on the environment in which they are expressed [Figure 3]. Experimental evidence using mouse eyes have shown that in the absence of normal glial cells, the apoptotic effect dominates. Microglial cells are thought to provide survival signals necessary for the neuroprotective effect of TNF- α. Insults such as ischemia, oxidative stress and optic nerve injury increases the expression of cell death signals and reduces the expression of the cell survival signals, thereby potentiating the harmful effects of TNF- α [61].

In contrast, normally functioning glial cells support the neuroprotective effects of TNF- α and TNF-R1. The ischaemic and hydrostatic stress in glaucoma activate microglial activity causing an inflammatory response. Activated glial cells produce TNF- α along with harmful compounds like NO and endothelin 1 (ET-1). In excessive microglial activation, up regulation of

TNF α - causes RGC apoptosis in the absence of normal glial support. If there is significant microglial insult early in the event, TNF α - continues to exert apoptosis even after the stimulus is removed, as has been shown in in-vivo studies with mice, where progression of RGC death was seen on immunostaining even after normal IOPs were reached [75].

13.3. Agmatine, an aminoguanidine

Current research targets TNF-α for neuroprotection by reducing RGC loss (Figure 3). Such agents need to have high selectivity and specificity for excessive TNF-α and TNF-1 expression while preserving local immunity. Agents such as Agmatine, an aminoguanidine, have been shown to protect RGCs against the apoptotic effects of TNF-α, but the effects on other receptors and pathways are yet to be established [44,45,75]. Agmatine has been used at a concentration of 60 mg daily in rat ocular hypertension model [31]. 10(-3) M agmatine solution 4 times a day has shown a high affinity for alpha 2 receptors on the ciliary body, where it exerts its IOP lowering effect which has been seen in the rat model [80]. Amnioguanidine also targets inducible nitric oxide synthase (iNOS) inhibitors [31,73].

13.4. Ethanrecept, the future in neuroprotection

Work done by Roh et. al (2012) demonstrated the ability of ethanrecept, a recombinant chimeric protein, to act as a TNFα inhibitor to reduce RGC loss in the wake of elevated TNFα [77]. This decoy protein selectively binds TNFα, sparing the RGC damage from this and other inflammatory agents such as microglia [77]. Ethanrecept is used in the treatment of juvenile idiopathic arthritis, rheumatoid arthritis, ankylosing spondylitis, and psoriatic arthritis, and has shown no IOP-lowering capabilities. The drug however shows promise as a neuroprotective agent for intravitreal use in the future.

13.5. Copolymer -1 (Cop-1), — A possible vaccination for neuroprotection?

The inflammatory process in neurodegenerative diseases such as alzheimer's and glaucoma has been found to be associated with pro-inflammatory activities mediated in part by T cell activity. Cop-1, a synthetic peptide polymer known to suppress autoimmune encephalomyelitis, modulates this T cell reaction by producing a Th2 anti-inflammatory phenotype with attenuation of normal inflammatory response in neurodegenerative diseases as well as increased neuroprotection [13, 81,82]. Cop-1, glatiramer acetate has been FDA approved in the treatment of multiple sclerosis, a demyelinating disease.

It had been noted experimentally that an eye that had recent glutamate injections had resulting large numbers of lymphocytes present, hence it was theorized that glutamate toxicity induces a T cell lymphocyte reaction [81]. Therefore, by immunizing against this with the correct antigen, theoretically could reduce the damage induced by the glutamate. Cop-1 immunization has shown some protection against glutamate toxicity and elevated IOP in mice retinal ganglion cells [81,82,83]. So T cell mediated immunoprotection may be a future option for glaucoma, however, much research is still to be done.

13.5.1. Opioids

Opioid receptor activation has been shown to reduce the ischemic damage to the retina as demonstrated by ERG [84]. Opioid receptor stimulation and the facilitation of the actions of endogenous opioids show promise in neuroprotection of RGCs in glaucoma [84,85]. In the mice model, glaucoma was induced by raising the IOP above the systolic blood pressure (155-160mmHg) for 45 minutes to induce ischemic retinal injury [84]. The opioid antagonist naloxone (3mg/kg) was given to mice intraperitoneally 24 hours before the ischemic event. Another study group of mice had morphine (0.01-10mg/kg given intraperitoneallly 24 hours before the ischemic injury. 7 days after the injury the retina of both groups were assessed by the ERG. The mice that has morphine had greater preservation of their ERG a and b wave amplitudes 7 days after the ischemic event. Further the protective effect of morphine on preservation of ERG amplitudes was dose related with the ED50 of 0.18mg/kg [84]. However, these strategies have not yet been tested in humans or undergone randomized controlled trials.

14. Stem cells

Much research is still yet to be done on stem cells and neuroprotection. Stem cells can supply neurotrophins and modulate matrix metalloproteinases after an injury which can be neuro-protective and limit neuronal damage [86]. However in a pre-clinical model of glaucoma, intravitreal stem cell injections have been shown to enhance the survival of the RGC [23].

15. Gene therapy

With emerging evidence for the molecular basis in glaucoma- pathophysiology, the disease may be interrupted by targeting key sites once the genetic expression is known. Studies of micro-RNA such as miRNA-125b has led to the understanding of the key sites for targeted down-regulation of messenger RNA which is thought to add to the oxidative stress induction of inflammation and astrogliosis in alzheimer's disease [78]. Alzheimer's disease, parkinson and glaucoma are thought to have a similar neurodegenerative basis (molecular and cellular pathways for neuronal cell loss) [78]. Hence gene therapy for glaucoma and other neurode-generative disorders may be where medical management is headed. Target sites include uveoscleral outflow site, surgical (trabeculectomy) site, ciliary apparatus, retina and optic nerve head (neuroprotection) [4].

Gene therapy would be helpful in preventing neurodegeneration using anti apoptotic genes, bcl-2 and bcl-x [2]. Another mechanism is blocking the apoptotic pathway with deprenyl (monamine oxidase inhibitor). It is proposed that it stabilizes the mitochondrial membrane potential, preventing the release of cytochrome c which can activate capsases (Figure 1) [2, 87].

Targeting antioxidant genes is a promising strategy for future management of glaucomatous neurodegeneration. Researchers used cloned extracellular superoxide dismutase (ECSOD) or catalase (CAT), carried on recombinant adeno associated virus intravitreally in mice. The mice were euthanized and optic nerve volume, myelin fibre area, axonal cell loss and RGC loss evaluated Inital response showed a 15 fold increase in ECSOD and 3.3-fold in CAT [88]. After six months the authors reported 29% reduction in RGC loss, 36% in ON demyelination, and reduction in axonal loss by 44% all compared to control eyes, indicating that antioxidant gene therapy will prove an invaluable adjunct to current glaucoma therapy.

15.1. Administering gene therapy

Administration of gene therapy must ideally be safe, repeatable, have low immunogenicity, and carry low infectious and mutagenic potential, modification of Koch's postulates [4]. Because viral vectors have the ability to maintain stable DNA within the target nucleus, they are preferred over non-viral vectors.

15.1.1. Viral vectors

Adenoviral vectors (Ad), non-enveloped replication-deficient recombinant viruses were the first to be used in gene therapy research [4,89]. They show high level of tropism for post mitotic and highly specialized cells, and have been known to reproduce TM cells with high accuracy. They have application in Muller cell and RPE cell replication as well. Studies have been done with Adenovirus (Ad) mediated intravitreal delivery of BDNF. However, repeated injections have been found to cause severe inflammation in experimental models [2, 90]

Adeno-associated Viruses (AAV). This is an integrating vector known to show efficient delivery to target tissues. AAVs do not carry viral genes, therefore they have no unwanted pathogenicity, immunogenicity, nor significant inflammation upon sub retinal application [2]. In the last 4 years the use of AAV vector in the delivery of gene therapy has met some success in human trials, but the effect is limited to RGC survival. Though the vectors may target trabecular meshwork cells, they are not very active there [89].

Herpes Simplex Virus (HSV). This virus has shown promise in glaucoma research and therapy as it is able to transduce trabecular meshwork,ciliary body epithelial, and retinal ganglion cells. The injected derivative however has been found to carry risks of inflammation, toxicity, and limited duration of gene expression [4].

Lentiviral vectors. These single strand RNA viruses can incorporate trabecular meshwork and RGC DNA by reverse transcription, with both neuroprotective and IOP lowering potential. Combining several enzymes such as cyclooxygenase and prostaglandin pathway enzymes increases their IOP-lowering properties. [90]

15.1.2. Non-viral vectors

Naked DNA Injection. Work done with naked DNA as plasmid vectors expressing chloramphenicol acetyl transferase has shown promise in the possible control of wound healing after trabeculectomy. The plasmid injected in the bleb or under collagen shield has resulted in a 30 fold increase in the activity of the enzyme. [4]

The use of short 21 siRNA by intracameral and intravitreal injection to silence the unwanted expression of glaucoma genes particularly in the trabecular meshwork is being studied. The effects are so far temporary, and such siRNAs need the assistance of developed nanoparticles, such as magnetic nanoparticles, to enter target cells [89]. Chemical approach include the use of *cationic lipids (liposomes)* used in vitro, and shows promise for in vivo application via intracameral route with the target tissue being trabecular meshwork [4].

16. Conclusion

The cause of glaucoma and ultimately retinal ganglion cell death is multifactorial. At present there is no cure for glaucoma and the mainstay of treatment medically and surgically is to control the IOP. However, this conventional approach of lowering IOP is merely a secondary or indirect approach to the real problem. Current studies show that glaucoma is a neurode-generative disease with neuroprotection and possibly neuroregeneration and neuro enhance-ment as the future treatment modality. Modified Koch's postulates have been applied in the experimental neuroprotective research. Ultimately the retinal ganglion cell death whether primary or secondary (bystander result) must be stopped and the neurons preserved. The clinical application of most of these experimental neuroprotective strategies still has yet to pass through randomized controlled clinical trials before they can be accepted. The future holds much promise as to possible effective neuroprotective strategies, however, much research is still yet to be done.

Author details

Lizette Mowatt[1,2*] and Maynard Mc Intosh[3]

*Address all correspondence to: lizettemowatt@yahoo.com

1 Faculty of Medical Sciences, University of the West Indies, Jamaica

2 University Hospital of the West Indies, Mona, Jamaica

3 St Joseph Hospital, Kingston, Jamaica

References

[1] Chang EE, Goldberg JL. Glaucoma 2.0: neuroprotection, neuroregeneration, neuroen-hancement. Ophthalmology. 2012 ;119:979-86.

[2] Kwon YH, Mansberger SL, Cioffi GA. Ganglion Cell Death in Glaucoma: Mechanisms and Neuroprotective Strategies. Ophthalmology Clinics of North America. 2000;13:465-479

[3] Naskar R, Dreyer EB New Horizons in Neuroprotection. Surv Ophthalmol 2001. 45 (Suppl 3):S250-S255

[4] Liu X, Rasmussen CA, Gabelt BT, Brandt CR, Kaufman PL. Gene therapy targeting glaucoma: where are we? Surv Ophthalmol. 2009 ;54:472-86

[5] Ebneter A, Chidlow G, Wood JP, Casson RJ. Protection of retinal ganglion cells and the optic nerve during short-term hyperglycemia in experimental glaucoma.Arch Ophthalmol. 2011;129:1337-44

[6] Halpern DL, Grosskreutz CL. Glaucomatous optic neuropathy: mechanisms of disease.Ophthalmol Clin North Am. 2002 ;15:61-8

[7] Bayer AU, Keller ON, Ferrari F, Maag KP. Association of glaucoma with neurodegenerative diseases with apoptotic cell death: Alzheimer's disease and Parkinson's disease.Am J Ophthalmol. 2002 Jan;133:135-7

[8] Guo L, Moss SE, Alexander RA, Ali RR, Fitzke FW, Cordeiro MF. Retinal ganglion cell apoptosis in glaucoma is related to intraocular pressure and IOP-induced effects on extracellular matrix. Invest Ophthalmol Vis Sci. 2005 ;46:175-82

[9] Yan X, Tezel G, Wax MB, et al. Matrix metalloprotineinases and tumour necrosis factor alpha in glaucomatous optic nerve head. Arch Ophthalmol 2000;118:666-73

[10] Agapova OA, Kaufman PL, Lucarelli MJ, et al. Differential expression of matric metalloproteinases in monkey eyes with experimental glaucoma or optic nerve transection. Brain Res 2003;967:132-43

[11] Hermandez MR, Pena JD, The optic nerve head in glaucomatous optic neuropathy. Arch Ophthalmol 1997;115:389-95

[12] Golubnitschaja O, Yeghiazaryan K, Liu R, Mönkemann H, Leppert D, Schild H, Haefliger IO, Flammer J. Increased expression of matrix metalloproteinases in mononuclear blood cells of normal-tension glaucoma patients. J Glaucoma. 2004;13:66-72

[13] Kuehn MH, Fingert JH, Kwon YH, Retinal Ganglion Cell Death in Glaucoma: Mechanisms and Neuroprotective Strategies. Ophthalmol Clin N Am 2005 ;18:383-395

[14] Ridet JL, Malhotra SK, Privat A, et al. Reactive Astrocyes; cellular and molecular cues to biological function. Trends Neurosci 1997:20:570-7

[15] Hernandez MR, Pena JD, Selvidge JA, et al. Hydrostatic pressure stimulates synthesis of elastin in cultured optic nerve head astrocytes. Glia 2000;32:122-36

[16] Ullian EM, Barkis WB, Chen S, et al. Invulnerability of retinal ganglion cells to NMDA excitotoxicity. Mol Cell Neurosci 2004;26:544-57

[17] Dreyer E, Zurakowski D, Schumer R, et al. Elevated glutamate levels in the vitreous body of humans and monkeys with glaucoma. Arch Ophthalmol. 1996;114:299–305

[18] Martin KRG, Levkovitch-Verbin H, Valenta D,Baumrind L, Pease ME, Quigley ,HA. Retinal Glutamate transporter changes in Experimental Gluacoma and after Optic Nerve Transection in the Rat. Invest Ophthalmol Vis Sci. 2002;43:2236–2243

[19] Vorwerk CK, Naskar R, Schuettauf F, et al. Depression of retinal glutamate transporter function leads to elevated intravitreal glutamate levels and ganglion cell death. Invest Ophthalmol Vis Sci. 2000;41:3615–3621

[20] Naskar R, Vorwek CK, Dreyer EB. Concurrent downregulation of a glutamate transporter and receptor in glaucoma. Invet Ophthalmol Vis Sci. 2000. 41:1940-4

[21] Harada T, Harada C, Nakamura Kazuaki, Quah HA, Okumura A,Nakamekata K, Saeki T, Aihara M, Yoshida H, et al.The potential role of glutamate transporers in the pathogenesis of normal tension glaucoma. J Clin Invest. 2007;117:1763–1770

[22] Sonkusare SK, Kaul CL, Ramarao P. Dementia of Alzheimer's disease and other neurodegenerative disorders—memantine, a new hope. Pharmacol Res. 2005;51:1–17

[23] Johnson KA, Conn PJ, Niswender CM. Glutamate receptors as therapeutic targets for Parkinson's disease. CNS Neurol Disord Drug Targets. 2009;8:475-91.

[24] Nandhu MS, Paul J, Kuruvila KP, Abraham PM, Antony S, Paulose CS. Glutamate and NMDA receptors activation leads to cerebellar dysfunction and impaired motor coordination in unilateral 6-hydroxydopamine lesioned Parkinson's rat: functional recovery with bone marrow cells, serotonin and GABA. Mol Cell Biochem. 2011 l; 353:47-57

[25] Hare WA, WoldeMussie E, Lai RK, Ton H, Ruiz G, Chun T, Wheeler L. Efficacy and safety of memantine treatment for reduction of changes associated with experimental glaucoma in monkey, I: Functional measures. Invest Ophthalmol Vis Sci. 2004;45:2625-39. Erratum in: Invest Ophthalmol Vis Sci. 2004;45:2878.

[26] Hare WA, WoldeMussie E, Weinreb RN, Ton H, Ruiz G, Wijono M, Feldmann B, Zangwill L, Wheeler L. Efficacy and safety of memantine treatment for reduction of changes associated with experimental glaucoma in monkey, II: Structural measures.Invest Ophthalmol Vis Sci. 2004;45:2640-51

[27] Wheeler L, The future of neuroprotection in glaucoma therapeutics. Acta Ophthalmologica, 2008;86: 0. doi: 10.1111/j.1755-3768.2008.6446.x-i1

[28] Gabelt BT, Rasmussen CA, Tektas OY, Kim CB, Peterson JC, Nork TM, Hoeve JN, Lütjen-Drecoll E, Kaufman PL Structure/function studies and the effects of memantine in monkeys with experimental glaucoma. Invest Ophthalmol Vis Sci. 2012 ; 53:2368-76

[29] Kapin M, DOshi R, Scatton B, DeSantis LM, Chandler ML. Neuroprotective Effects of Eliprodil in Retina Excitotoxicity and Ischemia. Invest Ophthalmol Vis Sci 1999;40:1177-1182

[30] Pang IH, Wexler EM, Nawy S, DeSantis L, Kapin MA.Protection by eliprodil against excitotoxicity in cultured rat retinal ganglion cells. Invest Ophthalmol Vis Sci. 1999;40:1170-6.

[31] Neufeld AH, Sawada A, Becker B.Inhibition of nitric-oxide synthase 2 by aminoguanidine provides neuroprotection of retinal ganglion cells in a rat model of chronic glaucoma. Proc Natl Acad Sci U S A. 1999;96:9944-8

[32] Neufeld AH, Hermandez MR, Gonzalez M: Nitric Oxide synthase in the human glaucomatous optic nerve head. Arch Ophthalmol 1997;115:497-503

[33] Nathan C, Xie QW. Nitric oxide synthases: roles, tolls and controls. Cell 1994;78:915-8

[34] Yuan L, Neufeld AH. Tumor necrosis factor-alpha: a potentially neurodestructive cytokine produced by glia in the human glaucomatous optic nerve head. Glia. 2000; 32:42-50

[35] Motallebipour M, Rada-Iglesias A, Jansson M, Wadelius C. The promoter of inducible nitric oxide synthase implicated in glaucoma based on genetic analysis and nuclear factor binding. Molecular Vision 2005; 11:950-7

[36] Agarwal R, Gupta SK, Agarwal P, Saxena R, Agrawal SS. Current concepts in the pathophysiology of glaucoma. Indian J Ophthalmol. 2009 ;57:257-66.

[37] Ellis DZ, Sharif NA, Dismuke WM. Endogenous regulation of human Schlemm's canal cell volume by nitric oxide signaling. Invest Ophthalmol Vis Sci. 2010;51:5817–5824

[38] Krauss AH, Impagnatiello F, Toris CB, Gale DC, Prasanna G, Borghi V, Chiroli V, Chong WK, Carreiro ST, Ongini E.Ocular hypotensive activity of BOL-303259-X, a nitric oxide donating prostaglandin F2α agonist, in preclinical models. Exp Eye Res. 2011 ;93:250-5

[39] Impagnatiello F, Borghi V, Gale DC, et al. A dual acting compound with latanoprost amide and nitric oxide releasing properties, shows ocular hypotensive effects in rabbits and dogs. Exp Eye Res.2011;03:243–249

[40] Fabrizi F, Mincione F, Somma T, Scozzafava G, Galassi F, Masini E, Impagnatiello F, Supuran CT.A new approach to antiglaucoma drugs: carbonic anhydrase inhibitors with or without NO donating moieties. Mechanism of action and preliminary pharmacology. J Enzyme Inhib Med Chem. 2012 ;27:138-47

[41] Woldemussie E, Wijono M, Pow D. Localization of alpha 2 receptors in ocular tissue. Vis Neurosci. 2007;24:745-756.

[42] Yoles E, Wheeler LA, Schwartz M. Alpha 2 adrenoreceptor agonists are neuroprotective in a rat model of optic nerve degeneration. Invest Ophthalmol Vis. Sci. 1999:40;65-73

[43] Wheeler LA, Lai R, WoldeMussie E. From the lab to the clinic: activation of an alpha-2 agonist pathway is neuroprotective in models of retinal and optic nerve injury. Eur J Ophthalmol. 1999;9:S17-S21.

[44] Pinar-Sueiro S, Urcola H, Rivas MA, Vecino E. Prevention of retinal ganglion cell swelling by systemic brimonidine in a rat experimental glaucoma model. Clin Experiment. Ophthalmol 2011:39;799-807

[45] Pan YZ, Li DP, Pan HL. Inhibition of glutamatergic synaptic input to spinal lamina II(o) neurons by presynaptic alpha(2)-adrenergic receptors. J Neurophysiol. 2002;87:1938–1947

[46] Dong CJ, Guo Y, Agey P, Wheeler L, and Hare WA. Alpha2 Adrenergic Modulation of NMDA Receptor Function as a Major Mechanism of RGC Protection in Experimental Glaucoma and Retinal Excitotoxicity. Invest. Ophthalmol. Vis. Sci. October 2008; 49: 4515-4522

[47] Gao H, Qiao X, Cantor LB, et al. Up-regulation of brain-derived neurotrophic factor expression by brimonidine in rat retinal ganglion cells. Arch Ophthalmol. 2002;120:797-803

[48] Lai RK, Chun T, Hasson D, et al. Alpha-2 adrenoceptor agonist protects retinal function after acute retinal ischemic injury in the rat. Vis Neurosci. 2002;19:175-185

[49] Tatton W, Chen D, Chalmers-Redman R, Wheeler L, Nixon R, Tatton N. Hypothesis for a common basis for neuroprotection in glaucoma and Alzheimer's disease:anti apoptosis by alpha 2 adrenergic receptor activation. Surv Ophthalmol 2003; 48 (Suppl 1), S25-37

[50] Osborne NN, Cazeviville C, Carvalho AL, Larsen AK, DeSantis L. In vivo and in vitro experiments show that betaxolol is a retinal neuroprotective agent. Brain Res. 1997:751;113-123

[51] Wood JP, Schmidt KG, Melena J, Chidlow G, Allmier H, Osborne NN. The beta adrenoreceptor antagonists metipranolol and timolol are retinal neuroprotectants:comparision with betaxolol. Exp Eye Res. 2003 76;505-516

[52] Osborne NN, Wood JP, Chidlow G, Casson R, DeSantis L, Schmidt KG. Effectiveness of levobetaxolol and timolol at blunting retinal ischemia is related to their calcium and sodium blocking activities: relevance to glaucoma. Brain Res Bull 2004.62:525-528

[53] Gross RL, Hensley SH, Wu S. Retinal Ganglion Cell Dysfunction Induced by Hypoxia and glutamate: Potential Neuroprotective Effects of beta blockers. Surv Ophthalmol 1999; 43[Suppl 1]: S162-S170

[54] Kaiser JH, Flammer J, Scumfig D, Hendrickson P, Long term follow up of glaucoma patients treated with beta blockers. Surv Ophthalmol 1994: 38 (Suppl):S156-S160

[55] Yu DY, Su EN, Cringle SJ, Alder VA, Yu PK, Desantis L.Effect of betaxolol, timolol and nimodipine on human and pig retinal arterioles.Exp Eye Res. 1998 ;67:73-81.

[56] Wood JP, De Santis L, Chao HM, Osborne NN. Topically applied betaxolol attenuates ischemia induced effects to the rat retina and stimulates BDNF mRNA Exp Eye Res. 2001: 72 ;79-86

[57] Cheon EW, Park CH, Kang SS, et al. Betaxolol attenuates retinal ischemia/reperfusion damage in the rat. Neuroreport 2003; 14:1913-1917

[58] Shih GC, Calkins DJ Secondary neuroprotective effects of hypotensive drugs and potential mechanisms of action. Expert Rev. Ophthalmol 2012:7:161-175

[59] Yamagishi R, Aihara M, Araie M. Neuroprotective effects of prostaglandin analogues on retinal ganglion cell death independent of intraocular pressure reduction. Exp Eye Res. 2011;93:265-70

[60] Kniep EM, Roehlecke C, Ozkucur N, Steinberg A, Reber F, Knels L, Funk RH. Inhibition of apoptosis and reduction of intracellular pH decrease in retinal neural cell cultures by a blocker of carbonic anhydrase. Invest Ophthalmol Vis Sci. 2006;47:1185-92

[61] Tezel G. Oxidative stress in glaucomatous neurodegeneration: mechanisms and consequences. Prog Retin Eye Res.2006;25:490-513

[62] Pai-Huei P, Ho-Shiang H, Yih-Jing L, Yih-Sharng C, Ming-Chieh M Novel role for the δ-opioid receptor in hypoxic preconditioning in rat retinas. Journal of Neurochemistry 2009; 108; 741–754

[63] Lam TT, Takahashi K, Tso MO. The effects of naloxone on retinal ischemia in rats.J Ocul Pharmacol. 1994;10:481-92.

[64] Riazi-Esfahani M., Kiumehr S., Asadi-Amoli F. et al. Morphine pretreatment provides histologic protection against ischemia-reperfusion injury in rabbit retina. Retina 2008; 28: 511–517

[65] Nakajima Y, Inokuchi Y, Nishi M, Shimazawa M, Otsubo K, Hara H. Coenzyme Q10 protects retinal cells against oxidative stress in vitro and in vivo. Brain Res. 2008 21;1226:226-33

[66] Nucci C, Tartaglione R, Cerulli A, Mancino R, Spanò A, Cavaliere F, Rombolà L, Bagetta G, Corasaniti MT, Morrone LA. Retinal damage caused by high intraocular pressure-induced transient ischemia is prevented by coenzyme Q10 in rat. Int Rev Neurobiol. 2007;82:397-406

[67] Osborne NN. Pathogenesis of ganglion "cell death" in glaucoma and neuroprotection: focus on ganglion cell axonal mitochondria. Prog Brain Res. 2008;173:339-52

[68] Hirooka K, Tokuda M, Miyamoto O, et al. The gingko biloba extract (EGB 761) provides a neuroprotective effect on retinal ganglion cells in a rat model of chronic glaucoma. Cur Eye Res 2004;28:153-7

[69] Marcocci L, Parker L, Dry-Lefaix MT, et al. Anti-oxidant action of gingko bilboa extract (EGB) 761. Methods Enzymol 1994;234:462-75

[70] Quaranta L, Bettelli S, Uva MG, et al. Effect of gingko bilboa extract on preexisting visual field damage in normal tension pressure. Ophthalmology 2003;110:352-62

[71] Mey J, Thanos S. Intravitreal injections of neurotrophic factors support the survival of axotomized retinal ganglion cells in adult rats in vivo. Brain Res. 1993;602:304-17

[72] Ghaffariyeh A, Honarpisheh N, Heidari MH, Puyan S, Abasov F. Brain-derived neurotrophic factor as a biomarker in primary open-angle glaucoma Optom Vis Sci. 2011 ;8:80-5

[73] Levin LA. Neuroprotection and regeneration in glaucoma Ophthalmol Clin North Am. 2005;18:585-96

[74] Pease ME, Zack DJ, Berlinicke C, Bloom K, Cone F, Wang Y, Klein RL, Hauswirth WW, Quigley HA. Effect of CNTF on retinal ganglion cell survival in experimental glaucoma. Invest Ophthalmol Vis Sci. 2009 May; 50: 2194–2200

[75] Agarwal R, Agarwal P. Glaucomatous neurodegeneration: An eye on tumor necrosis factor-alpha. Indian J Ophthalmol 2012;60:255-61

[76] Gabbita SP, Srivastava MK, Eslami P, Johnson MF, Kobritz NK, Tweed D, Greig NH, Zemlan FP, Sharma SP, Harris-White ME. Early intervention with a small molecule inhibitor for tumor necrosis factor-α prevents cognitive deficits in a triple transgenic mouse model of Alzheimer's disease. J Neuroinflammation. 2012;25:99. doi: 10.1186/1742-2094-9-99

[77] Roh M, Zhang Y, Murakami Y, Thanos A, Lee SC, Vavvas DG, Benowitz LI, Miller JW.Etanercept, a Widely Used Inhibitor of Tumor Necrosis Factor-α (TNF- α), Prevents Retinal Ganglion Cell Loss in a Rat Model of Glaucoma. 2012;7:e40065. Epub 2012 Jul 3. (last access August 6th 2012)

[78] McKinnon SJ. The Cell and Molecular Biology of Glaucoma: Common Neurodegenerative Pathways and Relevance to Glaucoma. Invest. Ophthalmol. Vis. Sci.2012; 53 :2485-2487

[79] Tezel G. TNF-alpha signaling in glaucomatous neurodegeneration Prog Brain Res. 2008;173:409-21

[80] Hong S, Kim CY, Lee WS, Shim J, Yeom HY, Seong GJ. Ocular hypotensive effects of topically administered agmatine in a chronic ocular hypertensive rat model. Exp Eye Res. 2010 ;90(1):97-103

[81] García E, Silva-García R, Mestre H, Flores N, Martiñón S, Calderón-Aranda ES, Ibarra A. Immunization with A91 peptide or copolymer-1 reduces the production of ni-

tric oxide and inducible nitric oxide synthase gene expression after spinal cord injury. J Neurosci Res. 2012;90:656-63. doi: 10.1002/jnr.22771

[82] Schori H, Kipnis J, Yoles E, WoldeMussie E, Ruiz G, Wheeler L.A and Schwartz M. Vaccination for protection of retinal ganglion cells against death from glutamate cytotoxicity and ocular hypertension: Implications for glaucoma Proc Natl Acad Sci U S A. 2001; 98: 3398–3403

[83] Nilforushan N. Neuroprotection in glaucoma.J Ophthalmic Vis Res. 2012;7:91-3

[84] Husain S, Potter DE, Crosson CE. Opioid receptor-activation: retina protected from ischemic injury. Invest Ophthalmol Vis Sci. 2009;50:3853-9

[85] Husain S, Abdul Y, Potter DE. Non-Analgesic Effects of Opioids: Neuroprotection in the Retina Curr Pharm Des. 2012 Jun 28. [Epub ahead of print] http://www.ncbi.nlm.nih.gov/pubmed/22747547 (last access August 5th 2012)

[86] Bull ND, Irvine KA, Franklin RJ, Martin KR. Transplanted oligodendrocyte precursor cells reduce neurodegeneration in a model of glaucoma. Invest Ophthalmol Vis Sci. 2009;50:4244–4253

[87] Tatton WG.Apoptotic mechanisms in neurodegeneration: possible relevance to glaucoma. Eur J Ophthalmol. 1999 Jan-Mar;9 Suppl 1:S22-9

[88] Qi X, Sun I, Lewin AS, et al. Long term suppression of neurodegeneration in chronic experimental optic neuritis:anti-oxidant gene therapy. Invest Ophthalmol Vis Sci 2007;48:5360-70

[89] Borrás T.Advances in glaucoma treatment and management: gene therapy. Invest Ophthalmol Vis Sci. 2012 4;53:2506-10.

[90] Di Polo A, Aigner LJ, Dunn RJ, et al. Prolonged delivery of brain derived neurotrophic factor by adenovirus infected Muller cells temporarily rescues injured retinal ganglion cells. Pro Natl Acad Sci USA. 1998;95:3978-83

Screening for Narrow Angles in the Japanese Population Using Scanning Peripheral Anterior Chamber Depth Analyzer

Noriko Sato, Makoto Ishikawa, Yu Sawada,
Daisuke Jin, Shun Watanabe, Masaya Iwakawa and
Takeshi Yoshitomi

Additional information is available at the end of the chapter

1. Introduction

Primary chronic angle-closure glaucoma (PACG) is a leading cause of blindness, and has particularly high prevalence rate in East Asia [1–3]. The Handan Eye Study [4] reported that the standardized prevalence of PACG is 0.5%, and two thirds of those with PACG were blind in at least one eye. Many cases of PACG are asymptomatic and often present with severe visual field loss at the first visit. The severe visual impairment from PACG is related to the insidious development of the disease. [5]

Primary angle closure suspect (PACS) is characterized by narrow or occludable angles without raised intraocular pressure (IOP) or glaucomatous optic neuropathy. Primary angle closure (PAC) is the eyes with narrow angles and the appositional closure, peripheral anterior synechiae (PAS) and/or raised IOP but without glaucomatous optic neuropathy. PACG is defined as the case of PAC with glaucomatous optic neuropathy. It has been estimated that 22% of the eyes with PACS progress to PAC and 28.5% progress from PAC to PACG over 5–10 years [6]. Prophylactic laser iridotomy (LI) is the first-line treatment for narrow angles, and may stop the progression of the angle closure process and prevent development of PACG. However, LI is less effective in controlling IOP if optic nerve damage with PAS has already occurred [7].

Assessment of angle width is essential for the diagnosis and managing angle closure [8–10]. Currently, the golden standard for angle assessment has been indirect visualization by gonioscopy. However, it is limited by its dependency on subjective interpretation and difficulties in manipulation techniques. Ultrasound biomicroscopy (UBM) generates high-resolution images of the angle, which can be used in quantitative analysis, and it adds useful information regarding causal mechanisms of angle closure. However, this method also requires trained and experienced technicians and is time consuming. Both gonioscopy and UBM require contact with the globe, and as a result, they can be unpleasant for the patient and can induce artifacts.

New devices for evaluating the anterior ocular segment in a more objective and quantitative manner have been introduced. Anterior-segment optical coherence tomography (AS-OCT) is a noninvasive technique allowing the measurement of the anterior ocular structures. A new generation of OCT, swept-source OCT (SS-OCT), has been recently introduced for the measurement of the anterior ocular segment. The SS-OCT is over tenfold faster than the time-domain OCT and gives a three-dimensional (3D) observation of the anterior ocular segment. The SS-OCT employs 1,310 nmin the nearinfrared light source and its scan rate is 30,000 A scan/s.

The scanning peripheral anterior chamber depth analyzer (SPAC) is a non-invasive device that objectively and quantitatively assesses the anterior ocular segment by employing the Scheimpflug camera principle. The SPAC measures the peripheral ACD and converts the measurements into numerical and categorical grades by comparison with a normative database. The SPAC has been proposed as a clinician-independent screening tool for angle closure.

In the study reported here, we review the advantages and limitations of newer anterior chamber imaging technologies, namely ultrasound biomicroscopy (UBM), anterior segment optical coherence tomography (AS-OCT), and scanning peripheral anterior chamber depth analyzer (SPAC). Additionally, the present study assessed the effectiveness and possibility of the SPAC in the glaucoma screening.

2. Ultrasound biomicroscopy (UBM) (Fig. 1)

UBM, which originally was used in ophthalmology to image the posterior segment (B-scan ultrasonography), is an objective alternative for anterior chamber angle assessment. Although ultrasound and UBM are based on the same principle, the frequencies are different. Objective and reproducible measurements of the anterior chamber structures can be obtained with cross-sectional imaging by UBM. Electric signals are converted by a radiofrequency signal generator coupled to a piezoelectric transducer into 50 MHz frequency ultrasonic sound waves, which are transmitted to the eye via saline solution that is held in a cup reservoir [11]. The examination may be performed through a viscous material such as sodium hyaloronate. UBM generates high-resolution images of the angle, which can be used in quantitative analysis, and it adds useful information regarding mechanisms of angle closure [11]. Although angle dimensions measured by UBM correlated significantly with gonioscopy in general [12], gonioscopic assessment sometimes resulted in an overestimation of the angle width in eyes with occludable angles [13]. Gonioscopy is the gold standard examination, because it allows direct viewing of the angle. Nevertheless, it may induce changes in the apposition of the iris depending on the technique and the lens.

The UBM measurement requires trained and experienced technicians and is time consuming. In addition, UBM require contact with the globe, and as a result, UBM can induce artifacts by inadvertent compression of the globe. Consequently, UBM is not suitable for glaucoma screening examination.

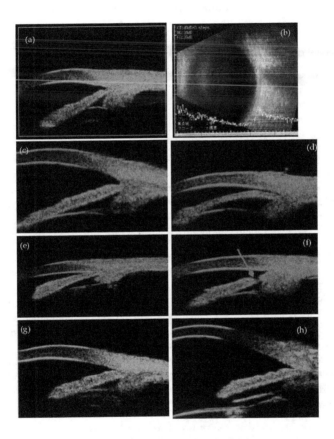

Figure 1. (a) UBM image of the normal anterior segment. This scan demonstrates all anterior segment structures, including anterior lens surface, iris, and ciliary body. In UBM, frequencies of 35-50 MHz and above provide over a threefold improvement in resolution compared with conventional ophthalmic ultrasound systems **(b)**. **b.** Conventional B-mode ultrasound image of the posterior segment. **c and d.** UBM image of the normal **(c)** and the PAC anterior segment **(d)**. Note the shallow anterior chamber depth of the PAC compared with the normal. **e and f.** UBM image of the anterior segment of the PACG patient before **(e)** and after laser iridotomy **(f)**. Note the increase of anterior chamber depth after laser iridotomy (LI). Arrow indicates the portion of the LI. **g and h.** UBM image of the anterior segment of the PACG patient before **(g)** and after cataract surgery (phacoemulsification and intraocular lens implantation) **(h)**. Note the increase of anterior chamber depth after cataract surgery.

3. Anterior-segment optical coherence tomography (AS-OCT)

AS-OCT is a non-contact imaging device allowing the visualization and measurement of the anterior ocular structures [11]. The Visante AS-OCT (Carl Zeiss Meditec Inc., Dublin, CA, USA) and the slit-lamp OCT (SL-OCT) (Heildelberg Engineering, Heildelberg, Germany) are the commercially available AS-OCT devices [11]. Compared with the OCT, the SL-OCT has a lower axial and transverse resolution of <25 µm and 20–100 µm, respectively. A major difference between the two devices is their scan speed, which is 2000 A-scans per s for Visante OCT, and 200 A-scans per s for SL-OCT. With a line scan of 256 and 215 A-scans, each image frame takes 0.13 and 1.08s for Visante OCT and SL-OCT, respectively [11]. Furthermore, the SL-OCT requires manual rotation of the scanning beam.

The advantages of the AS-OCT devices are non-contact, easy operation and a rapid image acquisition. The incorporation of automated analysis software allows for rapid estimation of the various anterior segment parameters, including corneal thickness, anterior chamber depth, etc.

Precise location of the scleral spur is a pre-requisite for reliable measurement of the angle. Limited by a relatively low-image resolution, the scleral spur may not always be visible even with the anterior segment OCT. Currently available software analysis programs require the manual localization of the scleral spur, which can at times be difficult, especially in closed angles or where there is a smooth transition from cornea to sclera [14]. Sakata et al. found that the sclera spur could not be detected in approximately 30% of the quadrants, this problem being worse in the superior and inferior quadrants [14].

It has been reported that AS-OCT is highly sensitive in detecting angle closure when compared with gonioscopy. Using gonioscopy as a reference standard results in AS-OCT having a sensitivity of 98.0% [15]. Several explanations have been suggested for the disparate findings between gonioscopy and AS-OCT [11]. The structures of the angle cannot be directly viewed by other techniques than gonioscopy (and may be SS-OCT in future), and therefore, cannot be identified. However, inadvertent pressure on the globe during gonioscopy may alter the configuration of the angle, leading to artificial widening of the angle. Another reason could be a difference in the definition angle closure. On gonioscopy, angle closure was defined as the apposition between the iris and the posterior trabecular meshwork, whereas on the AS-OCT, it was defined as any contact between the iris and the angle structures anterior to the sclera spur in 2-dimensional cross sections obtained by AS-OCT.

When this device is applied to the prospective observational case series, sensitivity and specificity are calculated as 98% (92.2%–99.6%) and 55.4% (45.2%–65.2%) [15]. The low specificity found with AS-OCT may limit the usefulness of these devices in screening for narrow angle.

A new generation of OCT [CASIA, Tomey, Nagoya, Japan], based on swept-source technology (SS-OCT) methods, has been recently developed for the assessment of the anterior ocular segment [16]. The SS-OCT is a variation of the Fourier-domain OCT, over tenfold faster than the time-domain OCT, and gives a three-dimensional (3D) image of the anterior ocular segment. Instead of using a spectrometer as in spectral-domain OCT, swept-source OCT uses a monochromatic tunable fast scanning laser source and a photodetector to detect wavelength-resolved interference signal [17]. The iris profiles and the angle configurations can be visualized three dimensionally and evaluated for 360° [16]. There might be apposition of the peripheral iris to the cornea that would be identified as a closed angle. SS-OCT imaging of the anterior segment could be useful to improve detection of angle closure, while the high cost of these devices may be a limiting factor for their use in screening examination.

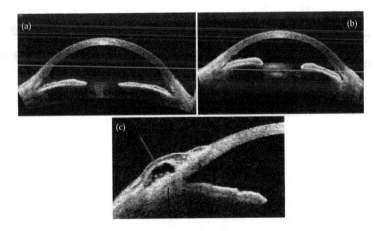

Figure 2. a and b. Transectional images of normal anterior segment **(a)** and plateau iris configuration **(b)** obtained using Visante AS-OCT (Carl Zeiss Meditec Inc., Dublin, CA, USA). Note the shallowperipheral anterior chamber depth of the plateau iris configuration compared with the normal. **c.** Transectional image of the conjunctival bleb after trabeculectomy using Visante AS-OCT.

4. Scanning peripheral anterior chamber depth analyzer

The scanning peripheral anterior chamber depth analyzer (SPAC) is a non-invasive device that objectively and quantitatively assesses the anterior ocular segment by employing the Scheimpflug camera principle [18]. The light from the slit lamp is in the visible spectrum and is projected from the temporal side at an angle of 60° from the optical axis. A camera records cross sectional slit images from the anterior cornea to the anterior iris, and does not rotate as Pentacam-Scheimpflug. The SPAC measures the peripheral ACD and converts the measurements into numerical and categorical grades by comparison with a normative database. SPAC quantitatively measures ACD in a noncontact fashion from the optical axis to the limbus in approximately 0.66 second and takes 21 consecutive slit-lamp images at 0.4 mm intervals. SPAC measurements ranged from 1 to 12, with 1 representing the shallowest anterior chamber. SPAC is equipped with an autofocusing system and a program for the detection of eyes with narrow angle, and usually completes measurement within 15 seconds for a pair of eyes by pressing the start button. The SPAC also reports 3 categorical grades for risk of angle closure: S (for "suspect angle closure", if there were ≥4 measured points exceeding the 95% confidence interval [CI]), P (for "potential angle closure", if there were ≥4 points exceeding the 72% CI), and no suffix (for "normal") [18].

It has been previously reported that the results of peripheral anterior chamber measurement by SPAC were well correlated with those by the van Herick technique as well as Shaffer's grading system and the ultrasound biomicroscope [19].

Pentacam-Scheimpflug (rotating scheimpflug imaging) uses the Scheimpflug principle in order to obtain images of the anterior segment [10]. It has a rotating Scheimpflug camera that takes up to 50 slit images of the anterior segment in less than 2 seconds [20]. Software is then used to construct a three-dimensional image. It calculates data for corneal topography (anterior and posterior corneal surface) and thickness, anterior chamber depth (ACD), lens opacification and lens thickness. It also provides data on corneal wavefront of the anterior and posterior corneal surface using Zernike polynomials. Compared with SPAC, Pentacam is highly expensive.

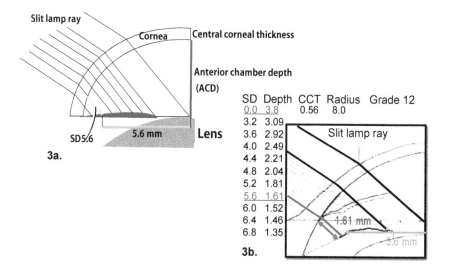

Figure 3. The SPAC automatically calculates central anterior chamber depths (ACD, red line) along the visual axis. SD5.6 (yellow line) means peripheral anterior chamber depth at 5.6 mm apart from the anterior pole of the lens. b. Printout of the results of SPAC measurement. The radius of curvature, the corneal thickness, and the anterior chamber depth are displayed. The SPAC anterior chamber depth value (corneal epithelium to anterior lens) was calculated by summing the corneal thickness and true anterior chamber depth measurements.

5. Application of anterior chamber imaging instruments for glaucoma

The ideal community-based screening test should be clinician-independent, quick, and noninvasive, and have high sensitivity and specificity. SPAC has an advanatage of detecting eyes at risk of ACG by non-physicians in public health screening [20]. When using gonioscopy as the gold standard [8,10], the performance of SPAC combined grade (P or S and/or ≤ grade 5) gave a sensitivity and specificity of 93.0% and 70.8%, respectively [19]. With sequential testing using both SPAC and van Herick, the specificity and sensitivity improves to 94.4% and 87.0%, respectively [21, 22]. Therefore, the SPAC examination in conjunction with the van Herick method is considered as a choice of the first-line screening tests for angle closure following precise examination by OCT, UBM, or gonioscopy (Fig. 4). Kashiwagi et al. [23] proposed the protocol of detecting angle closure glaucoma using SPAC in public health examination. Their protocol consisted of 2 phases: primary screening using SPAC measurements of ACD by nonphysicians and definitive examination by glaucoma specialists (Fig. 4), and was revealed useful for detecting eyes at risk of angle closure glaucoma [22].

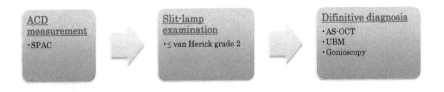

Figure 4. Flow chart for the detection and diagnosis of the narrow anterior chamber.

6. Research course

To investigate the frequency of eyes with a shallow anterior chamber at risk, the SPAC was used in subjects visiting a health screening center. In addition, the influences of age and sex on the distribution of central and peripheral ACD were also examined. Indeed, a productive approach would be to target high-risk groups, such as the elderly, far- sighted, and in particular, women.

7. Method used

Cross-sectional, observational, community-based study.

8. Participants

This was a cross-sectional study in an institutional setting [24]. Subjects older than 30 years were recruited at an annual community health checkup project held in the city of Akita (with a population of 325,537), the capital of Akita Prefecture, Japan. A total of 1,173 subjects participated in the comprehensive examinations from September 10, 2007 to October 26, 2007. Of these, 710 individuals underwent glaucoma screening. All of the participants were ethnically Japanese.

This study was performed after the approval by the Ethical Committee of Akita Prefecture Health Care Foundation. All study procedures adhered to the principles outlined in the Declaration of Helsinki for research involving human subjects, and all participants gave written informed consent for this research prior to their participation.

Exclusion criteria were (1) eyes with previous ocular surgery, trauma, or significant ocular disease; (2) eyes with any inborn aberrations, which might affect the morphology of the optic disc (eg, superior segmental optic disc hypoplasia).

9. Screening examination

The initial non-contact ocular examination was conducted by trained non-ophthalmologists and included measurement of refraction and keratometry (Topcon KR-8100PA, Tokyo, Japan), IOP by noncontact pneumotonometry (Topcon CT-90A, Tokyo, Japan), angle width (Scanning Peripheral Anterior Chamber Analyzer, Takagi Seiko, Nagano, Japan), non-mydriatic optic disc photography by stereoscopic fundus camera (30° angle, 3-DX/NM, Nidek, Gamagori, Japan), and confocal laser scanning tomography (Heidelberg Retina Tomograph II, software version 3.0, Heidelberg Instruments, Heidelberg, Germany). IOP was measured three times, and the mean value was adopted.

10. Definitive examination

When at least 1 finding suggested the presence of glaucoma, the subjects were recruited for definitive examination (Table 1). A definitive examination was performed when a subject was suspected to have glaucoma based upon the findings of the initial non-contact ocular examination. The definitive examination consisted of the following procedures: slit-lamp biomicroscopy, Goldmann applanation tonometry, gonioscopy, and optic nerve head evaluation using a Goldmann three-mirror lens (Haag-Streit International, Koeniz, Switzerland) and a visual field test with the Humphrey Field Analyzer II 24-2 SITA Standard Program (Carl Zeiss Meditec Inc, Dublin, CA, USA). Diagnosis of glaucoma was made based on optic disc appearance, including cup-to-disc ratio, rim width, nerve fiber layer defect, the visual field test, and the clinical records that were obtained through screening and definitive examinations. When present or suspected, glaucoma was categorized based upon the criteria of previous population studies (Table 2). In the definitive diagnosis, anomalous discs, including tilted discs, were carefully excluded. The final diagnosis of glaucoma was determined by 4 glaucoma specialists.

1) Intraocular pressure of 21mm Hg or higher in either eye
2) Presence of abnormalities in the stereoscopic fundus photographs, including one or more of the following glaucomatous changes:
1. Vertical cup/disc ratio of the optic nerve head was more than or equal to 0.6
2. Rim width at the superior portion (11-1 h), or inferior portion (5-7 h) was less than or equal to 0.2 of disc diameter ratio was
3. Difference in the vertical cup/disc more than or equal to 0.2 between both eyes
4. Nerve fiber layer defect or splinter disc hemorrhage was found
3) Failure to take stereoscopic fundus photographs

Table 1. Criteria for Definitive Examination Eligibility.

Category 1
The vertical cup-to-disc ratio of the optic nerve head is 0.7 or more, or the rim width at the superior portion (11-1 h) or the inferior portion (5-7 h) is 0.1 or less of the disc diameter, or the difference of the vertical cup-to-disc ratio is 0.2 or more between both eyes, or a nerve fiber layer defect is found, and the hemifield based visual field abnormality is compatible with optic disc appearance or nerve fiber layer defect.
Category 2
When the visual field test is not reliable or available, the cup-to-disc ratio of the optic nerve head is 0.9 or more, or the rim width at the superior portion (11-1 h) or the inferior portion (5-7 h) is 0.05 or less of the disc diameter, or the difference of the vertical cup-to-disc ratio is 0.3 or more between both eyes
Glaucoma suspect
When the cup-to-disc ratio of the optic nerve head is 0.7 or more portion (5-7 h) is 0.1 or less but more than 0.05 of the disc diameter but less than 0.9, or the rim width at the superior portion (11-1h) or the inferior, or the difference of the vertical cup-to-disc ratio is 0.2 or more but less than 0.3 between both eyes, or the nerve fiber layer defect is found, and the visual field test is not reliable or available or does not show hemi-field based compatible defect, the eye is diagnosed with suspected glaucoma

Table 2. Criteria for Glaucoma Diagnosis.

10.1. Category 1

The vertical cup-to-disc ratio of the optic nerve head is 0.7 or more, or the rim width at the superior portion (11-1 h) or the inferior portion (5-7 h) is 0.1 or less of the disc diameter, or the difference of the vertical cup-to-disc ratio is 0.2 or more between both eyes, or a nerve fiber layer defect is found, and the hemifield based visual field abnormality is compatible with optic disc appearance or nerve fiber layer defect.

10.2. Category 2

When the visual field test is not reliable or available, the cup-to-disc ratio of the optic nerve head is 0.9 or more, or the rim width at the superior portion (11-1 h) or the inferior portion (5-7 h) is 0.05 or less of the disc diameter, or the difference of the vertical cup-to-disc ratio is 0.3 or more between both eyes

10.3. Glaucoma suspect

When the cup-to-disc ratio of the optic nerve head is 0.7 or more portion (5-7 h) is 0.1 or less but more than 0.05 of the disc diameter but less than 0.9, or the rim width at the superior portion (11-1h) or the inferior, or the difference of the vertical cup-to-disc ratio is 0.2 or more but less than 0.3 between both eyes, or the nerve fiber layer defect is found, and the visual field test is not reliable or available or does not show hemi-field based compatible defect, the eye is diagnosed with suspected glaucoma

11. SPAC examination

All subjects underwent examination with SPAC. Paramedical staff correctively measured the ACD of 658 subjects (703 eyes of 354 men, 607 eyes of 304 women). SPAC examines the region from the optical axis to the temporal limbus in approximately 0.66 s, taking 21 consecutive slitlamp images at 0.4-mm intervals. The camera-captured cross-sectional slit-lamp images are immediately subjected to analysis, and the radius of curvature, the corneal thickness, and ACD values are displayed. The SPAC yields numeric and categorical grades that are calculated by comparison with the ACD values derived from a sample of Japanese subjects [18]. In our study, the range of ACD values of the patients was divided into 12 groups, each representing an equal increment in the ACD. Group 12 consisted of eyes with the deepest mean ACD values, whereas eyes with the shallowest mean ACD values were allocated to group 1.

Based on the data provided by SPAC, the following parameters were determined: distribution of ACD from the central and the peripheral region, distribution of the grades of ACD, and frequency of suspected (S) or possible (P) angle-closure eyes. The high risk of angle closure group includes eyes judged as S or P, or grade ≤5 by SPAC. These eyes were eligible for the definitive examination, The SPAC automatically calculates central ACD along the visual axis. Peripheral ACD means anterior chamber depth at 5.6 mm apart from the anterior pole of the lens (Fig. 3).

Of 1420 eyes of the 710 participants of the glaucoma screening study, reliable SPAC results were analyzed in 1310 eyes of 658 participants (Table 3). 104 eyes of fifty two participants were omitted from the study. The main reason for exclusion were that SPAC measurements could not be completed at the screening sites for various reasons, such as subjects' ocular or physical problems. 100 eyes were unable to fixate the fixation lamp due to poor visual acuity, and 2 subjects (4 eyes) were unable to keep their faces on the chin rest during measurement. Between the included and excluded subjects, the male/female ratio was not statistically different (P = 0.44, χ^2 test).

	30's	40's	50's	60's	70's	Total
Male	21	105	126	73	29	354
	(42, 3.2%)	(209, 16.0%)	(252, 19.2%)	(143, 10.9%)	(57, 2.2%)	(703, 53.7%)
Female	20	98	114	57	15	304
	(40, 3.1%)	(196, 15.0%)	(228, 17.4%)	(114, 8.7%)	(29, 2.2%)	(607, 46.3%)
Total	41	203	240	130	44	658
	(82, 6.3%)	(495, 37.8%)	(480, 36.6%)	(257, 19.6%)	(86, 6.6%)	(1310, 100%)

Table 3. Number of patients and eyes and the percentage of eyes (in parenthesis) examined by SPAC in each age group.

12. Data analysis

Descriptive statistical analysis for the determination of mean±standard deviation (SD) for continuous values was performed with SPBS software (Nankodo Publisher, Statistical Package for the Biosciences version 9.51, Tokyo, Japan). Data from both eyes of each individual were used, as it was more efficient and informative than data for single eyes. Comparisons of the different SPAC parameters between males and females or among each age group were analyzed with paired and unpaired t tests. Pearson correlation coefficients were calculated to assess the strength of the correlations between SPAC parameters and potential confounders. For all analyses, $P<0.05$ was considered statistically significant.

13. Results

13.1. Results of primary screening and definitive examination

A glaucoma specialist judged that 26 eyes of 19 subjects required the definitive examination, and all 19 subjects were enrolled in the definitive examination. The definitive examination revealed that 1 subject had PACG (0.08%), 1 subject had PAC (0.08%), and 1 had ciliary cyst (0.08%). None of all these eyes showed IOP elevation of more than 21mm Hg. Laser iridotomy was performed on PACG and PAC subjects. None of these subjects presented with subjective symptoms that are thought to demonstrate a strong association with angle closure.

13.2. Association of gender and age with SPAC parameters

Association of gender and age with SPAC parameters are summarized in Table 4.

In male subjects of 30 to 60 years of ages, the central and the peripheral anterior chamber depths were gradually decreased with ages. There were significant differences in these depths among 30, 40, and 50 age groups (p<0.0001). However, there was no significant difference in depths between 60 years and 70 years age group (Fig. 5). In female subjects, the ACD tended to be shallower in women than in men in each generation. The central and the peripheral anterior chamber depths were gradually decreased with ages. There were significant differences among each age group (p<0.0001) (Fig. 5). Correlation of anterior chamber depth and aging was statistically analyzed using linear regression equation ($y = ax + b$). Both central and peripheral ACD were significantly correlated with aging (p<0.0001) (Fig. 6). Regression equations were shown in Fig. 6.

		30's	40's	50's	60's	70's
	Grade	11.2 (1.7)	10.3 (1.0)	9.6 (0.9)	9.0 (0.9)	9.3 (0.9)
Male	Central ACD	3.6 (0.3)	3.4 (0.2)	3.3 (0.3)	3.2 (0.3)	3.3 (0.3)
	Peripheral ACD	1.6 (0.2)	1.3 (0.2)	1.1 (0.1)	1.0 (0.1)	1.2 (0.1)
	Grade	10.4 (1.2)	9.7 (1.0)	8.8 (0.9)	8.5 (0.9)	7.5 (0.8)
Female	Central ACD	3.5 (0.4)	3.3 (0.3)	3.2 (0.3)	3.1 (0.3)	2.9 (0.3)
	Peripheral ACD	1.4 (0.1)	1.1 (0.1)	1.0 (0.1)	0.9 (0.08)	0.9 (0.1)

Table 4. Average and standard deviation (parenthesis) of central and peripheral anterior chamber depth in male and female in each age group.

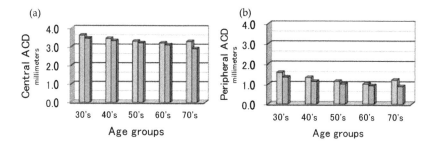

Figure 5. Average of central and peripheral anterior chamber depth at each age group. The central ACD (a) and the peripheral ACD (b) were measured at each age group in male (blue bars) and female (red bars). The y-axis represented anterior chamber depth (ACD) as millimeters. The decrease with age in each ACD was shown quantitatively in both men and women.

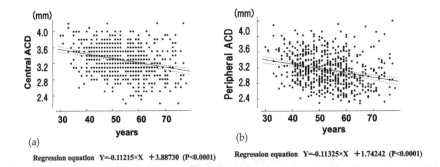

Regression equation Y=-0.11215×X +3.88730 (P<0.0001)   Regression equation Y=-0.11325×X +1.74242 (P<0.0001)

Figure 6. Correlation of the aging and the anterior chamber depth (a: central ACD, b: peripheral ACD) in all subjects. Although the distribution was wide, the central and peripheral ACD decreased with aging. There was a significant negative correlation between ACD and aging by lineal regression analysis.

13.3. Frequencies of eyes at risk

The high risk of angle closure group includes eyes judged as S or P, or grade ≤ 5 by SPAC. The prevalence of the high risk eyes was 1.7% and 2.3% among men and women, respectively. In particular, the prevalence of the high risk eyes was especially high in women 60 years age (6.1%) and 70 years age (6.9%). These data suggest that women older than 60 years may be vulnerable to possible angle closure. Women older than 60 years were at greater risk than male ($p<0.0021$) or female of younger age ($p<0.0001$) (Table 5). However, these eyes at risk did not show abnormalities in IOP or optic disc.

	30's	40's	50's	60's	70's	Total
Male	0/42	0/209	6/252	5/143	1/57	12/703
	(0%)	(0.51%)	(2.4%)	(3.5%)	(1.8%)	(1.7%)
Female	0/40	1/196	4/228	7/114	2/29	14/607
	(0%)	(0.05%)	(1.7%)	(6.1%)	(6.9%)	(2.3%)
Total	0/82	1/405	10/480	12/257	3/86	26/1310
	(0%)	(0.24%)	(2.1%)	(4.7%)	(3.5%)	(2.0%)

Table 5. Number and frequencies (percentage) of eyes at risk in each age group.

14. Discussion

The present study qualitatively demonstrates the decrease with age in the peripheral and the central ACD in both men and women in the Japanese subjects attending the health community checkup. Eyes at risk for angle closure were more frequent in women 60 years of age or older. Compared with other populations in Japan, the similar results were reported using SPAC [25] (Table 6). Kamo et al. [25] also reported that the frequency of eyes at risk for angle closure increased in women 50 years of age or older, and it is corresponding to our present results.

It has been reported that the prognosis of eyes with PACG especially acute angle closure is poor compared with that of eyes with PAC undergoing suitable treatment [6, 7]. Therefore, detecting eyes at risk of PACG or PAC is very important. The van Herick technique was employed for primary screening in previous epidemiologic studies of ACG eyes [21]. It has been reported that the results of peripheral ACD measurement by SPAC were well correlated with those by the van Herick technique as well as Shaffer's grading system and the ultrasound biomicroscope [22]. As the sequential testing using both SPAC and van Herick demonstrates high specificity and sensitivity [23], we considered that the SPAC examination in conjunction with the van Herick method is considered as a choice of the first-line screening tests for angle closure following precise examination by OCT, UBM, or gonioscopy. Further, almost all of the previous studies were conducted under the guidance of an ophthalmologist, and there are few reports of angle closure screening conducted as part of a public health examination that does not involve an ophthalmologist. Primary screening using SPAC measurements of ACD by nonphysicians seems to have possibility to induce cost-effective angle closure screening.

It seems that screening for PACG at least with SPAC and van Herick method should be performed in all the patients over 50 every 6 months and in those with shallow (peripheral) anterior chamber or high IOP, the angle should be further evaluated. LI should be performed in all PAC and PACG patients and those who do not respond to LI should undergo cataract surgery.

	40's	50's	60's	70's
Akita	0.24	2.1	4.7	3.5
Yamanashi[30]	0	2.7	4.1	2.8

Table 6. Comparison of frequencies of eyes at risk (judged as S or P by SPAC) between Akita (the present result) and Yamanashi in Japan.

Author details

Noriko Sato, Makoto Ishikawa*, Yu Sawada, Daisuke Jin, Shun Watanabe, Masaya Iwakawa and Takeshi Yoshitomi

*Address all correspondence to: mako@med.akita-u.ac.jp

Department of Ophthalmology, Akita Graduate University School of Medicine, Akita, Japan

References

[1] Quigley, H. A, & Broman, A. T. The number of people with glaucoma worldwide in 2010 and 2020. British Journal of Ophthalmology (2006). , 90(3), 262-267.

[2] Foster, P. J, & Johnson, G. J. Glaucoma in China: how big is the problem? British Journal of Ophthalmology (2001). , 85(11), 1277-1282.

[3] Resnikoff, S, & Pascolini, D. Etya'ale D, Kocur I, Pararajasegaram R, Pokharel GP et al. Global data on visual impairment in the year 2002. Bulletin of the World Health Organization (2004). , 82(11), 844-851.

[4] Liang, Y, Friedman, D. S, Zhou, Q, Yang, X. H, Sun, L. P, Guo, L, Chang, D. S, & Lian, L. Wang NL; Handan Eye Study Group. Prevalence and characteristics of primary angle-closure diseases in a rural adult Chinese population: the Handan Eye Study. Investigative Ophthalmology & Visual Science. (2011). , 52(12), 8672-9.

[5] Ang, L. P, Aung, T, Chua, W. H, Yip, L. W, & Chew, P. T. Visual field loss from primary angle-closure glaucoma: a comparative study of symptomatic and asymptomatic disease. Ophthalmology. (2004). , 111(9), 1636-1640.

[6] Thomas, R, Parikh, R, Muliyil, J, & Kumar, R. S. Five-year risk of progression of primary angle closure to primary angle closure glaucoma: A population-based study. Acta Ophthalmol Scand. (2003). , 81(4), 480-485.

[7] Alsagoff, Z, Aung, T, Ang, L. P, & Chew, P. T. Long-term clinical course of primary angle-closure glaucoma in an Asian population. Ophthalmology. (2000). , 107(12), 2300-2304.

[8] Aung, T, Nolan, W. P, Machin, D, Seah, S. K, Baasanhu, J, Khaw, P. T, et al. Anterior chamber depth and the risk of primary angle closure in 2 East Asian populations. Archive of Ophthalmology. (2005). , 123(4), 527-532.

[9] Casson, R. J, Baker, M, Edussuriya, K, Senaratne, T, Selva, D, & Sennanayake, S. Prevalence and determinants of angle closure in central Sri Lanka: the Kandy Eye Study. Ophthalmology. (2009). , 116(8), 1444-1449.

[10] Kurita, N, Mayama, C, Tomidokoro, A, Aihara, M, & Araie, M. Potential of the pentacam in screening for primary angle closure and primary angle closure suspect. Journal of Glaucoma. (2009). , 18(7), 506-512.

[11] Quek DTLNongpiur ME, Perera SA, Aung T. Angle imaging: Advances and challenges. Indian Journal of Ophthalmology. (2011). Suppl1): SS75., 69.

[12] Kaushik, S, Jain, R, Pandav, S. S, & Gupta, A. Evaluation of the anterior chamber angle in Asian Indian eyes by ultrasound biomicroscopy and gonioscopy. Indian Journal of Ophthalmology. (2006). , 54(3), 159-63.

[13] Narayanaswamy, A, Vijaya, L, Shantha, B, Baskaran, M, Sathidevi, A. V, & Baluswamy, S. Anterior chamber angle assessment using gonioscopy and ultrasound biomicroscopy. Japanese Journal of Ophthalmology. (2004). , 48(1), 44-49.

[14] Sakata, L. M, Lavanya, R, Friedman, D. S, Aung, H. T, Gao, H, Kumar, R. S, Foster, P. J, & Aung, T. Comparison of gonioscopy and anterior segment ocular coherence tomography in detecting angle closure in different quadrants of the anterior chamber angle. Ophthalmology. (2008). , 115(5), 769-774.

[15] Nolan, W. P, See, J. L, Chew, P. T, Friedman, D. S, Smith, S. D, Radhakrishnan, S, Zheng, C, Foster, P. J, & Aung, T. Detection of primary angle closure using anterior segment optical coherence tomography in Asian eyes. Ophthalmology. (2007). , 114(1), 33-39.

[16] Usui, T, Tomidokoro, A, Mishima, K, Mataki, N, Mayama, C, Honda, N, Amano, S, & Araie, M. Identification of Schlemm's canal and its surrounding tissues by anterior segment fourier domain optical coherence tomography. Investigative Ophthalmology & Visual Science. (2011). , 52(9), 6934-6939.

[17] Yun, S, Tearney, G, De Boer, J, Iftimia, N, & Bouma, B. High-speed optical frequency-domain imaging. Opt Express. (2003). , 11(22), 2953-2963.

[18] Kashiwagi, K, Kashiwagi, F, Toda, Y, Osada, K, Tsumura, T, & Tsukahara, S. A newly developed peripheral anterior chamber depth analysis system: principle, accuracy, and reproducibility. British Journal of Ophthalmology (2004). , 88(8), 1030-1035.

[19] Kashiwagi, K, Tsumura, T, & Tsukahara, S. Comparison between newly developed scanning peripheral anterior chamber depth analyzer and conventional methods of evaluating anterior chamber configuration. Journal of Glaucoma (2006). , 15(5), 380-387.

[20] Buehl, W, Stojanac, D, Sacu, S, Drexler, W, & Findl, O. Comparison of three methods of measuring corneal thickness and anterior chamber depth. Am J Ophthalmol (2006). , 141(7), 1417-12.

[21] Kashiwagi, K, Kashiwagi, F, Hiejima, Y, et al. Finding cases of angle-closure glaucoma in clinic setting using a newly developed instrument. Eye (2006). , 20(3), 319-324.

[22] Andrews, J, Chang, D. S, Jiang, Y, He, M, Foster, P. J, Munoz, B, Kashiwagi, K, & Friedman, D. S. Comparing approaches to screening for angle closure in older Chinese adults. Eye (Lond). (2012). , 26(1), 96-100.

[23] Kashiwagi, K, & Tsukahara, S. Case finding of angle closure glaucoma in public health examination with scanning peripheral anterior chamber depth analyzer. Journal of Glaucoma. (2007). , 16(7), 589-93.

[24] Ishikawa, M, Sawada, Y, Sato, N, & Yoshitomi, T. Risk factors for primary open-angle glaucoma in Japanese subjects attending community health screenings. Clinical Ophthalmology (2011). , 5(7), 1531-1537.

[25] Kamo, J, Saso, M, Tsuruta, M, Sumino, K, & Kashiwagi, K. Aging effect on peripheral anterior chamber depth in male and female subjects investigated by scanning peripheral anterior depth analyzer. J Jpn Ophthalmol Soc (2007). , 111(7), 518-525.

Chapter 11

The History of Detecting Glaucomatous Changes in the Optic Disc

Ivan Marjanovic

Additional information is available at the end of the chapter

1. Introduction

At the present time it is much easier to recognize and to assess glaucomatous changes at the optic nerve than it used to be. This is possible thanks to modern devices and imaging techniques that allow much faster and better diagnosing. Even today, the single most important thing in this matter is to know the characteristics of the normal -healthy optic disc (Figure 1.). The appearance of the optic disc, as in the other biological variables varies widely among healthy individuals. This fact complicates the recognition of the pathological changes.

Today modern glaucoma diagnostic is unimaginable without technological support, when it comes to discovering as well as for following up glaucoma optic neuropathy.

With standard clinical exam aside, there is a number of imaging devices that we use in everyday practice, and to mention a couple i.e. CVF, HRT, GDX, OCT, PACHIMETRY, FUNDUS PHOTOS, CDI… and we agree that without the help of this wide technological spectrum of supporting diagnostic devices we could not be able to diagnose the disease or to track the glaucoma changes. Just stop for a second and remember how it was in the old days? Let's take a glance of the old days and how it all started?

There was the time when ophthalmologist did not have those sophisticated imaging devices; they even did not have slit lamps… despite the fact that they were glaucomatologists!

This chapter is dedicated to the pioneers of ophthalmology and glaucomathology; their legacy for future glaucomatologists.

The term optic disc is frequently used to describe the portion of the optic nerve clinically visible on examination. This, however, may be slightly inaccurate as 'disc' implies a flat, 2 dimensional structure without depth, when in fact the 'optic nerve head' is very much a 3 dimensional structure which should ideally be viewed stereoscopically.

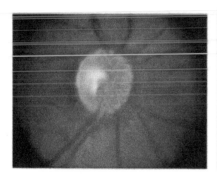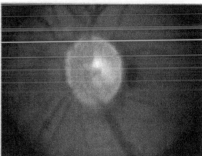

Figure 1. Healthy optic disc

Every disease has its history, as much in diagnosing-discovering it, as in quality and adequate treatment. History of the diseases categorized today under the term "glaucoma" may be divided into three major periods. First period is the earliest and it stretches from approximately 400 BC up until 1600 AD; during the course of this period the term "glaucoma" was used to refer to a general group of blinding ocular diseases without the distinctions that historians now can recognize. During the middle period from the beginning of the 17th century to the middle of the 19th century the cardinal signs of glaucoma, separately and in combination, were described in published texts. Finally, the third period starts with the introduction of the ophthalmoscope (Helmholtz, 1854) to the present.

1.   First period (400 BC to 1600 AD)

Etymology of the term glaucoma is that it derives from the Greek word "glaukos", which appears in the Homer's notes, where it is mentioned as -a sparkling silver glare, later used for colours such as sky-blue or green. As a diagnosis by physicians, glaucoma is first mentioned in Hippocrates' *Aphorisms* (Figure 2.),lists among the infirmities of the aged a condition he called "glaucosis" which he associated with "dimness of vision". Later Aristotel did not mention any diseases called glaucoma particularly, although he helped create the foundation for research into the pathology of the disease, thus giving his contribution to early glaucoma research.

It is interesting that most authors, by the Roman era, used the term *glaucoma* for what is now known as *cataract*. For example, Oribasius (325-400 AD) quotes Ruphus from Ephesus (1st century AD) as using the term for "that condition of the crystalline body in which the same loses its original colour and instead becomes blue-grey".

However, Archigenes, who practised at Rome in the time of Trajan (98-117 AD), used the term "ophthalmosglaucos" for a curable blindness that was not caused by cataract.

Archigenes revealed that he used the juice of the deadly nightshade, a mydriatic, in the treatment of this condition, adding, "the instilled juice of nightshade makes black the grey eyes."

Galen (129-216 AD), (Figure 3.) defined glaucoma as a condition in which changes in fluids of the eye caused the pupil to become grey. He also refers to the mydriatic effect of night-shade.

Aetius, the physician of the emperor Justinian (482-565) AD, and a great Ophthalmologist, identified two forms of glaucoma, one a curable condition of the lens and the other an in-curable condition that involved an effusion in which the pupil becomes thickly coagulated and dried.

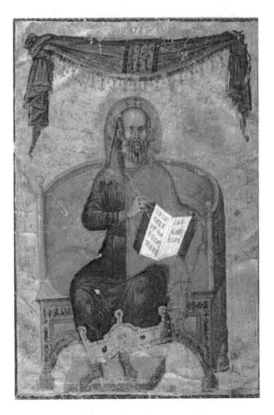

Figure 2. Hippocrates (c.460 B.C.-c. 370 B.C.), a famous Greek physician, and the father ofMedicine, who first used the term 'glaucosis' in his work 'Aphorisms' to describe,conditions correlated with blindness and possibly glaucoma

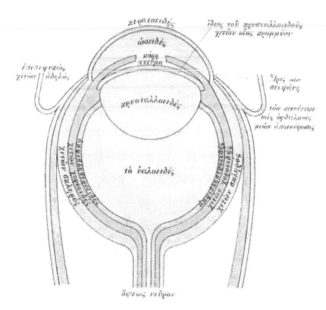

Figure 3. Anatomy of the Eye, according to Galen as the Arabs transferred to the West

2. Second period (1600 TO 1854)

This period is marked by the rising awareness among ophthalmologists that technology is a key to a proper diagnostic.

Glaucoma became more distinct when it comes to adult or elderly patients with the emergence of four characteristics: (1) the consistent failure of cataract operations to improve vision, (2) the clinical appearance of eyes in terminal stages of the disease, (3) a specific history indicating self-limited forerunners of the severe disease, and (4) the elevated intraocular pressure.

Important breakthrough in ophthalmology is marked with the anatomic findings of Brisseau (1707) and the introduction of the process of lens extraction by Daviel (1752). This led to a search for the site of glaucoma in other structures of the eye and to concentration on clinical signs that could be helpful in distinguishing between cataract and glaucoma. Since a majority of the eyes in which the diagnosis of glaucoma was made in the 18th century were in an advanced stage of visual loss and iris atrophy after one or several acute attacks or after a prolonged chronic course, the clinical picture was dominated by congestion (varicosities) of the anterior ciliary veins, a dilated, poorly reacting pupil, and a varying degree of nuclear lens opacity. On examination with the light sources of that period, a greenish reflection could often be obtained; since this seemed to point to the real location of the disease, it became a prominent sign listed in the literature of the 181h and early 191h centuries.

The clinical features of advanced glaucoma, occasionally preceded by attacks of blurred vision that recurred with a high degree of uniformity, was first recorded in St. Yves' "Treatise of the Diseases of the Eyes" (1741) and was described in more detail by Weller (1826).

It is a well known fact that elevation of the intraocular pressure as a distinct sign of ocular disease, recognizable by undue resistance of the eyeball to indentation by the physician's finger, was first clearly mentioned in the "Breviary" of the itinerant English oculist Banister (1626). In 1738 an equally clear reference to hardness of the eye appeared in the independent writings of Johann Platner, professor of anatomy, surgery, and therapeutics at the University of Leipzig. As a distinct clinical symptom, hardness of the eyeball was apparently generally known and accepted in the 1820s, as one may judge from the almost simultaneous but independent texts by Demours of France (1818), Guthrie of England (1823), and Weller of Germany (1826).

William Mackenzie[1] had a great influence on European and American ophthalmology through his personal teaching and through his textbook, between 1830. and 1854. He distinguished between acute and chronic glaucoma and gave a detailed description of the course of the latter from a stage 1 characterized just by a greenish hue reflected from the pupil to a stage 6 in which the eyeball, after perforation of a corneal ulcer in absolute glaucoma, has become atrophic. Mackenzie was well aware of the abnormal hardness of the glaucomatous eye from the second stage on; also, he apparently was the first to recommend a form of posterior sclerotomy to relieve the abnormal hardness.

Duke-Elder in his *System of Ophthalmology*, also, in detail described this second period[2].

2.   Third period (1854. to the present day)

With Eduard Jaeger, the grandson and son of distinguished Austrian ophthalmologist, began modern ophthalmology and modern ophthalmic exam. He was the first investigator who described and documented with the picture, ophthalmoscopic appearance of the glaucomatous disc in the literature. It was a picture from the monocular indirect ophthalmoscope, on which was described the glaucomatous disc as a swelling of the papillary tissues with respect to the surrounding retina[3].

Just a few months later, Albrecht von Graefe also described a prominence of the papilla in glaucoma[4]. His description of the optic disc, specially his description of the pulsation of the arteries in the glaucomatous eyes, became reliable and, at time, reliable indicator of elevated intraocular pressure. The ring-shaped zone around the disc was officialy named - *halo glaucomatosus*. At the von Graefe's clinic, after many examinations on rabbits with congenital fundus anomalies (i.e. coloboma of the uvea an optic nerve), examiners could not agree from ophthalmoscopic examinations whether observed parts of the fundus are elevated or depressed. The anatomic examination revealed tissue depression. This was confirmed by von Graefe's assistant, Adolf Weber[5], who will later in his life made significant contributions to the understanding of the mechanisms of glaucoma. His analysis of the monocular indirect ophthalmoscopy revealed several factors, partly optic and partly perceptual, which caused misinterpretations of relative depth in the fundus.

Later, pathological findings confirmed ophthalmoscopic findings of the optic disc depression, what was interpreted as an effect of the elevated intraocular pressure, or- *pressure excavation of the papilla*. This had profound effect on von Graefe's theory and made him examine all known symptoms of glaucoma and their link with elevated intraocular pressure. This research turned intraocular pressure from a simple symptom to an "essence" of glaucoma.

Early classification of glaucoma was made at von Graefe's clinic.

First type of glaucoma was acute or inflammatory, which characterized with self-limited prodromal attacks of misty vision (in 70 % of the cases), patient is seeing rainbows around the candle flame; attacks increased in severity, length and frequency until the real disease suddenly erupted in the form of an acute attack of inflammation and severe reduction of vision. Partial vision recovery with temporary remission mostly occurred spontaneously or responding on a treatment with large doses of opiates, antiphlogisthics and paracenthesis. Many penetrating exams were carried out during the remissions. After analysis of all phases of this type of glaucoma, von Graefe made a concept according which an acute glaucoma is:"achoroiditis or an iridochoroiditis, with diffuse impregnation of vitreous and aqueous with exudative material which caused the rise in pressure through an increase in volume."

Second type was the chronic glaucoma. Prodromal attacks were without any sign of irritation, congestion or swelling; lengthen gradually and fused in a chronic form, characterized with the anterior ciliary veins dilatation, shallow anterior chamber, iris atrophy, glaucomatous cupping, arterial pulsation in the fundus; followed with reduction in vision.

The third type von Graefe simply named amaurosis with excavation of the optic nerve, and for him it was not in a group of glaucomatous diseases[6]. Normal anterior segment, with optic disc excavation, which lead to the vision impairment.

Completing this classification, von Graefe used the designation *glaucomatous diseases* for a disorders or conditions which secondarily lead to glaucoma and thereby may result in blindness.

In the late period of his research (1861.), von Graefe declared that an exclusion of amaurosis with the optic disc excavation from the group of glaucoma diseases was a mistake[7]. This correction he credited to Doners of Utrecht, his friend, who found a palpable tension among many eyes with so-called amaurosis with optic nerve excavation to be significantly above normal. Doners, after his research, prepositioned a term *glaucoma simplex*, for the glaucoma without anterior segment manifestations and other complications, and *glaucoma with ophthalmia*, for those disorderswhere other manifestations appeared, especially in the anterior segment. The common cause of all glaucoma-the elevated intraocular pressure, Doners ascribed to a hyper secretion of intraocular fluid due to irritation of secretory nerves.

It is interesting that von Graefe discovered also an ocular hypertension patients among his amaurosis with optic nerve excavation cases. He accepted Doner's term glaucoma simplex.

His posterity, first of all Schnabel[8], had verb his amaurosis with optic nerve excavation, implying that it was an optic nerve disease unrelated to elevated intraocular pressure.

Theory of inflammation, that von Graefe's proposed as a cause of intraocular pressure rise and a name of that type of glaucoma held until the clinical discovery of the angle closure mechanism in the 20th century. Some of the alternative terms that were used are: "irritative" (de Wecker[9]), "congestive" (Hansen-Grut), and, much later, "uncompensated" (Elschnig).

The Anglo-Saxon literature preferred terms as acute, subacuteand chronic glaucoma

Finally, von Graefe in his last communication (1869), for the first time introduced a terms *primary* and *secondary glaucoma*.

2. Glaucoma – An optic nerve disease

In the late 1850s, German anatomist Heinrich Mueller[10] was the first who granted ophthal-moscopically observed depression of the optic disc. In his theory that was a result of an ab-normally increased vitreous pressure acting upon the lamina and forcing it to recede. Mueller and his followers assumed that the receding lamina had taken the entire papilla with it, placing the nerve fibres on a steadily increasing stretch or pressing them against the sharp edge of the excavation. Consequence of that was optic nerve atrophy.

Considering that this concept was not uniform for all glaucomatous eyes (in some cases pathologists confirmed the lamina cribrosa displacement, in others not), the theory was add to the basic pressure hypothesis and was widely accepted but also a new ophthalmoscopic and pathologic facts of glaucoma were revealed.

Austrian ophthalmologist Isidor Schnabel (1842-1908)[8] was the first to describe in detail the nerve fibre breakdown with the formation of cavities as a characteristic of the glaucoma-tous process in the optic nerve. It was the earliest sign and for a long time the only glaucom-atous change. In later stages the atrophy affected all portions of the optic nerve up to the entrance of the central vessels. In his opinion, cavernous atrophy was *the* glaucomatous atro-phy. Schnabel saw the mechanism of the glaucomatous optic nerve disease in a process of imbibition of pathologic fluid from the vitreous by the nerve fibres, a process independent of the intraocular pressure. His findings were partly confirmed and partly refuted by subse-quent investigators.

Another perspective on the origin and nature of the glaucomatous optic neuropathy was in-troduced by Priestley Smith[11]. The glaucomatous cup is not a purely mechanical result of exalted pressure, but is in part at least, an atrophic condition which, though primarily due to pressure, includes vascular changes and impaired nutrition in the area of the disc and around its margin which require a considerable time for their full development.

This Priestley Smith's original notion that the rise in pressure may cause damage to the tis-sues of the disc through its influence on blood circulation is valid until the present day.

3. Ocular hypertension – The mechanisms

Previously mentioned essence of glaucoma, recognized in the mid-1850s, attributed to excessive formation of intraocular fluid or hyper secretion and assumed to eider a type of choroiditis (von Graefe) or a secretory neurosis (Donders).

The clear concept of the eye mechanisms that were involved in the intraocular pressure production, in that time, was not plain. German anatomist Schwalbe[12] began in 1860s the experimental study of the fluid exchange of the eye, searching the lymphatics in the anterior segment. When the dye is injected into the anterior chamber of the eye, in aqueous solution or suspension, it appears promptly in veins on the surface of the globe! His conclusion was that the anterior chamber is a lymphatic space in open communication with anterior cilliary veins.

Theodor Leber[13] also injected dyes into the anterior chamber of the eye of a rabbit, and discriminated certain border structures. This disclosure stimulated many investigators of that time, including Leber, to investigate a cannular system and Schwalbe, to investigate the anterior chamber angle in animals. Thus Leber discovered normal outflow (on a fresh enucleated mammalian eye), he presented it as a filtration through the trabecular meshwork and a flow through ciliary and vortex veins.His conclusion was that the rate of outflow was, in principle, proportional to the perfusion pressure, except during an initial period, when the perfusion fluid took up the space occupied in the living eye by blood. He actually determined filtration coefficients, the forerunners of today's coefficients of aqueous outflow.

Since this outflow was from fresh enucleated eyes at the pressures prevailing in the living eye, Leber reasoned that the same process of outflow must also take place in the normal living eye. To maintain a stable in vivo pressure, the steady loss of fluid must be compensated for by steady formation of an equal amount of fluid, which Leber believed could also take place through a process of filtration. Thus, the filtration theory of aqueous formation and elimination was born. In a few human eyes enucleated in far-advanced stages of glaucoma, Leber found very low filtration coefficients which indicated abnormal resistance to aqueous outflow[14]. This finding fitted in well with the first detailed pathologic report on the condition of the chamber angle in far-advanced glaucoma[15]: "The most important finding in genuine glaucoma is the circular adhesion of the iris periphery to the periphery of the cornea or the obliteration of the space of Fontana."*

Although Kieser of Göttingen had clearly shown in 1804 that the spaces described by Fontana in the eyes of herbivores did not exist in man, the term "Fontana's space" was still used in the 1870s and 1880s for the intertrabecular spaces of the human corneoscleral meshwork. Only the detailed studies of the region begun by Schwalbe in 1870 and continued by others made the term "Fontana's space" clearly inapplicable to the human eye.

Considering that in either case glaucoma could result from an inflammatory or an obstructive process within the angle or from pressure from behind. It was realized almost immediately that the peripheral anterior synechiae could be either the cause or the effect of glaucoma. Pathologic specimens which supported these mechanisms were identified and reported. The theory that glaucoma was principally a disorder of aqueous outflow (referred to generally as the Leber-Knies theory) rapidly gained ground.

The essence of the Leber's (Leber-Knies) filtration theory has stood the test of time. Leber's best apprentice, Erich Seidel, in 1920's, made some necessary additions to this theory, including the effects of the colloidosmotic pressure of the plasma proteins and of active transfer processes in the formation of aqueous[16].

Interesting appendage is that the essence of the Leber's theory, the idea, admittedly without experimental proof, of a steady directional circulation of fluid through the chambers of the eye had been expressed by earlier observers, specifically William Porterfield, more than 100 years before Leber.

4. Glaucoma mechanisms

During 1880s and 1890s, it was observed that chronic inflammatory glaucomas composed two thirds of all glaucomas. Angle closure glaucomas were dominant. Priestley Smith measured the horizontal corneal meridian in normal eyes 11.6mm and in glaucomatous eyes 11.2mm[17], what expressed dominance of the angle closure glaucoma in that period. 1888. Priestley Smith also introduced the concept of a predisposition to glaucoma, which consists in progressive narrowing of the circumlental space with age, due to the steady growth of the lens in eyes with small corneas. Anatomicaly, the ciliary processes in states of hyperaemia are crowded forward, pressing the iris against the anterior angle wall. This based on a Smith's experiment on the animal that a small excess of pressure in the vitreous chamber (as little as 4 mm Hg) makes the lens and the suspensory ligament advance in such a manner as to close the angle of the anterior chamber.

Next step was the discovery of shallowness of the anterior chamber as an important role in the mechanism of the acute glaucoma (in the eyes with acute inflammatory glaucoma)[18]. The description of the mechanism: if the pupil dilates in an eye with shallow anterior chamber, the iris, particularly with its thicker portion, can occlude the filtration angle and, thereby, raise the intraocular pressure. If contraction of the sphincter frees the filtration space, the event remains a prodromal attack. At a certain level of intraocular pressure the ocular veins are compressed at their place of entry into the sclera; venous stasis develops with increased transudation; that, and not inflammation, is the true nature of glaucoma.[18]

The Revolution on this field came in 1920.when Curran [19](Kansas City) and Seidel [16] (Heidelberg), on the basis of astute clinical observations, independently announced the concept of the relative pupillary block.

Curran's paper[19]: "normally the aqueous passes through the pupil from the posterior to the anterior chamber, but it is here contended that in glaucoma this passage is impeded on account of the iris hugging the lens over too great a surface extent. Some of the aqueous gets through while some passes back, forcing the lens and the iris still more forward. "

5. Ophthalmoscopy

Ophthalmoscopy, the most important single invention in ophthalmology, that had shaped its evolution, was introduced by Hermann von Helmholtz in December of 1850.[20] [21]However, Jan Purkinje (known for the Purkinje images) had described the complete technique and published it in Latin in 1823,[22]but his audience apparently was not yet ready and his publication went unnoticed. A quarter of a century later, however, the situation changed.

The ophthalmoscope was not based on any radically new concepts. Rather, it combined the appropriate application of various known principles with recognition of its potential impact and presentation to an appropriate audience. Under the leadership of men like Bowman in London, Donders in Holland, and von Graefe and von Helmholtz in Germany, ophthalmology emerged as the first organ-based specialty in medicine.

Bowman (1816 to 1892) is known for Bowman's membrane and for his work in anatomy and histology.

Donders (1818 to 1889) clarified the principles of refraction and accommodation (1864) and defined visual acuity as a measurable quantity. His coworker Snellen developed the Snellen chart.

In Berlin, Albrecht von Graefe (1828 to 1870) was a leader in stimulating the clinical application of new techniques and the careful documentation of new findings. He is remembered for Graefe's knife and Graefe's Archives (1854) (one of the first ophthalmic journals), and he founded the German Ophthalmological Society (Heidelberg, 1857).

Several workers had tried to visualize the inside of the eye but had fallen short of putting it all together. Kussmaul (known for "Kussmaul'sairhunger") described the imaging principles in a thesis in 1845[23]but failed to solve the illumination problem. Cumming[24](1846) in England and Brücke[25](1847) in Germany had shown that a reflection from the fundus could be obtained by bringing the light source in line with the observer, but they failed to solve the imaging problem. Babbage,[26]the English mathematician, reportedly constructed an ophthalmoscope in 1847, but his ophthalmologist friend did not recognize the importance and did not publish it until 1854, when von Helmholtz' instrument was well known.

In the fall of 1850, von Helmholtz tried to demonstrate the inside of the eye to the students in his physiology class. On December 6, he presented his findings to the Berlin Physical Society[20]; on December 17, he wrote to his father[27]:

"I have made a discovery during my lectures on the Physiology of the Sense-organs, which was so obvious, requiring, moreover, no knowledge beyond the optics I learned at the Gymnasium, that it seems almost ludicrous that I and others should have been so slow as not to see it.... Till now a whole series of most important eye-diseases, known collectively as black cataract, has been terra incognita.... My discovery makes the minute investigation of the internal structures of the eye a possibility. I have announced this very precious egg of Columbus to the Physical Society at Berlin, as my property, and am now having an improved and more convenient instrument constructed to replace my pasteboard affair..."

Helmholtz' monograph on ophthalmoscopy was published in 1851 and soon was widely circulated. The next year there were several important improvements contributed by other workers. Rekoss,[28]von Helmholtz' instrument maker, added two movable disks with lenses for easier focusing. Epkens, working with Donders in Holland,[27] introduced a perforated mirror for increased illumination. Ruete[29] in Germany did the same and also developed the indirect method of ophthalmoscopy. With these basic components in place, future generations provided technical improvements. In 1913, Landolt[30] listed 200 different types of ophthalmoscopes.

5.1. Direct ophthalmoscopy

If the patient's fundus is properly illuminated, the field of view is limited by the most oblique pencil of light that can still pass from the patient's pupil to the observer's pupil (Figure 4.). In direct ophthalmoscopy the retinal point that corresponds to this beam can be found by constructing an auxiliary ray through the nodal point of the eye.[30] The point farthest from the centerline of view that can still be seen is determined by the angle α, that is, the angle between this oblique pencil and the common optical axis of the eyes.

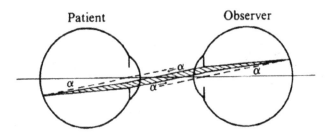

Figure 4. Field limits in direct ophthalmoscopy. The maximum field of view is determined by the most oblique pencil of rays (shaded) that can still pass from one pupil to the other.

Angle α, and therefore the field of view, is increased when the patient's or the observer's pupil is dilated or when the eyes are brought more closely together.

The more peripheral pencils of light use ever-smaller parts of each pupil. This means that, even if the patient's fundus is uniformly illuminated, the luminosity of the fundus image gradually decreases toward the periphery, so that there is no sharp limitation to the field of vision. In practice, therefore, the effective field of vision is determined by the illuminating system not by the viewing system. Most ophthalmoscopes project a beam of light of about one disc diameter.

5.2. Indirect ophthalmoscopy

Even with appropriate illumination, direct ophthalmoscopy has a small field of view (Figure 5.) shows that of four points in the fundus, points one and four cannot be seen because pencils of light emanating from these points diverge beyond the observer's pupil. To bring these pencils to the observer's pupil, their direction must be changed (Figure 6). This requires a fairly large lens somewhere between the patient's and the observer's eye. This principle was introduced by Ruete[29]in 1852 and is called indirect ophthalmoscopy to differentiate it from the first method, in which the light traveled in a straight, direct path from the patient's eye to the observer.

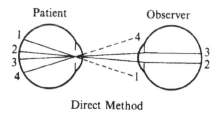

Direct Method

Figure 5. Limited field of view in the direct method. Peripheral pencils of light do not reach the observer's pupil.

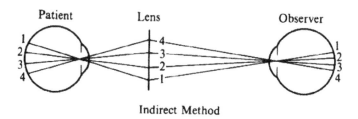

Indirect Method

Figure 6. Extended field of view in the indirect method. The ophthalmoscopy lens redirects peripheral pencils of light toward the observer.

The use of the intermediate lens has several important implications that make indirect ophthalmoscopy more complicated than direct ophthalmoscopy.

The primary purpose of the ophthalmoscopy lens is to bend pencils of light toward the observer's pupil. Figure 3 also demonstrates one of the most characteristic side effects of this arrangement: Compared with the image in direct ophthalmoscopy, the orientation of the image on the observer's retina is inverted. For the novice, this often causes confusion in localization and orientation. Figure 3 further shows that in this arrangement the patient's pupil is imaged in the pupillary plane of the observer. In optical terms the pupils are in conjugate planes.

The most important changes are related to the change from candle light to gas light, to external electric light and, finally, to built-in electric light sources.[31]

Although the older generation found it difficult to adapt to the new instrument, the younger generation did so eagerly. One of them was Eduard von Jaeger (1828 to 1884) from Vienna, best known for his print samples that were based on the print catalogue of the Vienna State Printing House. He was the son of a well-known ophthalmologist and an artistically gifted mother. In 1855, at the age of 27, he published his first atlas; he continued to add to his collection of authoritative fundus paintings until his death in 1884.[32]

6. Slit-lamp examination of the fundus

Although not generally considered as a method of ophthalmoscopy, fundus examination with the slit lamp offers an important addition to the traditional methods of direct and indirect ophthalmoscopy. It offers the advantage of high-power magnification through the microscope and flexible illumination with the slit-lamp beam. With appropriate contact lenses, it can offer higher magnification than direct ophthalmoscopy and a field several times wider than indirect ophthalmoscopy. These methods have become particularly important in combination with laser treatment.

Because the slit-lamp microscope has a fixed focus on a plane approximately 10 cm in front of the objective and because the image of the fundus of an emmetropic eye appears at infinity, the fundus cannot be visualized without the help of additional lenses. There are several options.

7. Negative lens

A negative lens placed in front of the objective of the microscope can move the microscope focus to infinity. The practical application of this principle was worked out by Hruby[33] [34]of Vienna (1942) with a lens known as the Hruby lens.

The optical principle is best understood if the lens is considered in conjunction with the eye, rather than as a part of the microscope. Parallel rays emerging from an emmetropic eye are made divergent by the Hruby lens and seem to arise from the posterior focal plane of that lens (Figure 7A.) For a -50-D lens, this would be 20 mm behind the lens (the usual Hruby lens is -55 D). The slit-lamp microscope is thus looking at a virtual image of the fundus in a plane somewhere in the anterior segment and must be moved a little closer to the patient than it would be for the regular external examination.

To estimate the field of view in this method, it may be assumed that only rays emerging parallel to the axis will reach the objective of the microscope and the observer's eye. When emerging from the eye, these rays must have been aimed at the anterior focal point of the Hruby lens. (Figure 7B), in which these rays are traced back to the retina, shows that the field of view (a) is proportional to the pupillary diameter as seen from the anterior focal point of the lens. This field is of the same order of magnitude as the field in direct ophthalmoscopy; it is largest when the lens is closest to the eye.

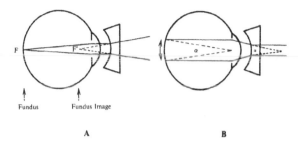

Figure 7. Hruby lens. A. The fundus image (F') is formed in the posterior focal plane of the lens. B. The field of view is proportional to the size of the pupil as seen from the anterior focal point of the lens.

With the lens close to the cornea, the fundus image will be close to the fundus plane and approximately actual size. The magnification to the observer is thus largely determined by the magnification of the microscope. At 16×, the magnification is about equal to that of direct ophthalmoscopy; at higher settings, the magnification is greater. Binocular viewing and slit illumination are advantages over direct ophthalmoscopy, even at similar magnification. Limitation to the posterior pole is a disadvantage.

8. Contact lens

When the Hruby lens is moved progressively closer to the eye, it will eventually touch the cornea and become a contact lens. If the curvature of the posterior lens surface equals the curvature of the anterior corneal surface, the image formation will not change, but two reflecting surfaces will be eliminated, and image clarity will increase.

The use of a contact lens for fundus examination was perfected by Goldmann[35]of Berne, Switzerland (1938). His contact lens is known for the three mirrors incorporated in it. These mirrors positioned at different angles make it possible to examine the peripheral retina with little manipulation of the patient's eye or of the microscope axis (Figure 8).

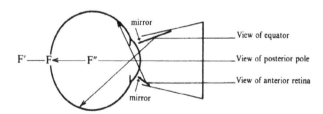

Figure 8. Three mirror contact lens by Goldmann. Two of the three mirrors are shown. They allow visualization of different parts of the fundus.

The refractive power of the cornea is eliminated in the contact lens. The only effective refractive element left would seem to be the far less powerful crystalline lens. The retina is situated well within the focal length of this lens, and the crystalline lens will therefore form a virtual image of the fundus (F) in a plane (F') behind the globe. How can the microscope focus on an image that far back? We overlooked one other refracting surface: the plano front surface of the contact lens. F' is seen through plastic and vitreous. To the observer in air F' appears at F", through the same effect that makes a swimming pool appear shallower than it is. Because of this, the microscope again must focus on a plane inside the globe. As with the Hruby lens, magnification is largely determined by the microscope.

Thus, contact lens fundus microscopy extends our range of examination methods to details beyond the reach of ordinary direct ophthalmoscopy.

9. "Indirect" slit-lamp microscopy

The use of the Hruby lens and Goldmann contact lens is comparable to direct ophthalmoscopy, because no real intermediate image is formed. The equivalent of indirect ophthalmoscopy can be achieved by focusing the microscope on the real image formed by a high-power plus lens.

El Bayadi[36]introduced the use of a +60-D lens for this purpose. The inverted image formed by this lens is situated 16 mm (0.0167 m) in front of it. A practical problem with some older slit lamps is that they cannot be pulled back far enough to observe this image.

Compared with the Hruby (-55 D) lens, the El Bayadi (+60 D) lens offers the same major advantage as does indirect ophthalmoscopy: a larger field of view. With proper placement of the lens, the field is about six disc diameters (40 degrees), compared with the one- or two-disc diameter field of the Hruby lens.

With a 60-D lens the aerial image is as large as the fundus; thus the magnification is approximately equal to the microscope magnification (similar to that with the Hruby lens).

10. Contact lens for the indirect method

Can the field of view be widened even further? This is possible by using a contact lens of very high plus power with some additional optical tricks.Figure 9 illustrates the RodenstockPanfunduscope, based on a design by Schiegel.[37]

The unit contains a high plus contact lens, which forms an inverted fundus image (F') located inside a second, spherical glass element.

In this arrangement, as in the previous example of a high myope (Figure 10), the image-forming and field-widening functions of the ophthalmoscopy lens are separated again. The contact lens forms the image; the spherical element serves to flatten the image and to redirect the diverging pencils of rays toward the observer. Because these elements are so close to the eye, the field of view can be very wide. Indeed, without moving the lens, the view reaches 200 degrees, that is, from equator to equator, 4 to 5 times the diameter (16 times the area) of regular indirect ophthalmoscopy or of the El Bayadi lens.

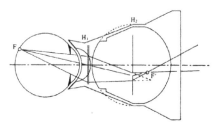

Figure 9. Contact lens arrangement for wide-angle indirect biomicroscopy. A high-power contact lens forms an inverted image (F') inside a spherical element, which redirects the light toward the observer.

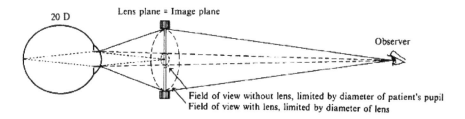

Figure 10. Indirect ophthalmoscopy of a high myope. The myopic eye forms its own aerial image (dotted lines) without the help of the ophthalmoscopy lens. Without the lens, only the central part of this image would be visible (dashed lines, limited by the patient's pupil). With lens (solid lines) the image is limited by the lens rim.

The size of the image inside the front lens is 70% of the retinal size; for detailed examination, therefore, 50% more microscope magnification is required than with the other slit-lamp methods. However, the principal use of this lens is not for its magnification but for its overview, an overview previously achievable only in fundus drawings or photocompositions.

Similar contact lens arrangements are used in specially designed fundus cameras that allow fundus photography of areas 100 degrees or more in diameter. With lenses such as these, the spectrum of our examining methods can be extended not only toward higher magnification than with direct ophthalmoscopy but also, at the other end, toward an overview of the fundus considerably beyond that obtainable with regular indirect ophthalmoscopy.

As the technology to calculate, design, and manufacture lenses with aspheric surfaces has improved, it has been possible to make lenses with higher powers and better light gathering abilities. The number and variety of lenses for indirect ophthalmoscopy and of contact lenses for slit-lamp microscopy has grown accordingly.

11. Related imaging techniques

11.1. Fundus photography

Fundus cameras have greatly improved the ability to document and follow fundus lesions. Eduard von Jaeger often spent countless hours drawing a single fundus, but today a photographic image is available in a fraction of a second. For reasons mentioned earlier, fundus cameras are built on the principle of indirect ophthalmoscopy. The observer's lens and retina are replaced by a camera lens and film. Because all components are enclosed in a rigid housing, more accessories can be built in. This includes a dual illumination system, which includes a constant light source for focusing and a flash for photography, and filters such as for fluorescein angiography. Rather than placing the viewing and illumination beams side by side, the illumination beam generally uses the periphery of the pupil and leaves the center for the observation beam.[38]

An angled glass plate that can be flipped to the right or to the left can be used to slightly deviate the observation beam to the right part or the left part of the patient's pupil to produce photo pairs that can be viewed stereoscopically.

Because newer lens designs have allowed the construction of wide-angle cameras, a special challenge has been to construct the optical system in such a way that the curved retina is imaged in a plane that can be captured on a flat film.

11.2. Adaptive optics

The optics of the eye are not perfect. Even if major errors are corrected with spherical and cylindrical lenses, small irregularities across the pupillary opening persist. The technique of adaptive optics was developed for astronomical telescopes to counteract image degradation by atmospheric irregularities. An adaptive optics system uses a grid to divide the pupillary opening into many small areas and determines a separate small correction for each area. The information is fed to a slightly deformable mirror with microactuators. Thus the image quality can be enhanced to the point at which the cone mosaic can be clearly visible. The setup is too laborious for use in routine photography. Because the corrective system has to be fixed in relation to the pupil, it cannot be implemented in glasses or contact lenses. However, the technique, also known as wavefront analysis, has found a place in the refractive sculpting of the cornea.[39]

12. Gonioscopy

Another important part of ophthalmic exam. First explored in by Trantas (1907.); then explored by Salzmann (1915-16.); Koeppe (1919-20.); and Troncoso (1925-30). Finally Otto Barkan (1887.-1958.) made gonioscopy a routine diagnostic method in the ophthalmologist's office, thereby bringing about the separation of the glaucomas due to the angle-closure mechanism from the open-angle glaucomas[40]that the elevation of the intraocular pressure depends of abnormal resistance to aqueous outflow caused by anatomic or functional changes within the outflow channels.

Not until the 1890s did open-angle glaucoma become well proved and accepted in theories.

Thanks to gonioscopy, started recognition of a type or types of glaucoma without obstruction of the angle by the iris.

13. Secondary glaucomas

In the first edition of the Graefe-SaemischHandbook of Ophthalmology (1877), Saemisch lists the following ocular diseases as frequently giving rise to secondary glaucoma: cicatricial ecstasies of the cornea, circular or total adhesions of the iris to the lens, iritis serosa, traumatic cataract, dislocations of the lens, intraocular tumours, hemorrhagic retinal processes (referring mainly, if not exclusively, to occlusions of the central retinal vein), and sclerectasia pastries (which probably referred to glaucoma in eyes with malignant myopia). Congenital hydrophthalmos was at the time also classified with the secondary glaucomas.

14. Tonometry

William Bowman introduced digital estimation of the ocular tension at the annual meeting of the British Medical Association in 1862. Estimation of the ocular tension by palpation became one of the ophthalmologist's special skills, and some ophthalmologists developed so much confidence in it that they viewed instrumental tonometry with suspicion.

The early beginning of instrumental tonometry, apparently made by von Graefe, who mentions preliminary trials of mechanical tonometers in a letter to Donders dated December 24, 1862. Unfortunately, none of these instruments, however, reached the drawing board stage.

The real beginning and the first tonometers actually produced and tested on human eyes were developed in Donders' clinic in Utrecht between 1863 and 1868. They were instruments for use on the sclera. The scleral curvature at the site of tonometer application was determined first; it then served as a reference plane for the measurement of the depth of the indentation.

Impression tonometry had its drawbacks. The principal flaw was that the indentation, by displacing a significant amount of intraocular fluid, changes the pressure which is intended to measure; this was clearly expressed for the first time by Adolf Weber in 1867. Weber was official inventor of the first applanation tonometer, which was intended to give a tension reading with only minimal fluid displacement. Despite its theoretic superiority, this instrument did not gain wide acceptance, because recognition of the point of perfect applanation without indentation proved to be difficult. Lately, the principles of applanation tonometry were explored by Maklakoff in 1885. andImbert and Fick, father and son, a few years later. It resulted a several new applanationtonometers, but only one of them, Maklakoff's model of 1892, has stood the test of time and has remained in use, mainly by groups in the USSR.

The beginning of the 20th century, digital tonometry was still a method of subjective assessment of the ocular pressure [41]. At that time neither applanation tonometer did not find widespread use in practice.Finally, in 1905.Schiøtz presented his impression tonometer and it did not take long for the instrument to acquire the epithet "the first clinically useful tonometer." First major comprehensive reports of the clinical value of Schiotz tonometer began to appear in 1910. The essence of today's knowledge of the intraocular pressure in the normal and in the diseased human eye was acquired between 1910. and 1920. through the use of Schiøtztonometers.

Disadvantages of digital and instrumental tonometry, realized by the pioneers of these methods, addressed to the properties of the eyeball wall, especially elasticity, affected estimation of the intraocular pressure. Early experimental attempts in that time, to measure these properties and to eliminate them revealed new variables. Schiøtz wrote in 1920: "I can not imagine any method available for living eyes by which errors due to variations of the envelope could be eliminated." [42]Thirty years later, the electronic form of his instrument came closest to yielding reasonable estimates of "ocular rigidity," the term introduced by Friedenwald for the resistance that the in vivo eyeball offers to a change in intraocular volume [43].

Correcting readings taken with the Schiøtz tonometer for deviation of the particular eye from average ocular rigidity, the coefficient of ocular rigidity lost some of its clinical importance through the tremendous progress in applanation tonometry that occurred in the early 1950s through the work of Goldmann, Perkins, and Maurice.

15. Goldman applanation tonometry

The technology to estimate intraocular pressure (IOP) has evolved tremendously since Sir William Bowman emphasized the importance of ocular tension measurements in 1826. In an address delivered at the annual meeting of the British Medical Association, Sir William underscored the critical role that digital estimation of ocular tension played in his practice. In his address, Sir William stated that "it is now my constant practice, where defective vision is complained of, to ascertain almost at the first instant the state of tension in the eye...It is easy enough to estimate the tension of the eye, though there is a right and a wrong way of doing even so simple a thing... With medical men, the touch is already an educated sense, and a very little practice should suffice to apply it successfully to the eye."[44]

Soon afterwards, digital tonometry became an essential clinical skill necessary to master by all ophthalmologists. When mechanical tonometry was first introduced in the late 1800s, many ophthalmologists felt so confident with their ability to estimate IOP by palpation that they viewed the new technology as inferior. Isador Schnabel, in an address to the Vienna Ophthalmological Society in 1908, was noted to state that although he did not object in principle to mechanical tonometry, he expected "...very little from this test since digital tonometry by an expert is a much more accurate test".[45]

Although Grafe is credited with the first attempts to create instruments that mechanically measured IOP in the early 1860s, his proposed instruments were neither designed nor built. Rather, it was Donders who designed the first instrument capable of estimating IOP – albeit not accurately – with mechanical tonometry in the mid 1860s. The principle behind Donders's instrument was to displace intraocular fluid by contact with the sclera. The ophthalmologist first measured the curvature of the sclera at the site of contact, and then used this measurement as a reference plane to measure the depth of indentation. Smith and Lazerat refined this technology in the 1880s, and the discovery of cocaine by Carl Koller in 1884 led the way to corneal impression tonometry soon thereafter. With the aid of a powerful corneal anesthetic agent, corneal tonometry became the definitive choice of IOP measurements because it offered a well – defined and uniform site of impression when compared with the sclera.

Impression tonometry's major shortcoming was that it displaced so much fluid upon contact with the eye that the measured readings were highly variable and mostly inaccurate. What was needed was a way to displace a minimal amount of fluid to record IOP. This breakthrough came when Adolf Weber designed the first applanation tonometer in 1867, which gave a highly defined applanation point without indentation. After two decades of skepticism, the value of applanation tonometry was re-discovered when Alexei Maklakoff and others introduced new versions of applanationtonometers. In early 20th century, there were about 15 models of tonometers in use. In fact, Maklakoff's 1892 model is the basis of applanation tonometry today. However, digital tonometry still remained the gold standard among most ophthalmologists in the early 1900s.

The first clinically useful mechanical tonometer was designed and introduced by Hjalmar-Schiotz in the early 1900s. The instrument was simple, easy to use, and highly precise. It was quickly accepted and became the new gold standard beginning the 1910s. Innovations in calibration led to its increased use, and a tremendous amount of knowledge about the normal and glaucomatous eye was quickly acquired. An adjustment for ocular rigidity was introduced by Goldmann in the 1950s, which led to the development of Goldmannapplanationtonometers. The Goldmanntonometers displace such little fluid that variations in ocular rigidity are mostly negligible. The electronic and non – contact tonometers used today rely heavily on the principles and instrumentation first introduced by Maklakoff, Schiotz and Goldmann.

Today, for the most part, digital tonometry has been replaced by sophisticated technologies to estimate IOP. Today's instruments are incredibly accurate and easy to use. Yet, there is sometimes no good substitute for digital tonometry. For example, some ophthalmologists may prefer digital tonometry when estimating IOP in patients with keratoprostheses. In these situations, fingers that have mastered Sir William's art are highly desirable. In fact, it is said that the famous Dr. Claus Dohlman, Harvard professor of Ophthalmology at the Massachusetts Eye and Ear Infirmary, remains as accurate in measuring IOP with his fingers as any ophthalmologist using the high-tech tonometers of today!

16. Perimetry

Modern diagnostic of glaucoma is unimaginable without perimetry. The merit for measurements of peripheral vision for the diagnosis and follow-up of ocular disease, as many
other things in ophthalmology, is attributed to Albert von Graefe. With a primitive
campimeter—a sheet of paper with radial rows of dots which served as stimuli—he was
probably the first (1856) to plot paracentral field defects in chronic glaucoma and to use
them in the evaluation of surgical results. Similar to von Graefe's device, Haffmanns
from Donder's clinic discovered the greater frequency in glaucoma simplex of serious involvement of the upper half of the field, which gave rise to an easily detectable nasal
step [46].

In 1857.Förster introduced the first perimeter, which placed accent on large targets, such
as the 10/330, which permitted only very gross measurements. The observations of that
time did suggest partial reversibility of field defects if the pressure was lowered substan-
tially by an iridectomy or sclerotomy. 1889. was a very important year for a development of techniques most appropriate for glaucoma. Bjerrum presented 2-meter screen,
the 2-meter test distance, and the 2- to 5-ram white test objects. He discovered the relative or absolute scotomas, circling the point of fixation and including the blind spot,
which became the hallmark of chronic glaucoma. Conceptually, it means the beginning
of the nerve fibre bundle theory of the glaucomatous optic nerve disease.

Further major step was the occurrence of small scotomas in the zone from 12° to 20° from
the point of fixation, in early glaucomas, presented by Peter [47]. These scotomas, in the beginning were not connected with the blind spot, but they reached it later via expansion.

The construction of smaller isopters, another early glaucoma characteristic, presented in
1920s, was clearly established with Bjerrum's technique. Bjerrum's technique also confirmed
the regression of early glaucomatous defects following normalization of pressure documented by instrumental tonometry. The close relationship between pressure and field of vision
was demonstrated further by Samojloff's observations [48]of temporary enlargement of the
blind spot concurrent with osmotically induced pressure elevations. By stereocampimetry
with minute targets, Evans was able to detect a gross form of parallelism between diurnal
pressure fluctuations and the size of paracentralscotomas[49].

Also in 1920s was noticed that among patients with glaucomatous defects close to the
point of fixation (late stages of glaucoma optic neuropathy), a surgical procedure, particularly iridectomy, could have an untoward effect and lead to further rapid shrinkage of
the visual field. The incrimination of the iridectomy referred originally to the period
when the alternative, the sclerotomy, had proved relatively free of unfavourable effects
on the visual field. Subsequent experience with filtering operations temporarily led to
the distinction between two classes of glaucoma operations: 1) the less risky: cyclodialysis and sclerotomy and 2) the riskier: iridectomy, sclerectomy, and trephination.

17. Glaucoma treatment

The early treatment of glaucoma has its course of history (Table 1. and Table 2.).

Main discoveries where:

1. A curative action of the iridectomy in certain glaucomas [44],

2. The development of the filtering operations [50], and

3. The discovery of the first three ocular hypotensive drugs: eserine, pilocarpine, and epinephrine [51].

Surgical Treatment of Glaucoma (1830-1920)

1830 Mackenzie[1] recommends scleral punctures to release vitreous and to relieve the pressure on the retina.

1857 von Graefe's iridectomy[6] almost overnight gains the position of *the* glaucoma operation.

1882 de Wecker, in a paper on the "filtering cicatrix"[9], expresses the concept that in the presence of elevated intraocular pressure, a properly executed corneoscleral incision can heal in a manner allowing intraocular fluid to "filter," ie, be driven by a pressure gradient through the loose scar tissue into subconjunctival spaces.

1891 Bader [52] finds the occurrence of an iris prolapse during or shortly after an iridectomy a favourable sign, auguring success of the operation.

1903 Herbert reports on a series of subconjunctival fistula operations in which he purposely leaves the iris in the operative incision. The report includes the first detailed description of the transformation of the epibulbar tissues that become exposed to the steady flow of aqueous [53].

1905 Heine first reports on the operation of cyclodialysis[54], based on Fuchs' [55] and Axenfeld's[56] observation of the association between postoperative choroidal detachment, a tear or tears in the insertion of the ciliary muscle at the scleral spur, and hypotony.

1906 Lagrange first reports on his iridosclerectomy[50].

1909 Freeland and Elliot independently substitute the trephine for Lagrange's scissors.

1913 At the first international review of glaucoma surgery the pronouncement is made that chronic glaucoma can only be arrested by establishing a filtering cicatrix in connection with the anterior chamber. The iridectomy loses its status of *the* glaucoma operation but still is first in favor for acute glaucoma [57].

1915 The abexterno incision is introduced by Foroni[58].

1920 Seidel demonstrates the transconjunctival passage of aqueous after trephining procedures[16].

Table 1. A summary of the early phases of the glaucoma surgical treatment.

Medical Treatment of Glaucoma (1863-1932)

1863	Argyll Robertson and von Graefe study the effect of extracts of the calabar bean on pupil and accommodation. Von Graefe finds the miotic effect useful in that it facilitates the iridectomy.
1876	Laqueur[59] reports "a definite drop of the elevated tension after repeated installations of physostigmine in five cases of glaucoma simplex and in one case of secondary glaucoma."
1876	Weber studies the mechanisms underlying the hypotensive effect of physostigmine in rabbits and in man and advises caution in its use because of the marked swelling and engorgement of the ciliary processes caused by the drug [60].
1877	Laqueur gives the first clear-cut account of the successful termination by use of physostigmine of attacks of acute glaucoma and of the prevention of recurrences [61].
1877	Weber introduces pilocarpine with the hope that it will replace the iridectomy in some of the chronic and simple glaucomas and that it will serve to make up for the insufficient effect of the latter in many other cases [62].
1898	The hypotensive effect of topically administered adrenal extracts is discovered.
1902	Darier reports significant lowering of pressure in some glaucomas, induced by adrenaline alone or in combination with physostigmine[51].
1909	Extensive clinical use of adrenaline has confirmed the beneficial results, but it has also brought to light the clear-cut untoward effects, ie, the drug may cause further elevation of pressure and even precipitate acute attacks in certain eyes.
1923	Hamburger reintroduces adrenaline; new, more potent, more stable preparations for topical use are becoming available. Untoward effects in certain eyes are rediscovered [63].
1932	Gonioscopy furnishes the answer to the unfavorable response of certain eyes to topical adrenaline.

Table 2. A summary of the early phases of the glaucoma medical treatment.

Author details

Ivan Marjanovic

Glaucoma Department, University Eye Clinic Clinical centre of Serbia and Belgrade University School of Medicine, Serbia

References

[1] Mackenzie W: Practical Treatise on the Diseases of the Eye. London: Longmarts, Reese, Orme Brown and Green, 1830, p 710.

[2] Duke-Elder S, Jay B: Introduction to Glaucoma and Hypotony. In Duke-Elder S(ed): System of Ophthalmology. St. Louis: Mosby, 1969, Vol XI, p 337.

[3] Albert DM: Jaeger's Atlas of Diseases of the Ocular Fundus. Philadelphia: Saunders, 1972, pp 67–79.

[4] von Graefe A: Vorläufige Notiz über das Wesen des Glaucoms. Arch Ophthalmol 1:371, 1854.

[5] Weber A: Ein Fall yon partieller Hyperämie der Chorioidea bei einem Kaninchen. Arch Ophthalmol 2:133, 1855.

[6] von Graefe A: Ueber die Wirkung der Iridectomie bei Glaucom. Arch Ophthalmol 3:456, 1857.

[7] von Graefe A: Weitere Zusätze über Glaucom und die Heil-wirkung der Iridectomie. Arch Ophthalmol 8:254, 1861.

[8] Schnabel I: Die Entwicklungsgeschichte der glaukomatösen Exkavation. Z Augenheilkd 14: 1, 1905.

[9] de Wecker L: La cicatrice à filtration. Ann Ocul 87:133, 1882.

[10] Mueller H: Anatomische Beiträge zur Ophthalmologie: Ueber Niveau-Veränderungen an der Eintrittsstelle des Sehnerven. Arch Ophthalmol 4:1, 1858.

[11] Smith P: Glaucoma: Its Causes, Symptoms, Pathology and Treatment. London: Churchill, 1879, p 91.

[12] Schwalbe G: Untersuchungen über die Lymphbahnen des Auges und ihre Begrenzungen. Arch mikrosk Anat 6:261, 1870.

[13] Leber T: Studien über den Flüssigkeitswechsel im Auge. von Graefe's Arch Ophthalmol 19:87, 1873.

[14] Bentzen CF, Leber T: Ueber die Filtration aus der vorderen Kammer bei normalen und glaukomatösen Augen. yon Graefe's Arch Ophthalmol 41:208, 1895.

[15] Knies M: Ueber das Wesen des Glaukoms. von Graefe's Arch Ophthalmol 22:163, 1876.

[16] Seidel E: Weitere experimentelle Untersuchungen über die Quelle und den Verlauf der intraokularen Saftströmung: VI. Die Filtrationsfähigkeit, eine wesentliche Eigenschaft der Skleralnarben nach erfolgreicher Elliotscher Trepanation, von Graefe's Arch Ophthalmol 107:158, 1921.

[17] Smith P: On the size of the cornea in relation to age, sex, refraction and primary glaucoma. Trans Ophthalmol Soc UK 10:68, 1890.

[18] Czermak W: Einiges zur Lehre vonder Entstehung und dem Verlaufe des prodromalen und acuten Glaukomanfalles. Prager med Wochenschr 22: 15, 1897.

[19] Curran EJ: A new operation for glaucoma involving a new principle in the etiology and treatment of chronic primary glaucoma. Arch Ophthalmol 49:131, 1920.

[20] Meeting of the PhysikalischeGesellschaft, Berlin, December 6, 1850 (von Helmholtz' paper, read by his friend Dubois-Raymond, has been lost).

[21] von Helmholtz H: Beschreibung eines Augenspiegels zur Untersuchung der Netzhaut im lebenden Auge, Berlin (1851). Translation in Arch Ophthalmol 46:565, 1951.

[22] Albert DM, Miller WH: Jan Purkinje and the ophthalmoscope. Am J Ophthalmol 76:494, 1973.

[23] Mark HH: The first ophthalmoscope? Arch Ophthalmol 84:520, 521, 1970.

[24] Cumming W: On a luminous appearance of the human eye, and its application to the detection of disease of the retina and posterior part of the eye. R Med Chir Soc Lond 29:283, 1846.

[25] Brücke E: Ueber das Leuchten der menschlichen Augen. Arch Anat Physiol Wissensch Med 25, 1847.

[26] Jones W: Report on the ophthalmoscope. Br Med Chir Rev 14:425, 1854.

[27] Rucker WF: A History of the Ophthalmoscope. Rochester, MN: Whiting, 1971.

[28] von Helmholtz H: Ueber eine neue einfachste Form des Augenspiegel. Arch Physiol Heilk 2:827, 1852.

[29] Ruete CGT: Der Augenspiegel und das Optometer für practische Aerzte. Gottingen, Prussia: Dieterich, 1852.

[30] Landolt E: Die Untersuchungsmethoden. Berlin, 1:234, 1913.

[31] Duke-Elder Sir Steward: System of Ophthalmology. Vol 7. Foundations of Ophthalmology: Heredity, Pathology, Diagnosis and Therapeutics. St. Louis: Mosby, 1962, 290–325.

[32] Albert DM: Jaeger's Atlas of Diseases of the Ocular Fundus. Philadelphia: Saunders, 1972.

[33] Hruby K: Spaltlampenmikroskopie des hinteren Augenabschnittes ohne Kontakglas. KIm Monatsbl Augenkeilkd 108:195, 1942.

[34] Hruby K: Spaltlampenmikroskopie des hinteren Augenabschnittes. Vienna: Urban and Schwarzenberg, 1950.

[35] Goldmann H: Zur Technik der Spaltlampenmikroskopie. Ophthalmologica 96:90, 1938.

[36] El Bayadi G: New method of slit lamp micro-ophthalmoscopy. Br J Ophthalmol 37:625, 1953.

[37] Schlegel HJ: Eine einfache Weitwinkeloptik zur spaltlampen-mikroskopischen Untersuchung des Augenhintergrundes. Doc Ophthalmol 26:300, 1969.

[38] Pomerantzeff O, Webb RH, Delori FC: Image formation in fundus cameras. IOVS 18:630, 1979.

[39] Roorda A: Adaptive optics ophthalmoscopy. J Refract Surg 16:S602, 2000.

[40] Barkan O: Glaucoma: Classification, causes and surgical control: Results of microgonioscopic research. Am J Ophthalmol 21: 1099, 1938.

[41] Draeger J: Geschichte der Tonometrie. Bibl Ophthalmol 56:1, 1961.

[42] Schi øtz H: Tonometry. Br J Ophthalmol 4:201, 249, 1920.

[43] Friedenwald JS: Calibration of tonometers. In Standardization of Tonometers, Decennial Report, Committee on Standardization of Tonometers. AmAcadOphthalmolOtolaryngol, 1954, p 95.

[44] Bowman W: Glaucomatous affections, and their treatment by iridectomy. Br Med J, Oct II, 1852, p 377-382.

[45] Schnabel I., Klin Montasbl Augenh 1908; 48:318.

[46] Haffmanns JHA: Zur Kenntnis des Glaukoms. Arch Ophthalmol 8: 124, 1862.

[47] Peter LC: A simplified conception of visual field changes in chronic glaucoma. Arch Ophthalmol 56: 337, 1927.

[48] Samojloff A: Die Grössenzunahme des blinden Fleckes nach subkonjunktivalen Kochsalzinjektionen. KlinMonatsblAugenheilkd 70:655, 1923.

[49] Evans JN: Transient fluctuations in the scotoma of glaucoma. Am J Ophthalmol 18:333, 1935.

[50] Kronfeld PC: The rise of the filtering operations. Survey Ophthalmol 17: 168, 1972.

[51] Spengler E: Kritisches Sammel-Referat über die Verwendung einiger neuerer Arzneimittel in der Augenheilkunde. Z Augenheilkd 13:33, 1905.

[52] Bader C: Sclerotomy in glaucoma. Trans 7th Internal Congr Med London, Section on Ophthalmol, 1881, p 98.

[53] Herbert H: Subconjunctival fistula operation in the treatment of primary chronic glaucoma. Trans Ophthalmol Soc UK 23:324, 1903.

[54] 54. Heine L: Die Cyklodialyse, eine neue Glaukomoperation. Dtsch med Wochenschr 31: 824, 1905.

[55] 55. Fuchs E: Ablösung der Aderhaut nach Operation. von Graefe's Arch Ophthalmol 53:375, 1902.

[56] Axenfeld T: Zur operativen Ablösung der Aderhaut, nebst einer Bemerkung zur Wirkung der Glaukomoperationen. KlinMonatsblAugenheilkd 41:122, 1903.

[57] Elliot RH, Lagrange F, Smith P: Report on glaucoma operations with special reference to the comparative results attained by iridectomy and its recent substitutes.
Trans 17th InternatCongr Med London, Section on Ophthalmol, 1913, p 57.

[58] Foroni C: Sclerectomia ab externo. von Graefe's Arch Ophthalmol 89:393, 1915.

[59] Laqueur L: Neue therapeutische Indikation für Physostigmine. Centralbl med Wissensch 14:421, 1876.

[60] Weber A: Ueber Calabar und seine therapeutische Verwendung. yon Graefe's Arch
Ophthalmol 22:215, 1876.

[61] Laqueur L: Ueber Atropin und Physostigmin und ihre Wirkung auf den intraokularen Druck. von Graefe's Arch Ophthalmol 23:129, 1877.

[62] Weber A: Die Ursache des Glaukoms. von Graefe's Arch Ophthalmol 23: 1, 1877.

[63] Löhlein W: Ueberblick über den heutigen Stand der Glaukomtherapie. Zentralbl Ge-
samte Ophthalmol 22:1, 1930.

Chapter 12

Recognizing a Glaucomatous Optic Disc

Vassilis Kozobolis, Aristeidis Konstantinidis and
Georgios Labiris

Additional information is available at the end of the chapter

1. Introduction

Glaucoma is an optic neuropathy with its hallmark being a characteristic loss of the ganglion cell axons which in turn leads to an excavation of the optic disc. Although optic disc cupping occurs in many other ocular diseases [1] the assessment of the optic nerve head with either optic disc photography or the newer modalities remains of utmost importance in the diagnosis and follow up of the glaucomatous process. The digital stereophotographs allow storage of optic disc photos for future comparison and offer qualitative assessment of the optic nerve head. The new imaging modalities can quantitatively and objectively analyze various parameters of the optic nerve head and the retinal nerve fiber layer in order to discriminate between glaucomatous and nonglaucomatous optic discs. They can also compare scans of the same patient overtime and detect any changes. As glaucoma is a progressive optic neuropathy patient's assessment overtime is of paramount importance in order to tract changes and monitor the progression of the disease.

1.1. New modalities for the imaging and analysis of the optic disc and retinal nerve fiber layer (RNFL)

1.1.1. Red-free photography of the optic disc and RNFL

Photography is not a new imaging technique [2,3]. However newer photographic methods allow stereographic assessment of the optic nerve head and more detailed visualization of the RNFL. Retinal nerve fiber layer is better visualized when the refractive media are clear and in pigmented fundi. Its defects can be broadly classified as localized and diffuse and the former are easier to identify.Red free photography of the RNFL is as accurate in distinguishing glaucomatous from nonglaucomatous patients as optical coherence tomography (OCT), scanning laser polarimetry (SLP) and confocal scanning laser ophthalmoscope (SCLO) [4,5]. Stereophotographs of the optic discs was proven to be as efficacious in detecting glaucoma as the objective analysis the optic nerve head with the new modalities [6,7].

The new imaging modalities on the optic disc and RNFL include the confocal scanning laser ophthalmoscopy (CSLO), optical coherence tomography (OCT) and scanning laser polarimetry (SLP). The first two technologies can analyze both the optic nerve head and RNFL while SLP analyzes the thickness of the RNFL only.

1.1.2. Confocal Scanning Laser Ophthalmoscopy (CSLO, fig 1)

The CSLO technology is used by the Heidelberg Retinal Tomograph (HRT, Heidelberg Engineering, Heidelberg, Germany). It is based on the principle of two conjugated pinholes. Laser light (670nm) enters through one pinhole and focuses on a plane of the retina or the optic disc. The reflected light passes through the confocal pupil and allows reflected light only from that specific plane to enter the photodetector. The focused laser light scans across the optic nerve head (ONH) and RNFL along the x and y axes at planes of different depth acquiring a series of images. This series is reconstructed to produce a three dimensional image. Each series consists of 16 images per mm and for a 4 mm depth scan 64 images are captured. A fundamental part of the SCLO technology is the reference plane. It is defined as a plane parallel to the retina and lies 50 μm below the temporal part of the scleral ring of Elsching. In ONH analysis structures above the reference plane are read as neuroretinal ring and structures below are read as disc cup. SCLO has a transverse resolution of 10 μm and an axial resolution of 300 μm. The field of view of the image is 15°×15°.

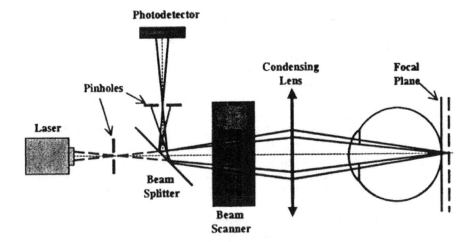

Figure 1. Light from the laser device passes through a pinhole sitting in front of it and focuses on a certain plane in the retina. The reflected light from the retina enters a confocal pinhole sitting in front of the photodetector. Only light

reflected from that specific plane (as determined by the position of the pinhole in front of the laser device) enters the photodetector. The focal plane can be changed by moving the pinhole of the laser device.

The HRT can analyze both the RNFL thickness and optic nerve head. A fundamental part of the analysis is the identification of the boundaries of the optic disc. The operator can draw a line along the edge of the optic disc. As the retinal vessels and peripapillary atrophy can make the exact identification of the boundaries difficult the examiner can use the 3-dimensional image of the optic nerve head in order to draw the line.

The RNFL thickness is measured at the edge of the optic nerve head for 360° and follows a double hump appearance as the RNFL is thicker in the superotemporal and inferotemporal sectors. The optic disc parameters analyzed are: the disc area, cup area, rim area, cup volume, rim volume, linear cup/disc ratio, mean cup depth. Mean cup depth, maximum cup depth, cup shape measure, height variation contour, mean RNFL thickness and RNFL cross-sectional area. The Moorfields regression analysis provides an overall assessment of the field of view and classifies it as "normal", "borderline" and "outside normal limits".

2. Strengths and limitations [8]

The advantages of the new version of CSLO (HRT 3) is the large normative database which includes subjects European, African and Indian ancestry and can analyze both optic nerve head and RNF. Its limitation is that some optic nerve head measurements rely on a reference plane based on a hand drown contour line around the disc margins. The Glaucoma Probability Score does not need a reference plane. HRT measurements can be influenced by intraocular pressure fluctuations [9].

2.1. Optical Coherence Tomography (OCT, fig 2)

Optical coherence tomography uses the principle of interferometry to construct high resolution cross-sectional images of the retina. An 800 nm laser light is split into two beams before entering the eye. The imaging beam consists of short pulses of light (the duration of each pulse is defined as the coherence length). One beam enters the eye and is reflected from the retina and the second beam is reflected from a reference mirror that moves back and forth along the Z axis. When the two reflected light beams constructively interfere they create a signal read by the interferometer. The time delay of the back scattered light from each layer of the retina differentiates the depth location of each layer (time-domain OCT). As a consequence in time domain OCT the instrument needs to perform two scans: a transverse scan across the eye (x axis) and a depth scan (z axis).The upgrade of time-domain OCT is the spectral-domain or Fourier-domain OCT (SD OCT/FD OCT). The SD OCT instead of the mechanical movement of the reference mirror analyzes with the aid of a mathematical equation (Fourier transform: $F_S(z) \propto FT\{A_S(K)\}$) multiple wavelengths reflected from the retina. SD OCT obtains retina scans much faster (as the movement of the reference mirror along the z axis is omitted and only the scanning of the beam along the x axis is used) and with a better resolution (5-6 μm axial resolution, 10-15 μm transverse resolution) than the time-domain OCT. For the analysis of the optic nerve head the OCT runs six scans across the optic disc in a spoke-like pattern (fig 3). The measurements of the area between the scans are interpolated from the values across the scans. The edge of the optic nerve head is automatically defined as the end of the retinal pigment epithelium (RPE)/choriocapillaris layer. A straight line is taken from one edge of the RPE to the other and a reference plane is set 150 µm above this line. Neuroretinal rim is defined as the area above the reference plane and cup the area below it.

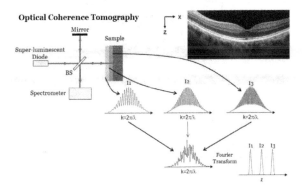

Figure 2. The beam from super-lumiscent diode laser source is split as it travels through the beam splitter (BS). One beam goes to the reference mirror (mirror) and the second beam in the tissue to be examined. The two beams are reflected back and they interfere as they enter the interfereometer (spectrometer in the figure). The mirror moves back and forth in order to create constructive interference at different depths (represented by different colors in the sample) of the examined tissue (z axis). The beam also travels across x axis in order to capture a slice of the sample.

3. Strengths and limitations [8]

OCT can analyze both the morphology of the optic disc and RNFL (fig 3,4). However automatic recognition of the edges of the optic disc as the end of the RPE layer can give incorrect measurements in patients with peripapillary atrophy. This is especially true for glaucoma patients who tend to have greater peripapillary atrophic areas that progress overtime. In this case what is incorrectly measured as optic disc area is the area of the optic nerve head plus the peripapillary atrophy. Furthermore as the information of the optic nerve head data between the scans are interpolated small defects of the neuroretinal rim may be missed.

3.1. Scanning Laser Polarimetry (SLP) (fig 5,6)

Scanning laser polarimetry is used in the GDx (GDX; Carl Zeis Meditec, Dublin, CA, USA). It is based on the principle of retardation. The RNFL has linear birefringence due to the parallel orientation of the microtubules in the axons of the RNFL. When polarized light travels through the RNFL the beam parallel to the RNFL slows down compared to the one that travels

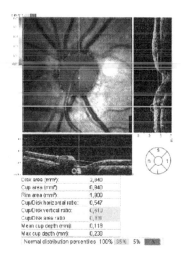

Disk area (mm²):	2,340
Cup area (mm²)	0,340
Rim area (mm²)	1,900
Cup/Disk horizontal ratio:	0,547
Cup/Disk vertical ratio:	0,610
Cup/Disk area ratio	0,331
Mean cup depth (mm)	0,119
Max cup depth (mm)	0,230

Normal distribution percentiles 100% 95% 5% 1%

Figure 3. Optic nerve head analysis of a normal optic disc. The disc margins are identified by the OCT but the examiner can accurately identify the true disc border by manually moving the blue squares. The parameters measured are shown in the figure

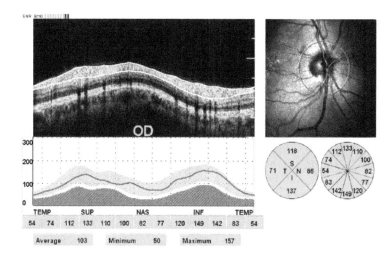

TEMP		SUP		NAS		INF		TEMP
54	74	112	133	110	100	82	77	120	149	142	83	54

Average	103	Minimum	50	Maximum	157

Figure 4. RNFL analysis with OCT. The numbers refer to RNFL thickness in μm. The green shaded area represents the normal RNFL thickness in the normative database of the OPKO spectral-domain OCT/SLO (Opko/OTI, Ophthalmic Technologies Inc, Toronto, Canada). Ninety five percent of the age-matched subjects with normal RNFL thickness will be included in the green area. On the other hand <5% of the subjects with normal RNFL thickness will fall in the yellow shaded area and <1% of the normal subjects will be in the red shaded area. In this patient the blue contour line of their RNFL thickness has the characteristic double hump appearance and falls in the green area. The RNFL thickness is normal for the age of this patient. The double hump pattern of the RNFL is due to the increased thickness of the fiber layer in the superotemporal and inferotemporal sector. The RNFL thickness is measured around a 3.46 mm diameter circle centered on the optic disc.

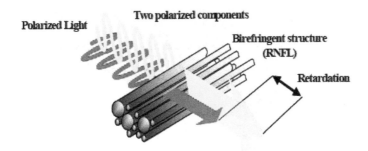

Figure 5. Polarized light that travels parallel to the RNFL slows down. This retardation is proportional to the thickness of the RNFL

perpendicular to the fiber layer. This difference in the speed between the two beams is called retardation and is proportional to the RNFL thickness. The scanning laser beam used is 785nm.

Because the corneal also exhibits birefringence the GDx has a variable corneal compensator (VCC) in order to subtract the retardation from the cornea and the only retardation measured is that derived from the RNFL. The newer GDx machines have an enhanced corneal compensator that offers better reproducibility of the measurements and is more accurate in the diagnosis of glaucoma [10]. The transverse resolution of the GDx is 45 μm.

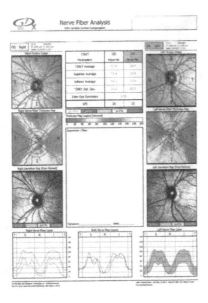

Figure 6. Printout of the RNFL analysis with the GDx VCC. The colored images at the top of the printout are the fundus photos. Below them is the thickness map. It is a color coded representation of the thickness of the RNFL within a 20° × 20°

(128×128 pixels) field centered on the optic disc. The warmer the colors the thicker the RNFL. Below the thickness map is the deviation map which represents the deviation of the RNFL thickness from the normal age matched value. At the bottom is the TSNIT (Temporal – Superior – Nasal – Inferior – Temporal) map which shows the RNFL thickness along the calculation ring. The latter is a ring 0.4 mm wide centered around the optic disc with the outer diameter being 3.2 mm and the inner 2.4 mm. The shaded areas (green for the right eye and purple for the left) represent the 95% of the normal values for this age group. The TSNIT contour line has a double hump appearance as for the OCT. The TSNIT parameters are the RNFL thickness along the calculation ring for the average, superior and inferior sector RNFL thickness. The TSNIT standard deviation is the modulation from peak to trough values of the double hump pattern. Because in glaucoma the superior and inferior sectors become thinned the difference between the peks and troughs decreases the TSNIT standard deviation value decreases as well. The intereye symmetry measures the symmetry between the eyes (values between -1 and 1). Normal eyes show good symmetry but the glaucomatous eyes tend to be asymmetrical as glaucoma can affect one eye more than the other. The Nerve Fiber Indicator is a global value based on the entire RNFL thickness map. The values range from 1-100 (1-30: normal, 31-50: borderline, >51: abnormal).

4. Strengths and limitations [7]

SLP can only measure data from RNFL. Areas of peripapillary atrophy give false information about the RNFL. A minority of the eyes examined show atypical retardation patterns (APRs) which are overcome by the GDx-ECC machines [11]. Atypical patterns are those which do not follow the normal histological distribution of the RNFL with the supero- and inferotemporal sectors being the thickest. APRs give falsely high RNFL measurements [12]. Newer SLP models are not compatible with the older ones. On the other hand RNFL analysis with SLP does not require a reference plane.

5. Sensitivity and specificity

Badala et al [4] compared the efficacy of stereoptic disc assessment and that of all three imaging modalities (OCT, GDx, HRT 3) in diagnosing glaucoma. The sensitivity at 95% specificity of the best performing parameter of each modality is: for the OCT (average RNFL thickness) 89%, for the GDx VCC (nerve fiber indicator) 78% and for the HRT 3 [Frederick S. Mikelberg (FSM) discriminant function] 70%. Optic disc stereophtographs are as accurate in detecting glaucoma as the other imaging modalities.

Retinal nerve fiber analysis with all the above modalities exhibit a characteristic double hump because the RNFL in thicker in the superotemporal and inferotemporal sectors compared to the nasal and temporal ones.

All of the above imaging modalities have been employed in the diagnosis and follow up of patients with various stages of glaucomatous optic neuropathy. Studies have shown that there is a discrepancy between the measurements of the optic disc parameters taken with OCT and HRT in glaucomatous eyes [13]. HRT II had higher values for disc and rim area while RTVue-100 OCT had higher values for cup area, cup-to-disc area ratio, and vertical and horizontal cup-to-disc ratio. Leite et al [14] compared three FD-OCT machines and reported that their performance in detecting glaucoma is similar. FD-OCT out-performed SD-OCT in detecting progression of the glaucomatous process [15] but they were comparable in detecting glaucomatous damage [16]. Lee et al [17] found that the best performing parameter for glaucoma detection of the GDx is the nerve fiber index and that for Cirrus OCT the inferior RNFL thickness. GDx was also more accurate in detecting glaucoma than the Cirrus OCT. Two recent studies [18,19] showed that the diagnostic accuracy for glaucoma of the HRT II is dependent on the disc size which is not the case for OCT and GDx.

The severity of the glaucomatous process also affects the accuracy of glaucoma diagnosis of the various imaging technologies. The more advanced the disease the more accurate the diagnosis of glaucomatous optic neuropathy [20,21]. OCT and SLP performed better than CSLO in discriminating between early glaucomatous eyes with or without visual field defects [22]. In eyes with early glaucoma the most accurate parameter is the inferior RNFL thickness which performs better than the most accurate parameter of the CSLO (vertical cup-to-disc ratio). In glaucoma suspect eyes the most accurate parameter for the OCT is the average RNFL thickness, for the SLP the nerve fiber indicator and for the CSLO the vertical cup-to-disc ratio. The first two parameters performed better than the vertical cup-to-disc ratio. Leung et al [23] confirmed that SD-OCT performed better than HRT in recognizing patients with glaucoma. RNFL thickness changes performed better than optic nerve head parameters as evaluated with CSLO. The nerve fiber index of the SLP was more accurate in diagnosing glaucoma than the rim volume parameter of the CSLO [24]. SLP was also superior in detecting glaucoma progression by analyzing RNFL thickness compared to CSLO analysis of the neuroretinal rim area [25].

6. Anatomy of the optic disc (fig 7)

The optic disc is the area in the posterior pole where the ganglion cell axons converge to exit the eye and travel towards the brain. Its margins are defined by a dense fibrous tissue, the Elsching's ring. The disc area is covered by the neuroretinal rim which contains the retinal ganglion cells axons and the disc cup in the center. The ganglion cells axons leave the eye by piercing the thinned part of the sclera called the lamina cribrosa. The axons are arranged in bundles and exit the eye via the pores of the lamina cribrosa to form the optic nerves. The size and shape of the neuroretinal rim and cup depend on the total size of the optic disc and the number of the axons that travel through it.

The following morphological features of the optic disc should be taken into account when assessing an optic nerve head [26]:

6.1. Optic disc size

The size of the optic disc shows great variability between different populations [27]. The range of the mean disc area measured in mm^2 for people of different ethnic backgrounds is: africans 1.84-2.50, whites 1.65-2.34, Indians 2.24-2.93, Asians 1.97-2.67 and latinos 1.95-2.56 [28].The size was shown to be independent of the age after the age of 10, the body height, gender and refractive errors between -5.00 and +5.00 D. In contrast the optic disc is smaller in high hypermetropes and larger in high myopes. Optic disc size abruptly increases for myopia above -8.00 diopters (D) and significantly decreases for hyperopia above +4.00 D [29] The optic disc area was found to have great variability between healthy individuals by many researchers [28,30,31]. For this reason the terms <<microdisc>> and <<macrodisc>> have been coined.

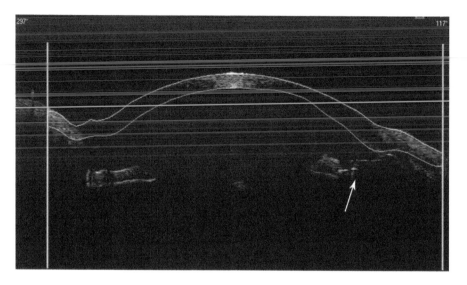

Figure 7. Normal optic disc. Note the presence of a small cup, thick neuroretinal rim, absence of peripapillary atrophy, equal distance of the exit of the trunk of the vessel from the superior and inferior sectors of the rim and normal arteriolar caliber.

Microdisc is a disc with a disc area two standard deviations less than the mean of the normal disc area and macrodisc is a disc with a disc area two standard deviations above the mean. The Blue Mountain Study [32] classified the discs as small (1.1 – 1.3), medium (1.4 – 1.7) and large (1.8 – 2.0) based on the vertical disc diameter measured in mm. The European Glaucoma Society classified the disc based on the disc area as small (<1.6mm^2), medium (1,6-2.8 mm^2) and large (>2.8 mm^2). Patients with primary open angle (POAG) and pigmentary glaucoma have normal disc size. In non-glaucomatous pathologies, optic disc drusen, pseudopapilledema, nonarteretic anterior ischemic optic neuropathy and tilted disc [33] are associated with small disc sizes while morning glory syndrome and optic disc pits with large discs. Furthermore larger discs have more axons in absolute number but less axons per disc area [34]. Patients with pseudoexfoliation glaucoma tend to have smaller discs and those with normal tension glaucoma larger discs [35,36]. Glaucoma, however, may occur in conjunction with abnormal disc size as well as with other disc pathologies.

6.2. Optic disc shape [26]

The optic disc is elongated along the vertical axis with the vertical axis being 7-10% longer than the horizontal. The disc shape as expressed by the ratio of minimal to maximal diameter shows less variability between individuals than the disc area. The disc shape is independent from sex, age, right and left eye and body weight and height and does not show interindividual variability for a refractive error less than -8.00D. In POAG patients the disc shape is not associated with the visual field defects. However for in high myopes >-12D it is more elongated.

Elongated optic discs were associated with increased corneal astigmatism. Overall disc shape bears little value in the diagnosis of glaucoma.

6.3. Neuroretinal rim shape and cup-to-disc ratio (C/D ratio)

It represents the quotient of the vertical cup diameter to the vertical overall disc diameter. In normal eyes the cup is horizontally elongated with the horizontal diameter being 8% longer than the vertical one. On the other hand the disc is vertically oval shaped. As a consequence the neuroretinal rim is thicker at superior and inferior poles. The mnemonic ISNT rule dictates that the neuroretinal rim is thicker in the inferior pole of the disc followed by the superior, the nasal and finally the temporal which is the thinnest. The C/D ratio also shows interindividual variability being higher in large discs and lower in smaller discs. Clinicians should bear in mind the opposite configuration of the cup and optic disc when assessing the disc for glaucomatous damage. They should also take into account that a high C/D ratio is not necessarily pathognomonic for glaucoma as it can occur in large diameter discs (fig 8,9). Conversely early glaucomatous damage can be overlooked in small discs with small cups.

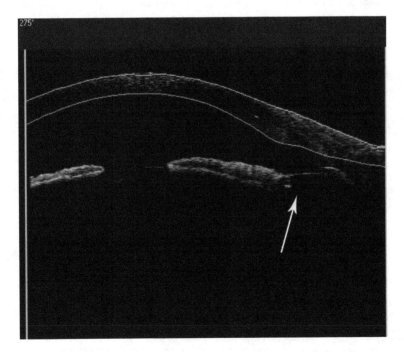

Figure 8. Large optic disc with a large cup. Neuroretinal rim shape respects **ISNT** rule (rim sectors wider to thinner (**I**nferior-**S**uperior-**N**asal-**T**emporal), there is no peripapillary atrophy and no optic disc haemorrhages are detected. The main vessels emerge with a dual trunk. The exit of each trunk lies at equal distance from the superior and inferior rim

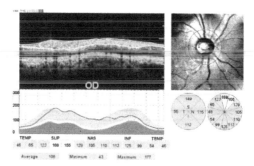

Figure 9. Retinal nerve fiber analysis (RNFL) with optical coherence tomography (OCT) of the same eye as in fig 8. The blue contour line represents the thickness of the RNFL of this patient and falls in the falls area. It is normal for this patient's age

In the early to moderate glaucoma the axons in the superotemporal and inferotemporal areas of the disc are affected usually first and this leads to an increase of the C/D vertical diameter faster than the horizontal causing an increased vertical C/D ratio with violation of the ISNT rule.

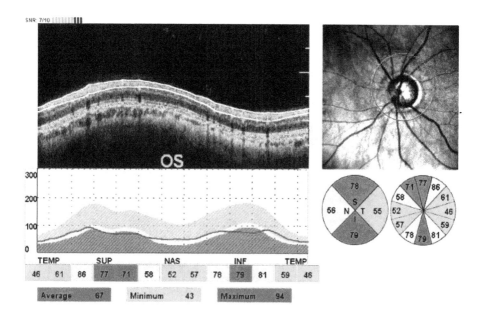

Figure 10. Typical RNFL loss in the superior and inferior RNFL sectors in a glaucoma patient. The RNFL contour line is flattened and crosses the red shaded abnormal area. Less than 1% of the normal subjects will have a similar RNFL thickness in the affected sectors as this patient has.

A large C/D ratio has been shown to be a risk factor for glaucoma progression [37], although Cioffi et al argued that it merely represents undetected damage [38].

6.4. Retinal Nerve Fiber Layer (RNFL)

The retinal nerve fiber layer is made up of the nonmyelinated axons of the retinal ganglion cells. They are more visible in the inferotemporal and superotemporal areas of the fundus and least visible in the horizontal nasal and temporal sectors. The visibility of the RNFL corresponds to the configuration of the neuroretinal rim which is thicker in the superior and inferior poles of the disc [26] giving a double hump configuration in the OCT RNFL analysis (fig 4). Defects in RNFL precede optic disc cupping in the corresponding sectors [39] as well as visual field defects with standard automated perimetry [40]. The most common sectors affected in glaucoma are the inferotemporal followed by the superotemporal [41]. This pattern of RNFL loss leads to the disappearance of the double hump configuration of the RNFL (fig 10,11). Nerve fiber defects are encountered in other optic nerve diseases such as optic disc drusen, toxoplasmic retinochoroidal scars, diabetic retinopathy and optic neuritis secondary to multiple sclerosis [26,42].

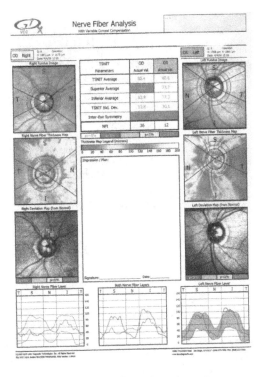

Figure 11. Thinning of the superior sector of the RNFL of the right eye due to glaucoma. Note the probabolity of each soperpixel (each superpixel includes 4 pixels) of the deviation to be normal. The purple pixel represent a 5% probabili-ty that the RNFL thickness in that superpixel is normal, the blue color represents a <2% probability, yellow <1% and

red <0.5%. The TSNIT map of the right eye has lost the double hump appearance, there is high inter-eye asymmetry as the left eye has not been affected by glaucoma and the NFI is high in the right eye.

6.5. Point of exit of the large vessel trunk on the optic disc

Research has shown that the area on the optic disc most susceptible to glaucomatous damage is the area that is the furthest away from the main vessel trunk (fig 12) [43]. The exit of the main vessel trunk is usually displaced superonasally which makes the inferotemporal quadrant more susceptible to the glaucomatous damage. The disc arterioles follow the contour of the neuroretinal rim. As the rim recedes in the glaucomatous process the arterioles tend to become displaced towards the periphery of the optic disc. If the rim becomes extremely thin the vessels may be pushed to the far periphery of the disc just next to the Elsching's ring and then they sharply angle on the retinal surface giving rise to the bayoneting sign (fig 13). The presence of a temporal cilioretinal artery has a protective role against the glaucomatous process [44]

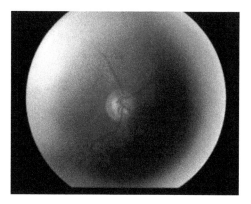

Figure 12. Right optic disc: The main vessel trunk emerges in the superotemporal disc quadrant. The neuroretinal rim is thinnest in inferior and nasal quadrants. The distance of the main vessel trunk to the inferior rim is longer compared to the distance to the superior rim. The glaucomatous damage is greatest in the inferior rim. There is no arteriolar narrowing

6.6. Optic disc haemorrhages (fig 14)

Optic disc haemorrhages are an independent risk factor for glaucoma and ocular hypertensive patients with disc haemorrhages are six times more likely to develop glaucoma than those patients without haemorrhages [45]. The frequency of disc haemorrhages in glaucoma eyes ranged from 9-20% [46,47]. Their frequency is not statistically different in glaucoma eyes with high or normal IOP [46]. Their prevalence in non-glaucomatous eyes ranges from 0.2% - 1.03% [48-51]

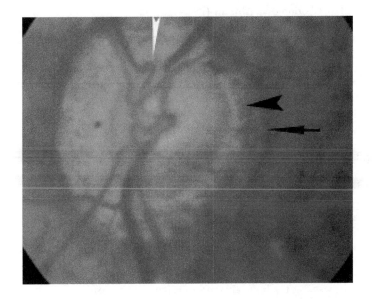

Figure 13. Large PPCA in advanced glaucoma with small alpha zone temporally (arrow) and a large beta zone (arrowhead). Bayoneting of the arterioles (white arrowhead)

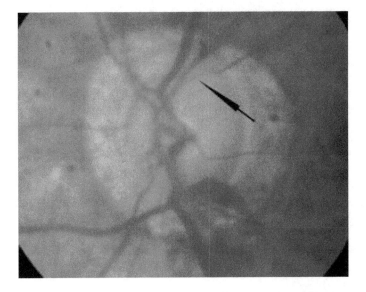

Figure 14. Optic disc haemorrhage in advanced glaucoma. Note the presence of focal arteriolar narrowing (arrow).

6.7. Peripapillary Chorioretinal Atrophy (PPCA, fig 13)

Peripapillary atrophy consists of an outer alpha zone with irregular hyper- hypopigmentation and an inner beta zone with visible large choroidal vessels and sclera. Alpha zone is present in most normal eyes but beta zone is more common in glaucoma eyes and tends to enlarge in eyes with progressing normal tension glaucoma [52]. They both tend to increase in size with advancing glaucoma damage [53]. The frequency of the beta zone varies between 59.5% and 69% in glaucoma patients and 17.4% and 24% in healthy subjects [53,54]. Beta zone is also larger in glaucomatous eyes (1.21 ±1.92 mm^2) compared to healthy ones (0.32 ± 0.99 mm^2) [54]. There is conflicting evidence as to whether the PPCA corresponds to areas of neuroretinal rim thinning. Uchida et al [55] reported that PPCA progression correlated to progressive disc damage and visual field defects. On the other hand See et al [56] showed that neuroretinal area decrease did not correlate with PPCA progression. The extent of PPCA positively correlated with the presence of optic disc haemorrhage in glaucoma eyes [57]. In this study beta zone was larger in the eyes with disc haemorrhage.

6.8. Retinal arterioles diameter

The diameter of retinal arterioles is decreased in both glaucomatous and non-glaucomatous optic nerve damage (fig 14). It merely represents the limited needs of the retina for oxygen rather the cause of the optic nerve damage [26]

7. Glaucomatous versus non-glaucomatous damage

Optic disc cupping is not pathognomonic for the glaucomatous optic neuropathy only [58]. Other diseases such as arteritic ischemic optic neuropathy (AION), optic neuritis, optic disc pit, colobomas, tilted disc, traumatic optic neuropathy, methanol toxicity, compressive lesions of the anterior visual pathways [59], disc drusen, long standing papilledema [26]. However nonglaucomatous disc damage produces optic disc rim pallor while glaucomatous damage produces focal or diffuse obliteration of the neuroretinal rim [60]. Glaucoma damage tends to produce deeper cups than the nonglaucomatous type [61]. In this study open angle glaucoma eyes had larger and deeper cups and smaller neuretinal rims compared to eyes with nonarteritic and arteritic AION. Contrary to glaucoma PPCA does not increase in nonglaucomatous damage [62].

Summary box

There is great variability among healthy subjects and people from different races in the morphology of the optic disc

which makes the diagnosis of glaucoma very complicated. The clinician should take into consideration various aspects

of the anatomy of the optic nerve head and the RNFL before deciding whether a patient has glaucoma or not

---

8. Congenital anomalies of the optic disc

8.1. Tilted disc

The tilted optic disc syndrome is caused by an oblique insertion of the optic nerves in the globe usually inferonasally. Its prevalence is around 0.5% and is commonly bilateral. It is associated with high myopia, astigmatism, visual field defects (usually superotemporal arcuate scoto-mas), small optic disc area, low best corrected visual acuity, peripapillary atrophy and choroidal neovascular membrane [63].

Tilted disc analysis with optical coherence tomography (OCT) showed decreased nerve fiber thickness of the superior, inferior and nasal sectors as well as on average, a thicker temporal sector and a more temporally positioned inferior and superior peak sectors (fig 15) [64]. Multifocal electroretinogram also revealed suboptimal macular function [65]

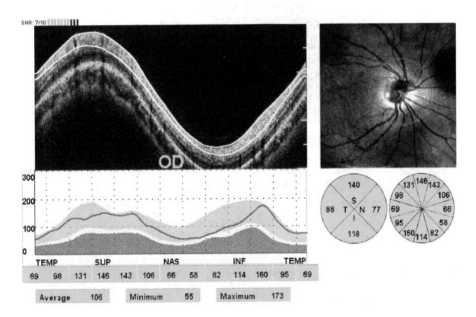

Figure 15. RNFL analysis with OCT in a patient with tilted disc. Slight thinning of the RNFL of the inferonasal sector. This patient has normal visual fields

8.2. Optic disc pit (fig 16)

Optic disc pits can be congenital or acquired. The former are a rare anomaly with a prevalence of 1:11,000 [66] and are associated with serous detachment of the macula which affects the vision and it can be treated with vitrectomy and gas tamponade. The acquired type is seen more often in pathological myopia and open angle glaucoma [67,68]. Their overall prevalence

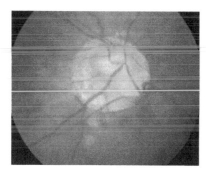

Figure 16. Peripapillary inferiorly located optic disc pit in a patient with primary open angle glaucoma.

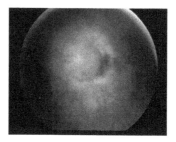

Figure 17. Morning glory syndrome. Visual acuity of this eye is hand movements with the other eye having similar clinical picture. The patient is registered blind.

in Blue Mountain Study is 0.19% [69]. The presence of optic disc pit in eyes with open angle glaucoma is a risk factor for progressive optic nerve head damage, advancing visual field defects and presence of disc haemorrhages. They more commonly seen in normal tension glaucoma than POAG and are associated with visual field defects close to fixation [70]

8.3. Morning glory syndrome (fig 17,18)

Morning glory syndrome is a rare developmental abnormality of the optic nerve. It is usually unilateral and can be complicated by serous retinal detachment and choroidal neovascularization. The OCT analysis of the RNFL shows large optic discs, increased thickness of the RNFL and decreased macular thickness [71]. Morning glory syndrome is associated with systemic diseases such as frontonasal dysplasia, neurofibromatosis 2 and PHACE (Posterior fossa abnormalities and other structural brain abnormalities -

Hemangioma(s) of the cervical facial region - Arterial cerebrovascular anomalies, Cardiac defects, aortic coarctation and other aortic abnormalities - Eye anomalies) syndrome

8.4. Optic disc colobomas

This disc anomaly results from incomplete closure of the embryonic fissure and it is usually unilateral. Possible ophthalmic complications include serous macular detachment, optic disc excavation despite normal IOP and choroidal neovascularization. It is also associated with multiple syndromes such as Patau, Edwards and cat eye syndromes and **CHARGE** (Coloboma of the eye - **H**eart defects - **A**tresia of the choanae - **R**etardation of growth and/or development - **G**enital and/or urinary abnormalitie - **E**ar abnormalities and deafness) syndrome. In uncomplicated cases (without serous macular detachment) OCT analysis of the RNFL shows normal fiber layer thickness [72]

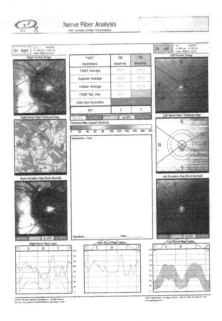

Figure 18. GDx VCC of the patient in fig 17. Note that the calculation ring is smaller than the optic nerve head and a meaningful analysis of the RNFL in this patient is not possible. The quality of the scan is poor due to nystagmus

8.5. Optic disc drusen

Optic disc drusen are hyaline bodies in the optic disc substance. Their prevalence is 3.4 – 24 per 1,000 and areusually bilateral [73]. They are usually located most commonly nasally and are difficult to visualize in childhood as they are buried but become more obvious in adolescence. Ophthalmic complications include choroidal and disc neovascularization and visual field defects. Disc drusen when buried can pose a diagnostic dilemma with papilledema. Disc drusen can be detected by fundus autofluorescence, B scan ultrasonography, computed tomography and recently OCT. Optical coherence tomography scans through the optic nerve head can directly show the drusen. Lee et al [74] reported that the RNFL thickness with spectral domain OCT was increased in all sectors in patients with papilledema as opposed to optic disc drusen in which the RNFL was thicker in the temporal quadrants compared to normal subjects. This can be explained by either a mechanical displacement of the retinal fibers by the drusen which usually lie in the nasal sector towards the temporal sectors or by the compression and subsequent atrophy of the nasal retinal fibers. In longstanding papilledema the retinal fibers are damaged and the average RNFL thickness is reduced. Disc drusen appear hyporeflective on OCT scans [75].

8.6. Optic nerve hypoplasia

Optic nerve hypoplasia is a congenital disorder that can be uni- or bilateral, segmental or total and the visual acuity can be normal or reduced to no light perception. It can be associated with many syndromes with the most common being de Morsier syndrome.

Two studies [76,77] found that in patients with superior segmental optic hypoplasia is associated with generalized reduction of the RNFL thickness involving all the sectors and not only the superior one.

9. Acquired optic disc disorders

9.1. Papilledema

Papilledema is the bilateral disc swelling secondary to increased intracranial pressure. Although bilateral it may be asymmetrical. It can be caused by space occupying lesions in the cavity of the skull, idiopathic intracranial hypertension, obstruction of the ventricles, impaired cerebrospinal fluid adsorption by the arachnoid villi, severe systemic hypertension, cerebral venous thrombosis, diffuse cerebral oedema following trauma.

Differential diagnosis includes: malignant hypertension, bilateral optic neuritis with optic nerve head involvement (papillitis), bilateral anterior ischemic optic neuropathy, diabetic papillopathy, Leber's hereditary optic neuropathy, pseudopapilledema (optic disc drusen, hypermetropia), and toxic optic neuropathy.

Optical coherence tomography is helpful in diagnosing early papilledema. Vartin et al [78] found that the peripapillary total retinal thickness rather than the conventionally calculated RNFL thickness as measured with spectral domain OCT differentiated early papilledema from normal subjects. Peripapillary total retinal thickness as a diagnostic tool for subtle papilledema was also reported by Skau et al [79]. OCT is useful in the follow up of patients with papilledema. Rebolleda et al [80] followed up patients with papilledema for 12 months following presentation and found that RNFL thickness decreased with time and visual field defects improved. Kupersmith et al [81] investigated different causes of optic disc swelling [papilledema, non-arteritic anterior ischemic optic neuropathy (NA-AION) and optic neuritis] with OCT and scanning laser polarimetry (SLP). Retinal nerve fiber thickness by OCT was increased in papilledema and NA-AION compared to eyes suffering from optic neuritis. This is due to greater disc edema in eyes with papilledema and NA-AION. SLP showed increased RNFL thickness in papilledema and optic neuritis. The authors concluded that OCT reveals increased retinal thickness due to axonal swelling but SLP shows the true damage of the axons.

Two studies investigated the morphology of the retinal pigment epithelium/Bruch's membrane (RPE/BM) complex and concluded that papilledema causes an inward (towards the vitreous cavity) bowing of the PRE/BM complex as opposed to patients with AION and optic neuritis [82,83]. The authors speculate that the increased pressure in the cerebrospinal fluid (CSF) caused the forward bowing of the RPE/BM complex. In the other types of disc swelling (AION, optic neuritis) pathophysiologically there is no high pressure of the CSF.

9.2. Optic Neuritis (ON) (fig 19)

Optic neuritis is the inflammatory process of the optic nerve. Anatomically it can affect the optic nerve head (papillitis), only the posterior part of the nerve (retrobulbar neuritis) or both.

Differential diagnosis includes: anterior ischemic optic neuropathy, compressive lesions of the optic nerve, Leber's hereditary optic neuropathy, central retinal vein occlusion, infiltration of the optic nerve head (sarcoidosis, tuberculosis, syphilis, leukemia)

Optical coherence tomography has been used in the diagnosis and follow up of patients with isolated optic neuritis or optic neuritis in clinically diagnosed multiple sclerosis (MS). It was found that as expected the patients with previous history of ON had thinner RNFL than normal subjects [84,85]. OCT can also demonstrate structural damage more accurately than standard automated perimetry. Noval et al reported that OCT can detect subtle RNFL changes in the presence of normal visual fields [86]. Interestingly Pro et al described RNFL thickening in the acute phase of ON even in patients without disc swelling [87]. OCT has been used in the follow up of patients with ON over time. Costello et al reported that the RNFL loss is more profound between the third and sixth month after the episode of ON [88]. The earliest damage in the RNFL is evident 2 months after clinical presentation and the RNFL damage halts 7 months after the episode of ON [89,90]. In patients suffering from multiple sclerosis, eyes unaffected by ON demonstrate lower RNFL thickness compared to normal subjects [91-95]. OCT findings have also been linked to visual function. Average RNFL thickness of less than 75μm predicted persistent visual dysfunction (90) and for every 1 line of reduced contrast sensitivity the RNFL thickness decreased by 4μm (91).

Secondary progressive MS was associated with greater RNFL decrease in both affected and unaffected by ON eyes (90, 92). Decreased RNFL thickness was also inversely associated with disease severity (the lower the RNFL thickness the more serious the disease) (95-97). Retinal nerve fiber thickness on OCT could not predict the risk of MS (96). In one study comparing the structural damage after optic neuritis it was found that only the modalities that measure RNFL thickness (OCT, GDx) were affected compared to disease free participants but the analysis of the optic disc with the HRT 3 was not statistically different compared to normal control group (99).

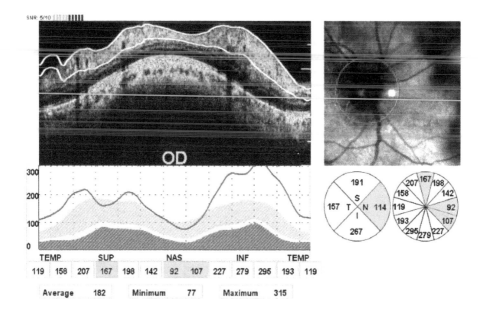

Figure 19. Swollen RNFL in a patient with papillitis secondary to multiple sclerosis.

9.3. Ischaemic optic neuropathy

Anatomically is classified as anterior and posterior and aetiologically as non-arteritic and arteritic. Predisposing factors for the non-arteritic anterior ischaemic optic neuropathy (NA-AION) is hypertension, diabetes mellitus, hyperlipidemia, sleep apnea, cataract surgery, erectile dysfunction, small crowded optic disc and long standing papilledema, while arteritic anterior ischaemic optic neuropathy (A-AION) is caused by giant cell arteritis. Posterior ischaemic optic neuropathy involves the retrolaminar part of the optic nerve. It can follow a heart or spine operation or be caused by giant cell arteritis or present as the posterior equivalent of non-arteritic AION. Differential diagnosis is as in optic neuritis.

Optical coherence tomography in the acute stages of AION shows diffuse thickening of the RNFL which turns into thinning as the disease becomes chronic (100,101) (fig. 20,21,22). Contreras et al (102) found that the superior RNFL quadrant was more affected and that for every 1μm of nerve fiber thickness loss there was 1 dB decrease of mean deviation in standard automated perimetry. OCT analysis of the RNFL showed RNFL thinning compared to healthy controls and the area of retinal axon loss correlated well with visual field defects (102-105). Macular thickness also correlated with visual field loss in eyes with NA-AION (106).

Research has shown that that AION and glaucoma affect the optic nerve differently. RNFL thickness in glaucoma and NA-AION eyes is not statistically different but it is markedly thinner compared to normal eyes (61,107). However when adjusting for mean deviation (MD) of visual fields RNFL was thicker in eyes with A-AION and NA-AION compared to open angle

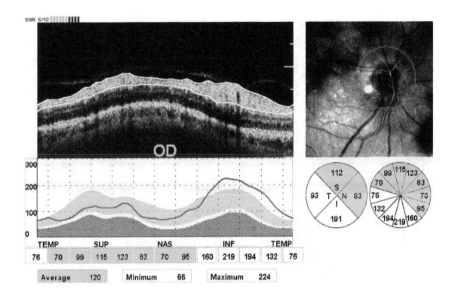

Figure 20. RNFL swelling in a patient with NA-AION 4 weeks following presentation.

glaucoma eyes. For the same level of MD, open angle glaucoma eyes had larger cup area, smaller rim area, larger cup/disc ratio, larger cup volume, smaller rim volume, and greater cup depth. When comparing the two types of AION, the non-arteritic type had smaller cup area, a larger rim area, and a smaller cup/disc ratio (61). In order to explain the discrepancy in the morphology of the optic nerve damage between both types of AION and glaucoma the authors suggest that glaucoma affects laminar connective tissue more than the prelaminar structures (as opposed to AION) and this causes the development of larger and deeper cups in glaucoma. The loss of laminar connective tissue leads in turn to retrodisplacement and thinning of the lamina cribrosa which causes the larger cup size in glaucoma. Both glaucoma and AION cause retinal gagglion cell loss but AION does not affect the laminar tissues.

9.4. Leber's Hereditary Optic Neuropathy (LHON)

LHON is a rare mitochondrial disorder that affects males and is associated with mutations of the maternal mitochondrial DNA. It presents with acute loss of vision between the ages 10 – 60 but most often in the age range 15-35. Early signs are optic disc hyperaemia and nerve fiber swelling. In the later stages optic atrophy dominates the clinical picture. Differential diagnosis is as in papilledema.

OCT demonstrated statistically significant increase of the RNFL thickness (mean, superior, inferior, nasal) in the early stage of the disease (6-8 weeks after initial presentation). Nine months after onset there is a decrease in RNFL thickness in all but nasal quadrants (108,109).

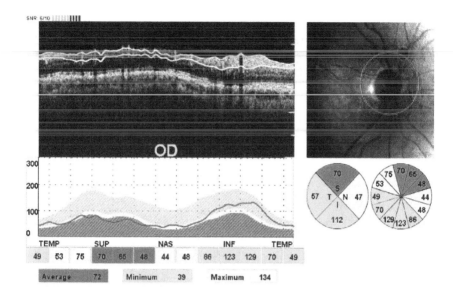

Figure 21. Same patient as in fig 20 3 months after initial presentation of NA-AION. Swelling of the RHFL has subsided and atrophy has begun to set in.

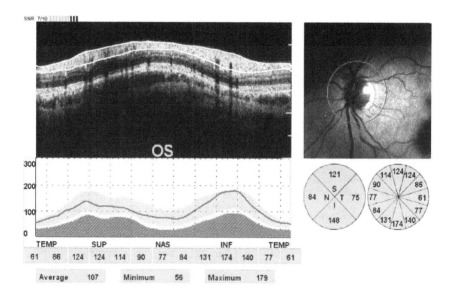

Figure 22. Fellow eye of the same patient as in fig 10 showing a crowded disc.

Unaffected male carriers had higher RNFL thickness in the temporal and inferior quadrants which was more pronounced in those with the 11778 mutation. Unaffected female carriers had a RNFL thickness increase in the temporal quadrant more pronounced in those with the 11778 mutation (110). Patients with the 11778 mutation tend to have increased RNFL thickness in the early stages of the disease and decreased thickness in the later stages compared to those with the 14484 mutation (111).

9.5. Optic atrophy

Optic atrophy is classified aetiologically as:

Primary (not associated with previous optic disc swelling. Most common causes are compressive lesions of the optic pathways up to the lateral geniculate bodies, hereditary disorders and multiple sclerosis).

Secondary (following longstanding swelling of the optic nerve head (papilledema, AION, papillitis)

Consecutive (following retinal diseases with widespread destruction of the retina such as retinitis pigmentosa, central retinal artery occlusion, vasculitis)

The new devices for the analysis of RNFL have been employed for the differential diagnosis of those types of optic atrophy in which the features of glaucomatous versus non-glaucomatous optic nerve damage are not clear. Autosomal dominant optic atrophy (ADOA, Kjer's optic neuropathy) is a rare hereditary disorder [it affects 1:35,000 people in the general population (112)] that can be misdiagnosed for normal tension glaucoma (113) and in this cases OCT provide useful information in order to reach the correct diagnosis. Several reports have shown that eyes with ADOA have reduced mean RNFL thickness and the quadrant most commonly affected being the temporal one (114-117). In contrast the glaucomatous process typically affects the inferior and superior sectors (118). There is also a reduction in macular thickness in patients with ADOA (119). Barboni et al (120) reported that the optic nerve heads in patients with ADOA have smaller size compared to normal controls.

Chiasmal compressive lesions produce a characteristic bitemporal hemianopia which is due to the preservation of the uncrossed fibers that originate from the temporal retina and enter the optic disc with the superior and inferior arcuate bands. The main damage therefore occurs in the nasal and temporal sectors of the disc and causes a characteristic ophthalmoscopic appearance named band atrophy. OCT has shown that not only the nasal and temporal sectors of the RNFL are affected but also the superior and inferior ones (121-123). OCT analysis of the optic nerve head could depict better than the Heidelberg Retina Tomograph the rim loss and subsequently the increased cup area in eyes with band atrophy (124).

Summary box

The new imaging modalities of the optic nerve head and RNFL thickness can describe with high accuracy the morphology of the above structures. However none of them has 100% accuracy in the diagnosis of glaucoma. RNFL thickness analysis seems to perform better than optic disc analysis. Clinical examination is of utmost importance before reaching the diagnosis of glaucomatous optic neuropathy

Acknowledgements

The authors have no proprietary interest in any of the products mentioned in the manuscript

Author details

Vassilis Kozobolis, Aristeidis Konstantinidis* and Georgios Labiris

*Address all correspondence to: aristeidiskon@hotmail.com

Eye Department, University Hospital of Alexandroupolis, Alexandroupolis, Greece

References

[1] Piette, S. D, & Sergott, R. C. Pathological optic-disc cupping.Curr Opin Ophthalmol. (2006). Feb;, 17(1), 1-6.

[2] Airaksinen, P. J, Drance, S. M, Douglas, G. R, Mawson, D. K, & Nieminen, H. Diffuse and localized nerve fiber loss in glaucoma. Am J Ophthalmol. (1984). Nov;, 98(5), 566-71.

[3] Airaksinen, P. J, & Nieminen, H. Retinal nerve fiber layer photography in glaucoma. Ophthalmolog (1985). , 92, 877-879.

[4] Badalà, F, Nouri-mahdavi, K, Raoof, D. A, Leeprechanon, N, Law, S. K, & Caprioli, J. Optic disk and nerve fiber layer imaging to detect glaucoma. Am J Ophthalmol. (2007). Nov;, 144(5), 724-32.

[5] Zangwill, L. M, Williams, J, Berry, C. C, Knauer, S, & Weinreb, R. N. A comparison of optical coherence tomography and retinal nerve fiber layer photography for detection of nerve fiber layer damage in glaucoma. Ophthalmology. (2000). Jul;, 107(7), 1309-15.

[6] Deleón-ortega, J. E, & Arthur, S. N. McGwin G Jr, Xie A, Monheit BE, Girkin CA. Discrimination between glaucomatous and nonglaucomatous eyes using quantitative imaging devices and subjective optic nerve head assessment. Invest Ophthalmol Vis Sci. (2006). Aug;, 47(8), 3374-80.

[7] Greaney, M. J, Hoffman, D. C, Garway-heath, D. F, Nakla, M, Coleman, A. L, & Caprioli, J. Comparison of optic nerve imaging methods to distinguish normal eyes from those with glaucoma. Invest Ophthalmol Vis Sci. (2002). Jan;, 43(1), 140-5.

[8] Gianmarco VizzeriSara M Kjaergaard, Harsha L Rao, Linda M Zangwill. Role of imaging in glaucoma diagnosis and follow-up. Indian J Ophthalmol. (2011). January; 59(Suppl1): SS68., 59.

[9] Bowd, C, Weinreb, R. N, Lee, B, Emdadi, A, & Zangwill, L. M. Optic disk topography after medical treatment to reduce intraocular pressure. Am J Ophthalmol. (2000). Sep;, 130(3), 280-6.

[10] Townsend, K. A, Wollstein, G, & Schuman, J. S. Imaging of the retinal nerve fibre layer for glaucoma. Br J Ophthalmol. (2009). Feb;, 93(2), 139-43.

[11] Yanagisawa, M, Tomidokoro, A, Saito, H, Mayama, C, Aihara, M, Tomita, G, Shoji, N, & Araie, M. Atypical retardation pattern in measurements of scanning laser polarimetry and its relating factors. Eye (Lond). (2009). Sep;, 23(9), 1796-801.

[12] Da Pozzo SMarchesan R, Canziani T, Vattovani O, Ravalico G. Atypical pattern of retardation on GDx-VCC and its effect on retinal nerve fibre layer evaluation in glaucomatous eyes. Eye (Lond). (2006). Jul;, 20(7), 769-75.

[13] Mesiwala, N. K, Pekmezci, M, Huang, J. Y, Porco, T. C, & Lin, S. C. Comparison of Optic Disc Parameters Measured by RTVue-100 FDOCT Versus HRT-II. J Glaucoma. (2011). Jun 22.

[14] Leite, M. T, Rao, H. L, Zangwill, L. M, Weinreb, R. N, & Medeiros, F. A. Comparison of the diagnostic accuracies of the Spectralis, Cirrus, and RTVue optical coherence tomography devices in glaucoma. Ophthalmology.(2011). Jul;, 118(7), 1334-9.

[15] Leung, C. K, Chiu, V, Weinreb, R. N, Liu, S, Ye, C, Yu, M, Cheung, C. Y, Lai, G, & Lam, D. S. Evaluation of retinal nerve fiber layer progression in glaucoma: a comparison between spectral-domain and time-domain optical coherence tomography. Ophthalmology.(2011). Aug;, 118(8), 1558-62.

[16] Leung, C. K, Cheung, C. Y, Weinreb, R. N, Qiu, Q, Liu, S, Li, H, Xu, G, Fan, N, Huang, L, Pang, C. P, & Lam, D. S. Retinal nerve fiber layer imaging with spectral-domain optical coherence tomography: a variability and diagnostic performance study. Ophthalmology. (2009). Jul;e1-2., 116(7), 1257-63.

[17] Lee, S, Sung, K. R, Cho, J. W, Cheon, M. H, Kang, S. Y, & Kook, M. S. Spectral-domain optical coherence tomography and scanning laser polarimetry in glaucoma diagnosis. Jpn J Ophthalmol. (2010). Nov;, 54(6), 544-9.

[18] Garudadri, C. S, Rao, H. L, Parikh, R. S, Jonnadula, G. B, Selvaraj, P, Nutheti, R, & Thomas, R. Effect of optic disc size and disease severity on the diagnostic capability of glaucomaimaging technologies in an Indian population. J Glaucoma. (2012). Sep;, 21(7), 475-80.

[19] Oddone, F, Centofanti, M, Tanga, L, Parravano, M, Michelessi, M, Schiavone, M, Villani, C. M, Fogagnolo, P, & Manni, G. Influence of disc size on optic nerve head versus retinal nerve fiber layer assessment for diagnosing glaucoma. Ophthalmology. (2011). Jul;, 118(7), 1340-7.

[20] Medeiros, F. A, Zangwill, L. M, Bowd, C, Sample, P. A, & Weinreb, R. N. Influence of disease severity and optic disc size on the diagnostic performance of imaging instruments in glaucoma. Invest Ophthalmol Vis Sci. (2006). Mar;, 47(3), 1008-15.

[21] Leite, M. T, Zangwill, L. M, Weinreb, R. N, Rao, H. L, Alencar, L. M, Sample, P. A, & Medeiros, F. A. Effect of disease severity on the performance of Cirrus spectral-domain OCT for glaucoma diagnosis. Invest Ophthalmol Vis Sci. (2010). Aug;, 51(8), 4104-9.

[22] Kanamori, A, Nagai-kusuhara, A, Escaño, M. F, Maeda, H, Nakamura, M, & Negi, A. Comparison of confocal scanning laser ophthalmoscopy, scanning laser polarimetry and optical coherence tomography to discriminate ocular hypertension and glaucoma at an early stage. Graefes Arch Clin Exp Ophthalmol. (2006). Jan;, 244(1), 58-68.

[23] Leung, C. K, Ye, C, Weinreb, R. N, Cheung, C. Y, Qiu, Q, Liu, S, Xu, G, & Lam, D. S. Retinal nerve fiber layer imaging with spectral-domain optical coherence tomography a study on diagnostic agreement with Heidelberg Retinal Tomograph. Ophthalmology. (2010). Feb;, 117(2), 267-74.

[24] Medeiros, F. A, Vizzeri, G, Zangwill, L. M, Alencar, L. M, Sample, P. A, & Weinreb, R. N. Comparison of retinalnervefiberlayer and optic disc imaging for diagnosing glaucoma in patients suspected of having the disease. Ophthalmology. (2008). Aug;, 115(8), 1340-6.

[25] Alencar, L. M, Zangwill, L. M, Weinreb, R. N, Bowd, C, Sample, P. A, Girkin, C. A, Liebmann, J. M, & Medeiros, F. A. A comparison of rates of change in neuroretinal rim area and retinalnerve fiber layer thickness in progressive glaucoma. Invest Ophthalmol Vis Sci. (2010). Jul;, 51(7), 3531-9.

[26] Jonas, J. B, Budde, W. M, & Panda-jonas, S. Ophthalmoscopic evaluation of the optic nerve head. Surv Ophthalmol (1999).

[27] Oliveira, C, Harizman, N, Girkin, C. A, Xie, A, Tello, C, Liebmann, J. M, & Ritch, R. Axial length and optic disc size in normal eyes.Br J Ophthalmol. (2007). Jan;, 91(1), 37-9.

[28] Samarawickrama, C, Hong, T, Jonas, J. B, & Mitchell, P. Measurement of normal optic nerve headparameters.Surv Ophthalmol. (2012). Jul-Aug;, 57(4), 317-36.

[29] Jonas, J. B. Optic disk size correlated with refractive error. Am J Ophthalmol. (2005). Feb;, 139(2), 346-8.

[30] Jonas, J. B, Gusek, G. C, Guggenmoos-holzmann, I, & Naumann, G. O. Variability of the real dimensions of normal human optic discs.Graefes Arch Clin Exp Ophthalmol. (1988). , 226(4), 332-6.

[31] Jonas, J. B, Gusek, G. C, & Naumann, G. O. Optic disc, cup and neuroretinal rim size, configuration and correlations in normal eyes.Invest Ophthalmol Vis Sci. (1988). Jul;, 29(7), 1151-8.

[32] Crowston, J G, Hopley, C R, Healey, P R, Lee, A, & Mitchell, P. The effect of optic disc diameter on vertical cup to disc ratio percentiles in a population based cohort: the Blue Mountains Eye Study Br J Ophthalmol. (2004). June;, 88(6), 766-770.

[33] You, Q. S, Xu, L, & Jonas, J. B. Tilted optic discs: The Beijing Eye Study.Eye (Lond). (2008). May;, 22(5), 728-9.

[34] Jonas, J. B, Schmidt, A. M, Müller-bergh, J. A, Schlötzer-schrehardt, U. M, & Naumann, G. O. Human optic nerve fiber count and optic disc size.Invest Ophthalmol Vis Sci. (1992). May;, 33(6), 2012-8.

[35] Tuulonen, A, & Airaksinen, P. J. Optic disc size in exfoliative, primary open angle, and low-tension glaucoma. Arch Ophthalmol. (1992). Feb;, 110(2), 211-3.

[36] Jonas, J. B, & Papastathopoulos, K. I. Optic disk appearance in pseudoexfoliation syndrome. Am J Ophthalmol. (1997). Feb;, 123(2), 174-80.

[37] Schulzer, M, Drance, S. M, & Douglas, G. R. A comparison of treated and untreated-glaucomasuspects. Ophthalmology. (1991). Mar;, 98(3), 301-7.

[38] Cioffi, G. A, & Liebmann, J. M. Translating the OHTSresults into clinical practice.J Glaucoma. (2002). Oct;, 11(5), 375-7.

[39] Airaksinen, P. J, & Alanko, H. I. Effect of retinalnervefibreloss on the opticnervehead-configuration in earlyglaucoma. Graefes Arch Clin Exp Ophthalmol. (1983). , 220(4), 193-6.

[40] Quigley, H. A, Addicks, E. M, & Green, W. R. Optic nerve damage in human glaucoma. III. Quantitative correlation of nerve fiber loss and visual field defect in glaucoma, ischemic neuropathy, papilledema, and toxic neuropathy.Arch Ophthalmol. (1982). Jan;, 100(1), 135-46.

[41] Leung, C. K, Choi, N, Weinreb, R. N, Liu, S, Ye, C, Liu, L, Lai, G. W, Lau, J, & Lam, D. S. Retinal nerve fiber layer imaging with spectral-domain optical coherence tomography: pattern of RNFL defects in glaucoma. Ophthalmology. (2010). Dec;, 117(12), 2337-44.

[42] Takahashi, H, Goto, T, Shoji, T, Tanito, M, Park, M, & Chihara, E. Diabetes-associated retinal nerve fiber damage evaluated with scanning laser polarimetry. Am J Ophthalmol. (2006). Jul;, 142(1), 88-94.

[43] Jonas, J. B, Budde, W. M, Németh, J, Gründler, A. E, Mistlberger, A, & Hayler, J. K. Centralretinal vessel trunkexit and location of glaucomatous parapapillary atrophy in glaucoma. Ophthalmology. (2001). Jun;, 108(6), 1059-64.

[44] Jonas, J. B, & Fernadez, M. C. Shape of the neuroretinal rim and position of the central retinal vessels in glaucoma. Br L Ophthalmol. (1994). , 99-102.

[45] Uhler, T. A, & Piltz-seymour, J. Optic disc hemorrhages in glaucoma and ocular hypertension: implications and recommendations.Curr Opin Ophthalmol. (2008). Mar;, 19(2), 89-94.

[46] Wang, Y, Xu, L, Hu, L, Wang, Y, Yang, H, & Jonas, J. B. Frequency of optic diskhemor-rhages in adult chinese in rural and urban china: the Beijing eye study. Am J Ophthal-mol. (2006). Aug;, 142(2), 241-6.

[47] Sonnsjö, B, Dokmo, Y, & Krakau, T. Disc haemorrhages, precursors of open angle glaucoma.Prog Retin Eye Res. (2002). Jan;, 21(1), 35-56.

[48] Yamamoto, T, Iwase, A, Kawase, K, Sawada, A, & Ishida, K. Optic disc hemorrhages detected in a large-scale eye disease screening project. J Glaucoma. (2004). Oct;, 13(5), 356-60.

[49] Healey, P. R, Mitchell, P, Smith, W, & Wang, J. J. Optic disc hemorrhages in a population with and without signs of glaucoma. Ophthalmology. (1998). Feb;, 105(2), 216-23.

[50] Wang, Y, Xu, L, Hu, L, Wang, Y, Yang, H, & Jonas, J. B. Frequency of optic disk hemorrhages in adult chinese in rural and urban china: the Beijing eye study. Am J Ophthalmol. (2006). Aug;, 142(2), 241-6.

[51] Tomidokoro, A, Iwase, A, Araie, M, Yamamoto, T, & Kitazawa, Y. Population-based prevalence of optic disc haemorrhages in elderly Japanese. Eye (Lond). (2009). May;, 23(5), 1032-7.

[52] Park, K. H, Tomita, G, Liou, S. Y, & Kitazawa, Y. Correlation between peripapillara-trophy and optic nerve damage in normal-tension glaucoma.Ophthalmology. (1996). Nov;, 103(11), 1899-906.

[53] Uhm, K. B, Lee, D. Y, Kim, J. T, & Hong, C. Peripapillaryatrophy in normal and primary open-angle glaucoma. Korean J Ophthalmol. (1998). Jun;, 12(1), 37-50.

[54] Xu, L, Wang, Y, Yang, H, & Jonas, J. B. Differences in parapapillary atrophy between glaucomatous and normal eyes: the Beijing Eye Study. Am J Ophthalmol. (2007). Oct;, 144(4), 541-6.

[55] Uchida, H, Ugurlu, S, & Caprioli, J. Increasing peripapillary atrophy is associated with progressive glaucoma.Ophthalmology. (1998). Aug;, 105(8), 1541-5.

[56] See, J. L, Nicolela, M. T, & Chauhan, B. C. Rates of neuroretinal rim and peripapillar-yatrophy area change: a comparative study of glaucoma patients and normal controls. Ophthalmology. (2009). May;, 116(5), 840-7.

[57] Ahn, J. K, Kang, J. H, & Park, K. H. Correlation between a disc hemorrhage and peripapillaryatrophy in glaucoma patients with a unilateral disc hemorrhage. J Glaucoma. (2004). Feb;, 13(1), 9-14.

[58] Roodhooft, J. M. Nonglaucomatous optic disk atrophy and excavation in the elder-ly.Bull Soc Belge Ophtalmol. (2003).

[59] Fournier, A. V, Damji, K. F, Epstein, D. L, & Pollock, S. C. Discexcavation in dominant optic atrophy: differentiation from normal tension glaucoma.Ophthalmology. (2001). Sep;, 108(9), 1595-602.

[60] Trobe, J. D, Glaser, J. S, Cassady, J, Herschler, J, & Anderson, D. R. Nonglaucomatous excavation of the optic disc. Arch Ophthalmol. (1980). Jun;, 98(6), 1046-50.

[61] Danesh-meyer, H. V, Boland, M. V, Savino, P. J, Miller, N. R, Subramanian, P. S, Girkin, C. A, & Quigley, H. A. Optic disc morphology in open-angle glaucoma compared with anterior ischemic optic neuropathies. Invest Ophthalmol Vis Sci. (2010). Apr;, 51(4), 2003-10.

[62] Jonas, J. B. Clinical implications of peripapillary atrophy in glaucoma. Curr Opin Ophthalmol. (2005). Apr;, 16(2), 84-8.

[63] You, Q. S, Xu, L, & Jonas, J. B. Tilted optic discs: The Beijing Eye Study.Eye (Lond). (2008). May;, 22(5), 728-9.

[64] Hwang, Y. H, Yoo, C, & Kim, Y. Y. Myopic optic disc tilt and the characteristics of peripapillary retinal nerve fiber layer thickness measured by spectral-domain optical coherence tomography. J Glaucoma. (2012). Apr-May;, 21(4), 260-5.

[65] Moschos, M. M, Triglianos, A, Rotsos, T, Papadimitriou, S, Margetis, I, Minogiannis, P, & Moschos, M. Tilted disc syndrome: an OCT and mfERG study. Doc Ophthalmol. (2009). Aug;, 119(1), 23-8.

[66] Gass, J. D. Serous detachment of the macula secondary to congenital pit of the optic nerve head. Am J Ophthalmol (1969). , 67, 821-841.

[67] Nduaguba, C, Ugurlu, S, & Caprioli, J. Acquiredpits of the optic nerve in glaucoma: prevalence and associated visual field loss. Acta Ophthalmol Scand. (1998). Jun;, 76(3), 273-7.

[68] Ohno-matsui, K, Akiba, M, Moriyama, M, Shimada, N, Ishibashi, T, Tokoro, T, & Spaide, R. F. Acquiredopticnerve and peripapillarypits in pathologicmyopia. Ophthalmology. (2012). Aug;, 119(8), 1685-92.

[69] Healey, P. R, & Mitchell, P. The prevalence of opticdiscpits and their relationship to glaucoma. J Glaucoma. (2008). Jan-Feb;, 17(1), 11-4.

[70] Ugurlu, S, Weitzman, M, Nduaguba, C, & Caprioli, J. Acquired pit of the optic nerve: a risk factor for progression of glaucoma. Am J Ophthalmol. (1998). Apr;, 125(4), 457-64.

[71] Srinivasan, G, Venkatesh, P, & Garg, S. Optical coherence tomographic characteristics in morning glory disc anomaly. Can J Ophthalmol. (2007). Apr;, 42(2), 307-9.

[72] Islam, N, Best, J, Mehta, J. S, Sivakumar, S, Plant, G. T, & Hoyt, W. F. Optic disc duplication or coloboma? Br J Ophthalmol. (2005). Jan;, 89(1), 26-9.

[73] Auw-haedrich, C, Staubach, F, & Witchel, H. Optic disk drusen. Surv Ophthalmol (2001). , 47, 515-532.

[74] Lee, K. M, Woo, S. J, & Hwang, J. M. Differentiation of optic nerve head drusen and optic disc edema with spectral-domain optical coherence tomography.Ophthalmology. (2011). May;, 118(5), 971-7.

[75] Wester, S. T, Fantes, F. E, Lam, B. L, Anderson, D. R, Mcsoley, J. J, & Knighton, R. W. Characteristics of optic nerve head drusen on optical coherence tomography images. Ophthalmic Surg Lasers Imaging. (2010). Jan-Feb;, 41(1), 83-90.

[76] Hayashi, K, Tomidokoro, A, Konno, S, Mayama, C, Aihara, M, & Araie, M. Evaluation of optic nerve head configurations of superior segmental optic hypoplasia by spectral-domain optical coherence tomography. Br J Ophthalmol. (2010). Jun;, 94(6), 768-72.

[77] Lee, H. J, & Kee, C. Optical coherence tomography and Heidelberg retina tomography for superior segmental optic hypoplasia. Br J Ophthalmol. (2009). Nov;, 93(11), 1468-73.

[78] Vartin, C V, Nguyen, A. M, Balmitgere, T, Bernard, M, Tilikete, C, & Vighetto, A. Detection of mild papilloedema using spectral domain optical coherence tomography.Br J Ophthalmol. (2012). Mar;, 96(3), 375-9.

[79] Skau, M, Milea, D, Sander, B, Wegener, M, & Jensen, R. OCT for optic disc evaluation in idiopathic intracranial hypertension. Graefes Arch Clin Exp Ophthalmol. (2011). May;, 249(5), 723-30.

[80] Rebolleda, G, & Muñoz-negrete, F. J. Follow-up of mild papilledema in idiopathic intracranial hypertension with optical coherence tomography. Invest Ophthalmol Vis Sci. (2009). Nov;, 50(11), 5197-200.

[81] Kupersmith, M. J, Kardon, R, Durbin, M, Horne, M, & Shulman, J. Scanning laser polarimetry reveals status of RNFL integrity in eyes with optic nerve head swelling by OCT. Invest Ophthalmol Vis Sci. (2012). Apr 18;, 53(4), 1962-70.

[82] Kupersmith, M. J, Sibony, P, Mandel, G, Durbin, M, & Kardon, R. H. Optical coherence tomography of the swollen optic nerve head: deformation of the peripapillary retinal pigment epithelium layer in papilledema. Invest Ophthalmol Vis Sci.(2011). Aug 22;, 52(9), 6558-64.

[83] Sibony, P, Kupersmith, M. J, & Rohlf, F. J. Shape analysis of the peripapillary RPE layer in papilledema and ischemic optic neuropathy. Invest Ophthalmol Vis Sci.(2011). Oct 10;, 52(11), 7987-95.

[84] Parisi, V, Manni, G, Spadaro, M, Colacino, G, Restuccia, R, Marchi, S, Bucci, M. G, & Pierelli, F. Correlation between morphological and functional retinal impairment in multiple sclerosis patients. Invest Ophthalmol Vis Sci. (1999). Oct; , 40(11), 2520-7.

[85] Trip, S. A, Schlottmann, P. G, Jones, S. J, Altmann, D. R, Garway-heath, D. F, Thompson, A. J, Plant, G. T, & Miller, D. H. Retinal nerve fiber layer axonal loss and visual dysfunction in optic neuritis. Ann Neurol. (2005). Sep; , 58(3), 383-91.

[86] Noval, S, Contreras, I, Rebolleda, G, & Muñoz-negrete, F. J. Optical coherence tomography versus automated perimetry for follow-up of optic neuritis. Acta Ophthalmol Scand. (2006). Dec; , 84(6), 790-4.

[87]   Pro, M. J, Pons, M. E, Liebmann, J. M, Ritch, R, Zafar, S, Lefton, D, & Kupersmith, M.
       J. Imaging of the optic disc and retinal nerve fiber layer in acute optic neuritis. J Neurol
       Sci. (2006). Dec 1; 250(1-2):114-9.

[88]   Costello, F, Coupland, S, Hodge, W, Lorello, G. R, Koroluk, J, Pan, Y. I, Freedman, M.
       S, Zackon, D. H, & Kardon, R. H. Quantifying axonal loss after optic neuritis with
       optical coherence tomography. Ann Neurol. (2006). Jun; , 59(6), 963-9.

[89]   Costello, F, Hodge, W, Pan, Y. I, Eggenberger, E, Coupland, S, & Kardon, R. H. Tracking
       retinal nerve fiber layer loss after optic neuritis: a prospective study using optical
       coherence tomography. Mult Scler. (2008). Aug; , 14(7), 893-905.

[90]   Costello, F, Hodge, W, Pan, Y. I, Freedman, M, & Demeulemeester, C. Differences in
       retinal nerve fiber layer atrophy between multiple sclerosis subtypes. J Neurol Sci.
       (2009). Jun 15; 281(1-2):74-9.

[91]   Fisher, J. B, Jacobs, D. A, Markowitz, C. E, Galetta, S. L, Volpe, N. J, Nano-schiavi, M.
       L, Baier, M. L, Frohman, E. M, Winslow, H, Frohman, T. C, Calabresi, P. A, Maguire,
       M. G, Cutter, G. R, & Balcer, L. J. Relation of visual function to retinal nerve fiber layer
       thickness in multiple sclerosis. Ophthalmology. (2006). Feb; , 113(2), 324-32.

[92]   Henderson, A. P, Trip, S. A, Schlottmann, P. G, Altmann, D. R, Garway-heath, D. F,
       Plant, G. T, & Miller, D. H. An investigation of the retinal nerve fibre layer in progressive
       multiple sclerosis using optical coherence tomography. Brain. (2008). Jan; 131(Pt 1):
       277-87.

[93]   Pueyo, V, Martin, J, Fernandez, J, Almarcegui, C, Ara, J, Egea, C, Pablo, L, & Honrubia,
       F. Axonal loss in the retinal nerve fiber layer in patients with multiple sclerosis. Mult
       Scler. (2008). Jun; , 14(5), 609-14.

[94]   Pulicken, M, Gordon-lipkin, E, Balcer, L. J, Frohman, E, Cutter, G, & Calabresi, P. A.
       Optical coherence tomography and disease subtype in multiple sclerosis. Neurology.
       (2007). Nov 27; , 69(22), 2085-92.

[95]   Sepulcre, J, Murie-fernandez, M, Salinas-alaman, A, García-layana, A, Bejarano, B, &
       Villoslada, P. Diagnostic accuracy of retinal abnormalities in predicting disease activity
       in MS.Neurology. (2007). May 1; , 68(18), 1488-94.

[96]   Toledo, J, Sepulcre, J, Salinas-alaman, A, García-layana, A, Murie-fernandez, M,
       Bejarano, B, & Villoslada, P. Retinal nerve fiber layer atrophy is associated with physical
       and cognitive disability in multiple sclerosis. Mult Scler. (2008). Aug; , 14(7), 906-12.

[97]   Spain, R. I, Maltenfort, M, Sergott, R. C, & Leist, T. P. Thickness of retinal nerve fiber
       layer correlates with disease duration in parallel with corticospinal tract dysfunction
       in untreated multiple sclerosis. J Rehabil Res Dev. (2009). , 46(5), 633-42.

[98]   Costello, F, Hodge, W, Pan, Y. I, & Metz, L. Kardon RH Retinal nerve fiber layer and
       future risk of multiple sclerosis. Can J Neurol Sci. (2008). Sep; , 35(4), 482-7.

[99]   Bertuzzi, F, Suzani, M, Tagliabue, E, Cavaletti, G, Angeli, R, Balgera, R, Rulli, E,
       Ferrarese, C, & Miglior, S. Diagnostic validity of optic disc and retinal nerve fiber layer

evaluations in detecting structural changes after optic neuritis. Ophthalmology. (2010). Jun;, 117(6), 1256-1264.

[100] Savini, G, Bellusci, C, Carbonelli, M, Zanini, M, Carelli, V, Sadun, A. A, & Barboni, P. Detection and quantification of retinal nerve fiber layer thickness in optic disc edema using stratus OCT. Arch Ophthalmol. (2006). Aug;, 124(8), 1111-7.

[101] Alasil, T, Tan, O, Lu, A. T, Huang, D, & Sadun, A. A. Correlation of Fourier domain optical coherence tomography retinal nerve fiber layer maps with visual fields in nonarteritic ischemic optic neuropathy. Ophthalmic Surg Lasers Imaging. (2008). Jul-Aug;39(4 Suppl):S, 71-9.

[102] Contreras, I, Noval, S, Rebolleda, G, & Muñoz-negrete, F. J. Follow-up of nonarteritic anterior ischemic optic neuropathy with optical coherence tomography. Ophthalmology. (2007). Dec;, 114(12), 2338-44.

[103] Bellusci, C, Savini, G, Carbonelli, M, Carelli, V, Sadun, A. A, & Barboni, P. Retinal nerve fiber layer thickness in nonarteritic anterior ischemic optic neuropathy: OCT characterization of the acute and resolving phases. Graefes Arch Clin Exp Ophthalmol. (2008). May;, 246(5), 641-7.

[104] Aggarwal, D, Tan, O, Huang, D, & Sadun, A. A. Patterns of ganglion cell complex and nerve fiber layer loss in nonarteritic ischemic optic neuropathy by Fourier-domain optical coherence tomography. Invest Ophthalmol Vis Sci. (2012). Jul 3;, 53(8), 4539-45.

[105] Deleón-ortega, J, Carroll, K. E, Arthur, S. N, & Girkin, C. A. Correlations between retinal nerve fiber layer and visual field in eyes with nonarteritic anterior ischemic optic neuropathy. Am J Ophthalmol. (2007). Feb;, 143(2), 288-294.

[106] Papchenko, T, Grainger, B. T, Savino, P. J, Gamble, G. D, & Danesh-meyer, H. V. Macular thickness predictive of visual field sensitivity in ischaemic optic neuropathy. Acta Ophthalmol. (2012). Sep;90(6):e, 463-9.

[107] Horowitz, J, Fishelzon-arev, T, Rath, E. Z, Segev, E, & Geyer, O. Comparison of optic nerve head topography findings in eyes with non-arteritic anterior ischemic optic neuropathy and eyes with glaucoma. Graefes Arch Clin Exp Ophthalmol. (2010). Jun;, 248(6), 845-51.

[108] Barboni, P, Carbonelli, M, & Savini, G. Ramos Cdo V, Carta A, Berezovsky A, Salomao SR, Carelli V, Sadun AA. Natural history of Leber's hereditary optic neuropathy: longitudinal analysis of the retinal nerve fiber layer by optical coherence tomography. Ophthalmology. (2010). Mar;, 117(3), 623-7.

[109] Barboni, P, Savini, G, Valentino, M. L, Montagna, P, Cortelli, P, De Negri, A. M, Sadun, F, Bianchi, S, Longanesi, L, Zanini, M, De Vivo, A, & Carelli, V. Retinal nerve fiber layer evaluation by optical coherence tomography in Leber's hereditary optic neuropathy. Ophthalmology. (2005). Jan;, 112(1), 120-6.

[110] Savini, G, Barboni, P, Valentino, M. L, Montagna, P, Cortelli, P, De Negri, A. M, Sadun, F, Bianchi, S, Longanesi, L, Zanini, M, & Carelli, V. Retinal nerve fiber layer evaluation

by optical coherence tomography in unaffected carriers with Leber's hereditary optic neuropathy mutations.Ophthalmology. (2005). Jan;, 112(1), 127-31.

[111]   Seo, J. H, Hwang, J. M, & Park, S. S. Comparison of retinal nerve fibre layers between 11778 and 14484 mutations in Leber's hereditary optic neuropathy. Eye (Lond). (2010). Jan;, 24(1), 107-11.

[112]   Yu-wai-man, P, Griffiths, P. G, Burke, A, Sellar, P. W, Clarke, M. P, Gnanaraj, L, Ahkine, D, Hudson, G, Czermin, B, Taylor, R. W, Horvath, R, & Chinnery, P. F. The prevalence and natural history of dominant optic atrophy due to OPA1 mutations. Ophthalmology. (2010). Aug;117(8):1538-46, 1546

[113]   Fournier, A. V, Damji, K. F, Epstein, D. L, & Pollock, S. C. Discexcavation in dominant optic atrophy: differentiation from normal tension glaucoma.Ophthalmology(2001). Sep;, 108(9), 1595-602.

[114]   Barboni, P, Savini, G, Parisi, V, & Carbonelli, M. La Morgia C, Maresca A, Sadun F, De Negri AM, Carta A, Sadun AA, Carelli V. Retinal nerve fiber layer thickness in dominant optic atrophy measurements by optical coherence tomography and correlation with age.Ophthalmology. (2011). Oct;, 118(10), 2076-80.

[115]   Milea, D, Sander, B, Wegener, M, Jensen, H, Kjer, B, Jørgensen, T. M, Lund-andersen, H, & Larsen, M. Axonal loss occurs early in dominant optic atrophy. Acta Ophthalmol. (2010). May;, 88(3), 342-6.

[116]   Kim, T. W, & Hwang, J. M. Stratus OCT in dominant optic atrophy: features differentiating it from glaucoma. J Glaucoma. (2007). Dec;, 16(8), 655-8.

[117]   Yu-wai-man, P, Bailie, M, Atawan, A, Chinnery, P. F, & Griffiths, P. G. Pattern of retinal ganglion cell loss in dominant optic atrophy due to OPA1 mutations. Eye (Lond).(2011). May;, 25(5), 596-602.

[118]   Bowd, C, Weinreb, R. N, Williams, J. M, et al. The retinal nerve fiber layer thickness in ocular hypertensive, normal, and glaucomatous eyes with optical coherence tomography. Arch Ophthalmol (2000). , 118, 22-6.

[119]   Ito, Y, Nakamura, M, Yamakoshi, T, Lin, J, Yatsuya, H, & Terasaki, H. Reduction of inner retinal thickness in patients with autosomal dominant optic atrophy associated with OPA1 mutations. Invest Ophthalmol Vis Sci. (2007). Sep;, 48(9), 4079-86.

[120]   Barboni, P, Carbonelli, M, Savini, G, Foscarini, B, Parisi, V, Valentino, M. L, Carta, A, De Negri, A, Sadun, F, Zeviani, M, Sadun, A. A, Schimpf, S, Wissinger, B, & Carelli, V. OPA1 mutations associated with dominant optic atrophy influence optic nerve head size. Ophthalmology. (2010). Aug;, 117(8), 1547-53.

[121]   Monteiro, M L R, Leal, B C, Rosa, A A M, & Bronstein, M D. Optical coherence tomography analysis of axonal loss in band atrophy of the optic nerve. Br J Ophthalmol. (2004). July; , 88(7), 896-899.

[122]   Kanamori, A, Nakamura, M, Matsui, N, Nagai, A, Nakanishi, Y, Kusuhara, S, Yamada, Y, & Negi, A. Optical coherence tomography detects characteristic retinal nerve fiber

layer thickness corresponding to band atrophy of the optic discs. Ophthalmology. (2004). Dec;, 111(12), 2278-83.

[123] Monteiro, M. L, Moura, F. C, & Medeiros, F. A. Diagnostic ability of optical coherence tomography with a normative database to detect band atrophy of the optic nerve. Am J Ophthalmol. (2007). May;, 143(5), 896-9.

[124] Nagai-kusuhara, A, Nakamura, M, Tatsumi, Y, Nakanishi, Y, & Negi, A. Disagreement between Heidelberg Retina Tomograph and optical coherence tomography in assessing optic nerve head configuration of eyes with band atrophy and normal eyes. Br J Ophthalmol. (2008). Oct;, 92(10), 1382-6.

Permissions

The contributors of this book come from diverse backgrounds, making this book a truly international effort. This book will bring forth new frontiers with its revolutionizing research information and detailed analysis of the nascent developments around the world.

We would like to thank Shimon Rumelt, for lending his expertise to make the book truly unique. He has played a crucial role in the development of this book. Without his invaluable contribution this book wouldn't have been possible. He has made vital efforts to compile up to date information on the varied aspects of this subject to make this book a valuable addition to the collection of many professionals and students.

This book was conceptualized with the vision of imparting up-to-date information and advanced data in this field. To ensure the same, a matchless editorial board was set up. Every individual on the board went through rigorous rounds of assessment to prove their worth. After which they invested a large part of their time researching and compiling the most relevant data for our readers. Conferences and sessions were held from time to time between the editorial board and the contributing authors to present the data in the most comprehensible form. The editorial team has worked tirelessly to provide valuable and valid information to help people across the globe.

Every chapter published in this book has been scrutinized by our experts. Their significance has been extensively debated. The topics covered herein carry significant findings which will fuel the growth of the discipline. They may even be implemented as practical applications or may be referred to as a beginning point for another development. Chapters in this book were first published by InTech; hereby published with permission under the Creative Commons Attribution License or equivalent.

The editorial board has been involved in producing this book since its inception. They have spent rigorous hours researching and exploring the diverse topics which have resulted in the successful publishing of this book. They have passed on their knowledge of decades through this book. To expedite this challenging task, the publisher supported the team at every step. A small team of assistant editors was also appointed to further simplify the editing procedure and attain best results for the readers.

Our editorial team has been hand-picked from every corner of the world. Their multi-ethnicity adds dynamic inputs to the discussions which result in innovative outcomes. These outcomes are then further discussed with the researchers and contributors who give their valuable feedback and opinion regarding the same. The feedback is then collaborated with the researches and they are edited in a comprehensive manner to aid the understanding of the subject.

Apart from the editorial board, the designing team has also invested a significant amount of their time in understanding the subject and creating the most relevant covers. They scrutinized every image to scout for the most suitable representation of the subject and create an appropriate cover for the book.

The publishing team has been involved in this book since its early stages. They were actively engaged in every process, be it collecting the data, connecting with the contributors or procuring relevant information. The team has been an ardent support to the editorial, designing and production team. Their endless efforts to recruit the best for this project, has resulted in the accomplishment of this book. They are a veteran in the field of academics and their pool of knowledge is as vast as their experience in printing. Their expertise and guidance has proved useful at every step. Their uncompromising quality standards have made this book an exceptional effort. Their encouragement from time to time has been an inspiration for everyone.

The publisher and the editorial board hope that this book will prove to be a valuable piece of knowledge for researchers, students, practitioners and scholars across the globe.

List of Contributors

Nicola Calandrella, Simona Giorgini and Gianfranco Risuleo
Department of Biology and Biotechnology "Charles Darwin"- Sapienza University of Rome, Rome, Italy

Yoko A. Ito and Michael A. Walter
Department of Medical Genetics, University of Alberta, Edmonton, AB, Canada

Adriana Silva Borges- Giampani and Jair Giampani Junior
Federal University of Mato Grosso, Brazil

A.A. Zilfyan
Scientific-Research Center, Yerevan State Medical University, Yerevan, Armenia
"Shengavit" Medical Center, Yerevan, Armenia

Barkur S. Shastry
Department of Biological Sciences, Oakland University, Rochester, MI, USA

Ghanshyam Swarup, Vipul Vaibhava and Ananthamurthy Nagabhushana
Centre for Cellular and Molecular Biology, Council of Scientific and Industrial Research, Hyderabad, India

Najwa Mohammed Al- Dabbagh, Sulaiman Al-Saleh and Nourah Al-Dohayan
Department of Ophthalmology, Riyadh Military Hospital Riyadh, Saudi Arabia

Misbahul Arfin, Mohammad Tariq and Abdulrahman Al-Asmari
Research Center, Riyadh Military Hospital Riyadh, Saudi Arabia

Sotiria Palioura and Demetrios G. Vavvas
Department of Ophthalmology, Massachusetts Eye and Ear Infirmary, Harvard Medical School, Boston, MA, USA

Demetrios G. Vavvas
Angiogenesis Laboratory Retina Service, Department of Ophthalmology, Massachusetts Eye and Ear Infirmary, Harvard Medical School, Boston, MA, USA

Lizette Mowatt
Faculty of Medical Sciences, University of the West Indies, Jamaica
University Hospital of the West Indies, Mona, Jamaica

Maynard Mc Intosh
St Joseph Hospital, Kingston, Jamaica

Noriko Sato, Makoto Ishikawa, Yu Sawada, Daisuke Jin, Shun Watanabe, Masaya Iwakawa and Takeshi Yoshitomi
Department of Ophthalmology, Akita Graduate University School of Medicine, Akita, Japan

Ivan Marjanovic
Glaucoma Department, University Eye Clinic Clinical centre of Serbia and Belgrade University School of Medicine, Serbia

Vassilis Kozobolis, Aristeidis Konstantinidis and Georgios Labiris
Eye Department, University Hospital of Alexandroupolis, Alexandroupolis, Greece